THE HERITAGE
OF
HOMŒOPATHIC
LITERATURE

*Who would object to a library because it is too large?
If you have good catalogues you always have a better
chance of finding what you are looking for than in a
small one.
— Constantine Hering, MD*

*Despite the enormous quantity of books,
how few people read!
— Voltaire*

Finally! A technology so simple everyone can use it!

Announcing the new **B**uilt-in **O**rderly **O**rganized **K**nowledge device (**BOOK**).

The **BOOK** is a revolutionary breakthrough in technology: no wires, no electric circuits, no batteries, nothing to be connected or switched on. It's so easy to use even a child can operate it. Just lift its cover!

Compact and portable, it can be used anywhere— even sitting in an armchair by the fire— yet it is powerful enough to hold as much information as a CD-ROM. Here's how it works…

Each **BOOK** is constructed of sequentially numbered sheets of paper (pages) (recyclable), each sheet capable of holding thousands of bits of information. These pages are locked together with a custom–fit device called a binder, which keeps the sheets in their correct sequence. Opaque Paper Technology (OPT) allows manufacturers to use both sides of the sheet, doubling the information density and cutting costs in half. Experts are divided on the prospects for further increases in information density; for now, **BOOK**s with more information simply use more sheets. This makes them thicker and harder to carry, and has drawn some criticism from the mobile crowd.

Each sheet is scanned optically, registering information directly into your brain. A flick of the finger takes you to the next sheet. The **BOOK** may be taken up at any time and used by merely opening it. The **BOOK** never crashes and never needs rebooting, though like other display devices it can become unusable if dropped overboard. The "browse" feature allows you to move instantly to any sheet, and move forward or backward as you wish.

Many come with an "index" feature, which pinpoints the exact location of any selected information for instant retrieval. An optional "BOOKmark" accessory allows you to open the **BOOK** to the exact place you left it in a previous session-- even if the **BOOK** has been closed. BOOKmarks fit universal design standards; thus, a single BOOKmark can be used in **BOOK**s by various manufacturers. Conversely, numerous bookmarkers can be used in a single **BOOK** if the user wants to store numerous views at once. Only the number of sheets in the **BOOK** limits the number. You can also make personal notes next to **BOOK** text entries with an optional programming tool, the Portable Erasable Nib Cryptic Intercommunication Language Stylus (PENCILS).

Portable, durable, and affordable, the **BOOK** is being hailed as the entertainment and education wave of the future. The **BOOK's** appeal seems so certain that thousands of content creators have committed to the platform. Look for a flood of new titles soon.

—*Anon. found on the internet, 1997*

THE HERITAGE OF HOMŒOPATHIC LITERATURE

An Abbreviated Bibliography and Commentary

by

Julian Winston

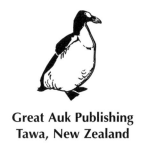

Great Auk Publishing
Tawa, New Zealand

Copyright © 2001 by Julian Winston

Great Auk Publishing
PO Box 51-156
Tawa, Wellington 6230
NEW ZEALAND
e-mail: jwinston@actrix.gen.nz

All rights reserved. No part of this book may be reproduced by any mechanical, photographic, or electronic process, or in the form of a phonographic recording, nor may it be stored in any retrieval system, transmitted, or otherwise be copied for public or private use without the written permission of the publisher.

First Printing, December 2001

Printed by Data Reproductions Corporation
Auburn Hills, Michigan, USA

Book Design by Julian Winston

This book was designed on a Macintosh 7600 using QuarkXpress,
Adobe Photoshop, and a Hewlett Packard Scanjet IIcx

ISBN 0–473–07996-8

single copies may be had from the publisher or through homœopathic booksellers

for multiple copies or bulk orders contact the publisher at the above address

THE COVER:

A selection of volumes from the personal library of the author
Photograph by David Hamilton

**This book is dedicated to the memory of
Thomas Lindsley Bradford, MD
without whom I would have never even begun**

With every year it is becoming more difficult to obtain reliable facts concerning the history of Homœopathy in America.

The stalwart and self-denying Fathers of our Faith have nearly all finished their labor of usefulness. It is in their books and pamphlets that the homœopathic physician of the future may read the history of their earlier struggles to proclaim the law of Hahnemann.

This volume is as complete a collection of data regarding the progress of Homœopathy in America as it has been possible to make.

If any of the statistics are incorrect it is not from carelessness. The difficulty in obtaining reliable information concerning the earlier books, pamphlets, magazines, and institutions has been very great. Many letters have been written, libraries have been ransacked, all the Homœopathic literature of the United States and some of the foreign has been carefully collated.

When doubt has occurred regarding any information, it has been omitted.

If this book be the means of teaching the junior members of the Homœopathic profession in the United States what a debt they owe to the Fathers of American Homœopathy, if it awakens a greater love for the scholarly books of the past, if it serves to bring us, as a School, nearer to the truth that the Homœopathy of Hahnemann is the real and only Law of Healing, then its mission will have been accomplished.

Thomas Lindsley Bradford, MD
Philadelphia, May, 1892

Excerpted from the Preface to *Homœopathic Bibliography*

Acknowledgements

There are a number of people without whose help this book would not exist.

Jacques Imberechts, MD, who asked if I could assemble a listing of original publication dates; Fran Treuherz, FSHom, and Bill Kirtsos, who scoured their libraries for missing information; the staff at the The Glasgow Homeopathic Library— Mary Gooch, Sandra Davies, Moira Gantiner— for being there, half-way around the world with immediate replies to questions; Sharon Stevenson and Jane Hansen at the National Center for Homeopathy in Alexandria, VA for searching out replies to my specific questions; Elias Carlos Zoby, VMD, who traded some invaluable information with me; Maria Helena, Librarian at the Associação Paulista de Homeopatia in Brazil; Jitka Drabkova, of the Czech Republic; Alexander Kotok, who provided a picture of the first Russian *Organon*; Joseph W. Audette ND, AP, and Jean Claude Ravalard, who found information that had previously eluded me; Juan Manuel Martinez, MD who provided needed information about the work of Ortega; Ian Miller at C. W. Daniel and John Churchhill at Beaconsfield for historical information about publishing in the UK and helping me sort out publication dates; Klaus-Henning Gypser, MD, with whom I discussed many of the topics in this work and who was kind enough to read and annotate the first draft of the manuscript; Paul Herscu, ND, who looked at the final manuscript and made enough suggestions that I re-did whole sections; Sylvain Cazalet of Homéopathe International who gave me good information and provided useful leads; Dr. Alejandro Flores García of the Centro de Homeopatía Flores in Mexico; Félix Anton of the Instituto Homeopatico y hospital de San José in Madrid; Gaby Rottler, DVM, who found a number of German titles for which I was searching and translated many things into English; Christina Schultz who offered to look at a preliminary manuscript and said, "How about some comments from you?"; Richard Moskowitz, MD and Andre Saine, ND, who looked at the first draft and gave me invaluable suggestions; Jay Yasgur, RPh, who not only proof-read, but by offering many corrections in grammar and style, served as editor; Christopher Ellithorp, who proofed the work, added 68 books to the list, and offered comments on many others; Thomas Lindsley Bradford, MD, who sat over my shoulder as I worked, and my wife Gwyneth Evans, RCHom, who read and corrected the manuscript, gave me invaluable advice, and listened to my endless prattling about it all.

Foreword

When Julian Winston phoned me in March of this year and related his idea of a "book about books," I was very surprised to hear that the first draft had been finished— just two years after his marvelous *Faces of Homœopathy*, the most interesting publication in the whole field of homœopathy I have seen for many years.

On the following pages the reader can expect a broad overview concerning homœopathic literature, written by an experienced pen. Naturally for an American author, books and periodicals in English are primarily referenced, but German titles of greater importance are also mentioned— such as the writings of Hahnemann, Bönninghausen, or Jahr.

Everybody dealing with homœopathy as practitioner, scientist, or historian will find a lot of very useful information in these pages. Due to the chronological arrangement of entries the development of our literature is seen at first glance. The homœopathic community is very much indebted to the author for his efforts in compiling this book. He has done the same as Claude Rozet did in 1984 for the French homœopathic publications. When will Germany follow?

Klaus-Henning Gypser, MD
Glees, Germany
April 2001

Table of contents

Preface

    Acknowledgements . . . . page iv
    Foreword . . . . page v
    Table of Contents . . . . page vi
    An Appreciation of our Literature. . . . . page vii
    Author's Preface. . . . . page xi
    Introduction. . . . . page xi

The Organon. . . . . page 1

Principles . . . . page 9

Materia Medica . . . . page 23
    Comparative Materia Medica . . . . page 47
    Regional Materia Medica . . . . page 49
    Materia Medica with Repertory . . . . page 50

Repertory . . . . page 53
    Computer Repertories . . . . page 77

Therapeutics . . . . page 79

Domestic Manuals . . . . page 99

Veterinary Manuals. . . . . page 113

Anatomy, Pathology, and Diagnosis . . . . page 121

Pharmacy . . . . page 127

Popular Books . . . . page 137

Critical Works . . . . page 145

History . . . . page 149

Biography . . . . page 159

Other Books . . . . page 165

Journals. . . . . page 179

Appendices. . . . . page 189

    The Homœopathic Armamentarium . . . . page 190
    Publishers listing . . . . page 195
    Books by publication date . . . . page 197
    Books by author . . . . page 217
    Glossary . . . . page 237
    Graph of all books . . . . page 238

Final Thoughts . . . . page 239

An Appreciation of Our Literature

Julian Winston is to be thanked and commended yet again for taking such pains to compile this monumental bibliography of our homœopathic literature, which spans its entire history from Hahnemann to the present. You may ask why he does it, or whether it's worth all that effort. After all, who really needs or uses all this stuff, other than a few antiquarians like myself, who like old vests and get their kicks browsing through used book-stores?

A few weeks ago, when told of some old homœopathic books looking for an owner, a colleague of mine felt only mildly interested in them, since so much of her library was already on computer that she saw little point in collecting old books merely to watch them continue mouldering on her shelves. When Julian asked me to write something about his latest labor of love, I thought of her words and how I could answer them for the movement as a whole, since what we do is linked inseparably to the printed word, and also to how readers can gain access to it, from the leatherbound tomes of Hahnemann's day to the advanced software of today.

Indeed, my own enduring fascination with homœopathy was kindled in no small part from its almost religious devotion to text. With our literature consisting essentially of glosses and emendations of Hahnemann, and even our arguments buttressed by scriptural quotations on every side, I realized early on that homœopaths are veritable "People of the Book," like Jews with the Old Testament, Christians with the New, or Muslims with the Qu'ran, all of them deriving fresh inspiration from a set of quasi-eternal truths revealed to a distinctly human writer at a definite point in historical time.

Our homœopathic literature is thus no mere repository of information, but also the communal efforts of flawed human writers to approach the Divine, such that each book, even one that is no longer used, becomes a kind of historical monument to the Word, which if not quite immutable at least doesn't change every year or two, as the concepts and methods of modern "scientific" medicine are explicitly designed to do. It tickles my fancy to imagine a day in the far-distant future when medicine as we know it no longer survives, and an archaeologist unearths a huge trove of artifacts — tools of incorruptible stainless steel, instruments for diagnosis and surgery and the like — while the only enduring traces of homœopathy will be the idea of it, as expressed in words and preserved for all time in these sacred texts.

On the other hand, a bibliography for today must also and above all be useful, not only to scholars and antiquarians, but also to students and practitioners, who bear the responsibility of applying the words to their Hahnemannian task of curing and healing the sick. That is why it need not and cannot include every last volume or article written on the subject, why it necessarily involves a selection.

It is here in particular that we are all most deeply indebted to Julian, who in addition to his many other talents is a splendid archivist, scholar, and librarian, in that his omnivorous appetite for all things homœopathic extends not only to hunting, gathering, preparing, and serving up all this stuff, but also to tasting, devouring, and digesting it for our benefit, quite

The Heritage of Homœopathic Literature

possibly even more than his own. While he stops well short of including every last domestic manual, for example, there are more than enough here to satisfy every conceivable taste, and he's earned my thanks for leaving the rest out.

The result is a leisurely guided tour down the main highways and through many forgotten back alleys of our literature, according to the inclinations of his fancy, the mature likes and dislikes of a connoisseur, and his own unashamedly personal opinions about everything and everyone you can think of, as well as quite a few you will discover for the first time. The travelogue is a perfect companion piece to *The Faces of Homœopathy*, his equally idiosyncratic ramble through our history, and it deserves to be savored just as he wrote it, with each section in more or less chronological order, as well as by sampling assorted tidbits, as in a book of reference.

Quite apart from its considerable entertainment value, its practical usefulness was brought home to me while reviewing Catherine Coulter's new book on cancer, which is firmly rooted in the organopathic tradition, sorely maligned by classical fundamentalists from Hahnemann himself to many in our own time. From reading Burnett, a 19th Century prescriber, and Clarke, his student and disciple of a generation later, I knew that they had long ago successfully treated patients with cancer and other advanced organic pathology. Although they give only the most tantalizing clues and hints about how they proceeded, their books at least made me ready and eager to investigate Ramakrishnan's method, much more than I might have been without knowing that history.

Not counting the Preface and Introduction, the bibliography proper is divided into fifteen sections (the Organon, Materia Medica, Repertory, Therapeutics, etc.), plus six appendices (all books arranged by date, by author, and Woodbury's "five-foot shelf" of indispensable books, published in 1931, a glossary, and a visual charting of the publications). I can't begin to enumerate even a small fraction of the wonderful snippets, tangents, anecdotes, and curmudgeonly rants contained in these pages. But I'll mention a few surprises that caught my eye and made me want to read them, in some cases for the first time.

Several were in the section on Therapeutics, that neglected and despised bastard child of pure homœopathy and pathological diagnosis, which still does useful service in many more cases than most purists would care to admit. The crowning achievement of a long and illustrious career, Jahr's *Therapeutic Guide*, also known as *Forty Years' Practice*, was the digest of his clinical experience, and contains a lot of useful information that is still relevant today. It is the mature and perfected version of his earlier *Clinical Guide* (1850), used by Mary Baker Eddy, the founder of Christian Science, who was quite a skillful prescriber and had homœopathic physicians visit her, by the back door of course, when she herself was ill. I've had copies of both books for years, and Julian's mini-review has given me the impetus I needed to begin reading them at last.

Worthy successor to Hering's *Domestic Physician* (1838), the first of its kind, Laurie's *Domestic Medicine* went through at least 12 editions in less than 50 years, and helped many a pioneer family in their pilgrimage to the west by covered wagon. I have the 4th American edition (1849), and Julian's plug for it has gotten me to take it off the shelf.

In the Philosophy section, *A New Synthesis*, by Guy Beckley Stearns and Edgar Evia (1942), was a cutting-edge essay into homœopathic research that prophesied and actually began the development of kinesiology, made original contributions to radionics, and dared to sketch out a philosophy of these still esoteric frontiers of homœopathy at a time when such matters were a lot further beyond the pale of respectable science even than they are today. I've already bitten off a lot more than I'll most likely be able to chew, and these are only the beginning.

As perceptive and opinionated as ever, Julian is one of a very small and select group whose favorites and pet peeves, passions and prejudices are always worth paying careful attention to, because he has thought them through and given cogent reasons for what he thinks. Though they may infuriate some, his broadsides against Sankaran and other "illuminists" are often witty, always thought-provoking, and do make some attempt to give credit where it is due. But don't expect a neutral, detached attitude. He's passionate about homœopathy, he has a point of view, and isn't afraid to play favorites and advocate for what he believes. That is precisely what makes this collection so valuable. Like any good librarian, he has included virtually everything of importance; like every discerning critic, he displays our subject through the medium of his own sensibility, and in doing so he reveals us to ourselves.

When all is said and done, I suppose that my friend and colleague was right to the extent that the new software does in fact contain the best of the old volumes, such that the originals are best preserved and stored for posterity in some museum where those of us who simply like the look and feel of them can kvell to our hearts' content. The obvious bridge for keeping the old world of bound volumes connected with the new world of computer software would be the modern research library, equipped with the most up-to-date technology, and a well-trained professional staff to locate, reprint, and reproduce selected items from the literature for the benefit of scholars and practitioners alike, so the Word may continue to be made flesh as of old. If we ever get our act together to create such an institution, Julian should logically be its first librarian.

Richard Moskowitz, MD, DHt
Watertown, MA
June, 2001

Preface

While cleaning up the desktop on my computer in August 2000 I came across a file of material that I had written in 1984 about homœopathic literature. I had given it to Ken Pober, MD, then editor of the *Hahnemannian*, the journal of the Homeopathic Medical Society of the State of Pennsylvania in 1989. The paper was printed there, over several issues.

When I was asked to speak about "repertories" in Australia in October 2000, I took the repertory section of that article and expanded it. That accomplished, I began to think about doing the same for the rest of the material. The time between the thought and the action was less than a day.

During the last 16 years, my knowledge of the literature has grown, and so has my library. This volume began as the article I wrote in 1984 and has been amended, edited, and, as you can imagine, reworked.

A story is told of a visitor who, upon seeing his host's huge library, exclaimed, "That's a lot of books! Have you read them all?" To which the host replied, "If I had read them all why would I have them?"

Working on this volume has given me the opportunity to renew my acquaintance with many old friends on my shelves as well as to meet many new ones, some of whom I did not even know I possessed.

While looking through all of the books mentioned here, many of the authors express the sentiment that they hope their work is found useful by the profession. I second that!

Julian Winston
Tawa, NZ November 2001

Introduction

When T. L. Bradford compiled his *Homœopathic Bibliography* in 1892, he listed 872 authors and over 3,000 written works. His book covered only those works which had been printed in the USA until that time, although he did have a full listing of most of the foreign publications of Hahnemann's work. It is a valuable and unique volume, and long out of print. There is no such analogous volume for the works produced in the UK and for those authors whose works were not issued in an American printing.

Bradford's listing, because of his cut-off date of 1891, is far from complete. Many of our basic authors— Kent, Nash, Boger, Clarke, to name a few— are not fully represented.

An effort to update the Bradford work was undertaken by Francisco Cordasco in 1991. His work, though useful, was unfortunately incomplete. At the time of its publication, a brief perusal by Chris Ellithorp and I of our personal libraries as well as those of Boericke and Tafel and the National Center for Homeopathy, yielded over 200 volumes published between 1892 and 1925 that Cordasco had overlooked and even yielded a few that Bradford had missed. To put together a complete bibliography of all the works in English would be a daunting task. Yet, an abridged listing of some of the major works would serve several purposes, among others:

- first, to remind veteran homœopaths, and to show the newer homœopaths, the vastness of our literary heritage;

- second, to avoid the false impression given by some references that, for example, Nash's *Leaders* was written and published in 1984— the date of the Jain reprint; and

- third, to inspire homœopaths and others to seek out these works and use them for the valuable information which is buried within.

When the first homœopathic school was founded in Allentown, Pennsylvania in 1835, all the instruction was in German, the language of the homœopathic literature at the time. Within a year of its founding, Hering had diligently translated Jahr's *Manual* into English.

The practice of homœopathy IS universal, and books have been written about it in almost all languages. Although much of the German, Italian, French, and Spanish literature remains untranslated, most books that have generally been considered "important" have been translated into English. To encompass ALL of the literature in one listing would be an overwhelming task. I have mostly confined my exploration to works in the English language, and hope that my efforts will inspire others to formulate similar listings for other languages.

I have attempted to list all the "major" works and many of the "minor" ones as well. I have included monographs of 915 works produced from 1810 until 2000. Of course, this is a listing established through *my* bias, and gleaned from Bradford's *Bibliography* and several libraries including my own. While Bradford lists 64 "domestic manuals," I have included only the 32 best known; of the 135 works on "therapeutics" found in Bradford, I have listed but 47 of the major works— this is, after all, an *abbreviated* bibliography. I trust that in mentioning a few of my favorites I have not excluded too many of yours.

There was a temptation to include in this listing pictures and biographical information about the authors. I have resisted doing so. For those interested in the authors, many of them have extensive biographies in my book, *The Faces of Homœopathy: An Illustrated History of the First 200 Years*, and in Jay Yasgur's to be published *111 Great Homeopaths*. This present book will remain a simple bibliography of our magnificent heritage.

In an effort to understand the progression of our heritage, I have decided to list the works in their chronological order rather than by author, although in some cases, several books (with different time frames) are grouped together under the authors most known work.

I have included the first publication date and the date/s of the subsequent editions, if known. It is unfortunate that many of the publishers in the UK did not include the date of publication on the title page or elsewhere in the volume. Often the date was given by the author in the preface, but not always. A number of works were written and published in the UK before they were published in the USA. I have attempted to find the dates of the original publication. Because there is no equivalent to Bradford's *Homœopathic Bibliography* for books in the UK, this was often difficult. Even if the book did exist in one of the several large homœopathic libraries in the UK, it is often labeled as "nd" (no date), and, for those few volumes, I had to settle for the date of the publication in the USA or provide an approximate date.

The Literature

From its inception, the science of homœopathy has been a verbal discipline. The subjective symptoms— so important in the selection of the remedy and listed in the homœopathic materia medica and repertory— are recorded in "the words of the patient." In a brilliant essay in his book *Planet Medicine*, Richard Grossinger outlines the beginnings of homœopathy and points out that one must understand the man, Hahnemann, to understand the system he developed. Hahnemann was well versed in over a half-dozen languages. After he abandoned the practice of medicine, he spent much of his time earning his living as a translator. The subjects which he translated were not confined to those of medicine and allied fields. He spent a third of the time between the ages of 30 to 34 translating the French classic *The Story of Abelard and Heloise* from English into German. Says Grossinger, "There is a reason, though, why homeopathy spoke clear and advanced words from the beginning. Its fluency came from somewhere. Out of the labyrinth of ancient languages and remote peoples, and the ignored work of obscure botanists and physicians of different nations, Hahnemann made a synthesis utterly different from any of its parts."

Grossinger goes on to point out that, "Translation involves a highly scientific and disciplined meditation on the structure of language, the roots of meaning and the transformation between codes" and that the science of homœopathy is more akin to those transformations than it is to "medicine." The "advanced words" that Grossinger speaks of come not only from Hahnemann, but from his pupils and disciples as well. The very nature of uncovering medicinal qualities of substances— the homœopathic proving— has as its root the precision of the written word. The edifice upon which homœopathy stands is not one of objective symptoms, the pathology lab, and test tubes but one of individualized subjective symptoms, written words and the store of homœopathic literature.

In any discussion of homœopathic literature, the obvious starting place is Hahnemann's *Organon of Rational Healing*. With this book in hand, one could learn everything about homœopathy. Hahnemann explains all that is needed: how to prepare the medicines; how to conduct a proving to determine medicinal value; how to document information; how to take a case; how to properly select the remedy and dosage; how to determine the course of action in subsequent consultations; how to relate to patients; and how to determine the relevance of adjunct therapies. This is all held together by a treatise on the meaning of health and disease, and establishes a framework in which the health care practitioner can work. The only things missing, of course, are the details, and those are what our literary heritage is all about.

The Structure

With the sheer mass of our literature, how does one establish categories? When Benjamin Woodbury discussed (in 1931) the "Five-Foot Book Shelf" that homœopaths should own (see the first appendix), he divided the works into four categories: Materia Medica, Philosophy, Repertory, and Therapeutics and Practice. These divisions can be further refined, but, nevertheless, they all remain interrelated. Many materia medicae contain repertories. Many books on therapeutics are almost specialized materia medica. The boundaries of the categories often blur. That said, I have developed a visual construct of our literature, seen on the next page. It all flows from the *Art and Practice of Medicine* which includes anatomy, physiology, hygienic measures, diet, prevention, and surgery. From this base came the *Organon*, the book that outlines the principles from which flows the therapeutics. Once that is in place, we have the "entity" of homœopathy, which is the subject of this work. The categories in the shaded blocks are those which have chapter headings in this work.

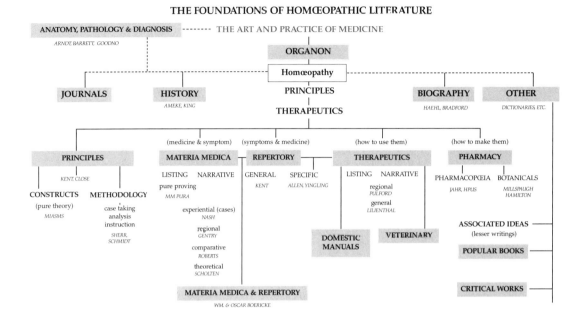

The Selection

In the mass of our literature, how does one select the "gems"? Some lie on the surface, large and bright, waiting to be picked up. Others have to be dug out. Some appear like diamonds upon first glance, but are found to be just glass imitations of little value. Others look like plain rocks and have to be cleaned and polished to find the value hidden within.

Authors write because they believe they have something to share. Many of them who had been teachers (Hughes, Dudgeon, Hale, Kent) merely condensed and refined lectures given to their students. Others (Kent, Pulford, Worcester, W. A. Allen, Neidhard) developed books for their own needs and were urged by many to "present it to the profession." Others (Hering, Malan, Laurie, Johnson) wished to help those who were not trained professionally, achieve a level of competence to tide them through times until a physician could be found. Others (Speight, Green, Panos, Dooley) have written because they needed something to explain to their patients what they were doing. Many wrote simply to relieve an "itch" caused by their muse.

During the last two centuries, some books have become "classics" and it is those that we immediately identify— the materia medica of Hering, the repertory of Kent, the philosophy of Close. Most were acclaimed at the time they were written. Unlike the visual arts, homœopathy does not sport a Van Gogh or Matisse. Almost none of our literature was recognized as "great" after its authors died, although a number of books were published posthumously celebrating the greatness which was collectively recognized.

Yet, there were hidden gems buried in the mound that were recognized in the past and have simply been covered up. If this book can get one person to discover a work previously unknown and find that single "ah ha!" then it has served its purpose.

There is certainly the need to separate the wheat from the chaff. We need to look to those books that give us reliable information for use in practice. But even some of our most reliable works have flawed translation errors and the slip of the type-setter. Which are reliable? Why?

The Heritage of Homœopathic Literature

Which should be consigned to the shredder? Which are simply of "historical" value?

I have not listed all the books that have been published. Some neither I nor others have ever seen— they exist only as an entry in Bradford. Most were probably not "gems," otherwise they would have been preserved and we would know more about them, but the rare "gem" has been lost as well. Although full descriptions of the content of such books are not available through Bradford's work, I have included many of those obscure works if only to give a picture of exactly how high is the mound in which we are digging.

Some in Bradford's, although I have not included them, certainly open up many questions. In 1878 Edward Fowler wrote a 12-page pamphlet called *Medical Science against Exclusive Homeopathy: A reply to Edward Bayard's Plea for Pure Homeopathy against Eclectic Homeopathy*. What did Bayard say? What was Fowler's rejoinder? Who was Troy Dye, the subject of an 1879 paper, *The Real Insanity of Troy Dye*? What was the slander against Dr. D. J. Earon of Manitowac, WI which caused him to write 16 pages in 1859, *Refutation of Slander Against D. J. Earon, MD*? What exactly did L. D. Fleming write in 1846 in his *Self Pollution; The Cause of Youthful Decay*?

I have chosen to look only at "books." Our literature does include many journals and volumes of papers presented at various homœopathic meetings. Although Bradford listed many of those published papers, to find and document all of them since 1892 would require superhuman effort. I will briefly discuss the journals, but to describe the content is a task I will leave for someone else to tackle.

There are certain pitfalls encountered in including our more recent books. Which ones will become the "standards"? Are we too close to judge? The physical task of preparing a manuscript and printing it has changed drastically in the last 20 years. One can publish with only a computer and laser-printer. More and more written work is being created making choices that much more difficult.

One filter I have used is to see which books are being sold by the major homœopathic booksellers and to notice which books the homœopaths I know are buying. A second filter, of course, is my subjective view as to which ones speak clearly.

I have chosen to ignore most of the small pamphlets written by prescribers like Dr. Farokh Master, Dr. Fayazuddin, Dr. Kamthan, Dr. Ibarra, and numerous other authors. While some of these works are valuable, the inclusion of all of them would have made this work much larger and perhaps cumbersome. A brief perusal of a catalog by a contemporary Indian homœopathic publisher shows more that 1000 titles listed.

Most homœopaths I know suffer from a unique disease— "desires to buy more books." Every conference has a book seller, and almost everyone leaves with one more book… which, too often, remains unused on the shelf. Later, the homœopath decides they have too many unread books, and offers them for sale. Then they get gobbled up by a younger, budding homœopath who, by this time, has succumbed to the aforementioned dreaded disease. But this disease has a serious side-effect. Many people buy books in a search for shortcuts to find the remedy, and when they find the answer does not lie in that book, it gets relegated to the shelf, later to be sold. In these times of desire for instantaneous gratification, homœopathy is an anachronism. It requires effort. It moves slowly. And it requires a mind that can, as Grossinger said, make a "synthesis that is different from any of its parts."

To do this requires reading the literature to understand the whole— not merely looking for the remedy. With the advent of placing the books in electronic media and being able to search them for symptoms, the literature is slowly being lost.

A dear friend and homœopath, who loves his books, summed it up as this:

"The main issue people have not deeply understood is that the literature gives you the background- it places you in the material. The second step is to have a good teacher who can use that material and guide you in taking it to the next level.

"The way the material is being used now is to search through it, rather than to read it. Searching does not give you breadth or background.

"The sad thing is that people are so far away from understanding the problem that they can not even differentiate the two skills."

It is my hope that this book will kindle the desire to re-acquaint ourselves with our magnificent literary heritage.

The Information

Monographs are presented in chronological order in the categories listed in the above diagram. If you cannot find your favorite materia medica under "Materia Medica" then look for it in another category. Perhaps, because it is both a materia medica and a repertory, I have placed it in the latter category.

The date is the date of first publication. When subsequent editions are known those dates appear within the initial entry and not as a separate entry.

The publisher's name is listed. Since many publishers were, essentially, "homœopathic" publishers, a full citation is not supplied. An appendix gives full information about the publishers. The publishing information is followed by the number of pages in the first edition. This is often followed by a brief summary of what the book contains. I have occasionally taken a quote from the introduction to allow the author to voice his/her intent. With some, I provide a quote from reviews or other noteworthy sources.

Some books, like provings and specialized repertories, need no descriptions; the title is self explanatory.

Several people who have seen my preliminary manuscript have asked me to provide some sort of commentary, evaluation, or notation— and I have done so where I felt it to be of benefit. For those books where I have an opinion to express, my commentary is in italics.

I have indicated, after the author's name, a "✱" if the book appears in Woodbury's listing of books for the "five foot book shelf," and a "✔" if it is still listed as being in print.

I have attempted to end each monograph at the bottom of the page. In those few instances where the monograph is lengthy, this has not been possible. When a monograph carries over to another page, it is indicated by the "✈ " at the bottom corner.

There are several appendices:
- The full text of the article from 1931 called "The Homœopathic Armamentarium" by Dr. Benjamin C. Woodbury, Jr., and an addendum bringing it up to date.
- A listing of all the publishers and their location that are mentioned in the text.
- A complete listing of all books ordered by publication date.
- A complete listing of all books in alphabetical order by author.
- A glossary of some of the terms used.
- A graph, visually depicting literature production by year.

I end with some "Final Thoughts" about the historical record of our literature.

The Organon

The Organon

What can one say? The *Organon* developed slowly out of Hahnemann's thinking and experimentation. It appeared 20 years after Hahnemann's seminal experiment with Cinchona, 14 years after his "Essay on a New Principle For Ascertaining The Curative Powers of Drugs, and Some Examination of the Previous Principles," and five years after his essay on "The Medicine of Experience," in *Hufeland's Journal*.

Written while he was living in Torgau, it is a masterful exercise in explaining the need for the system and then showing, step by step, how to use it. The Greek word *Organon* denotes "an instrument for acquiring knowledge; a body of methodological doctrine comprised of principles for scientific or philosophical procedures or investigation," and Hahnemann's work certainly fulfilled that requirement.

Hahnemann's use of the title *Organon*, certainly has classical roots. The *Organon* is the name given to the six logical treatises of Aristotle. Francis Bacon (1561-1626) called his work *Novum Organum*, (The New Organon) in the belief that he had discovered new principles of inductive logic. Based on the example of these two previous works, Hahnemann called his work the *Organon Der Rationellen Heilkunde— the Organon of Rational Healing*. By the second edition, the title was changed to *Organon Der Heilkunst— The Organon of the Medical Art*.

The *Organon* went through six editions. The sixth edition was readied for printing in 1842, but Hahnemann died before it could be printed. In a letter written in 1842 he says, "After 18 months work I have just finished the sixth edition of my *Organon* which is the most complete existing edition of my book." By March of 1843, a few months before his death, Hahnemann wrote, "I draw your attention to the last edition of the *Organon* which, if it please God, will be published in the near future, in the French version at least. You will find it satisfactory in every respect. The German version will be difficult on account of my mortal enemy, Trinks." It was never published. The exact details of the feud between Hahnemann and his ex-pupil Carl Trinks were never disclosed.

Melanie Hahnemann kept the manuscript and only made its presence known when several other versions were being claimed to be "the sixth." Melanie began negotiations for publication in Germany, but the Prussian/Austrian war in 1865 intervened.

In 1865 negotiations to obtain the book were conducted between Melanie and Hering, Lippe, and Raue, but nothing materialized.

During the Franco-Prussian War of 1870-71, all of Hahnemann's papers were moved from Paris to Westphalia and watched over by Melanie's adopted daughter who had married Karl Bönninghausen.

Carroll Dunham was negotiating for the purchase of the *Organon* in 1877, but he died before completing the process. In 1877, Dr. Bayes, from the London School of Homeopathy asked to publish the manuscript. Melanie said that she would be willing to supervise the translation so there could be "no malicious or deceptive alterations of the text," and she asked for a sum, the yearly interest of which would equal her yearly professional income. The matter was then dropped.

In 1880, Dr. H. N. Guernsey met Madam Bönninghausen while in Europe and he attempted to raise $10,000 from the American homœopathic community for the purchase of the work, but funds were not forthcoming.

Just before the turn of the century, Dr. Richard Haehl contacted the Bönninghausen family, and Dr. William Boericke offered to buy the book were it ever available. Hahnemann's papers were again nearly lost during the military occupation of Westphalia during the period of 1914-18. Shortly after this, Haehl negotiated the purchase of the *Organon* from the Bönninghausen family.

Drs. William Boericke and James William Ward paid the $1,000 being asked, and Dr. Haehl brought the manuscript to the United States. No French edition was ever found. The sixth edition finally appeared in print in Germany in 1921 and in the United States in 1922. The original manuscript now resides in the School of Medicine at the University of California in San Francisco.

note: all the information above was gleaned from Haehl's two volume biography of Hahnemann.

The Organon

1810: *ORGANON DER RATIONELLEN HEILKUNDE:* Samuel Hahnemann, MD
Arnoldischen Buchhandlung; 222 pages.
The first edition.

1819: *ORGANON DER HEILKUNST:* Samuel Hahnemann, MD
Arnoldischen Buchhandlung; 222 pages.
The second edition. The first to say "Aude Sapere" (dare to know/experience) on the title page.

1824: *ORGANON DER HEILKUNST:* Samuel Hahnemann, MD
Arnoldischen Buchhandlung; 282 pages.
The third edition.

1824: *ORGANON DE L'ARE DE GUÉRIT, OU THEORIE FONTEMENTALE DE LA METHODE HOMŒOPATHIQUE:* Samuel Hahnemann, MD
Arnold, Dresden; 271 pages.
First French edition. Translated by Dr. Ernst G. de Brunnow.

1824: *ORGANO DELL'ARTE MEDICA*: Samuel Hahnemann, MD
Dalla Tipografia Zameraja, Napoli; 440 pages
Italian edition. Translated from the second German edition by Dr. Giuseppe Gaimari.
Rapou speaks of an earlier edition in 1823. The translator was Professor Hernando Quanranta. No other information about that edition has been found.

1827: ORGANON DER GENEESKUNST: Samuel Hahnemann, MD
Gebroeders Diederichs, Amsterdam; 318 pages.
Translation of the third German. Translated by Pierre Joseph de Moor. There were no homœopathic physicians in Holland when it was published.

c. 1828: *ORGANON*: Samuel Hahnemann, MD
First Danish edition. Translated by Hans Christian Lund.
This work was mentioned by Haehl and Bradford. Although Lund translated a number of Hahnemann's "lesser" writing, there is no evidence that this work ever existed.

1829: *ORGANON DER HEILKUNST:* Samuel Hahnemann, MD
Arnoldischen Buchhandlung; 307 pages.
The fourth edition.

1830: *ORGANON (ELETMUVE) A GYOGYMUVESZSEGNEK VAGY HAHNEMANN SAMUEL, HOMEOPATHIA-JA (HANSONSZEUVE):* Samuel Hahnemann, MD
Wigand Ottonal, Pesten; 123 pages.
First Hungarian edition. Translated by Dr. Georges Forgo, Professor Bugath and Dr. Paul Balogh.

1833: *ORGANON DER HEILKUNST:* Samuel Hahnemann, MD
Arnoldischen Buchhandlung; 222 pages.
The fifth edition.

1833: *THE HOMŒOPATHIC MEDICAL DOCTRINE OR THE ORGANON OF THE HEALING ART*:
Samuel Hahnemann, MD
W. F. Wakeman, Dublin, Ireland; 332 pages.
Translated from the 4th German edition by Charles H. Devrient, with notes by Samuel Stratten, MD. The first English translation. It was reprinted, in a full leather binding, by Classics of Medicine Library, NY, **1995**.

1834: *EXPOSION DELA DOCTRINE MÉDICAL HOMŒPATHIQUE OU ORGANON DE L'ART DE GUÉRIR*: Samuel Hahnemann, MD
Pharmacopée Homœpathique, Bruxelles; unknown pages.
First Belgian edition. Translated from the fourth German by A. J. L Jourdan.

1835: *ORGANON VRACHEBNOGO ISKUSSTVA ILI OSNOVNAIA TEORIA SPOSOBA GOMEOPATICHESKOGO LECHENIIA DOKTORA SAMUILA GANEMANA*: Samuel Hahnemann, MD
Tipografia ("printing house") at the Moscow University, Moscow; 461 pages.
First Russian edition. Translated by Baron Wrassky. (*Organon of medical art or The principal theory of a homeopathic method of treatment of Dr. Samuel Hahnemann.*)

1835: *ORGANON FÖR LÄKEKONST:* Samuel Hahnemann, MD
Elmena et Granberg, Stockholm; 276 pages.
First Swedish edition. Translated by Peter Jacob Liedbeck.

1835: *EXPOSICION DE LA DOCTRINA MÉDICA HOMEOÁTICA Ú ORGANON DEL ARTE DE CURAR*:
Samuel Hahnemann, MD
D. M. Calero, Madrid; 230 pages.
The first Spanish edition. Translated from the 5th German and 2nd French by Doctor López Pinciano, a pseudonym of Dr. Ramón Ysaac López Pérez, of Valladolid. Other Spanish editions followed.

1836: *THE ORGANON OF HOMŒPATHIC MEDICINE:* Samuel Hahnemann, MD
Academical Bookstore; 212 pages.
The first American edition. From the British translation of the 4th German edition, with improvements and notes from the 5th edition, edited by Constantine Hering.

1843: *THE ORGANON OF HOMŒPATHIC MEDICINE:* Samuel Hahnemann, MD
William Radde; 212 pages.
The 2nd American edition. A reprint of the 1836 edition. It was printed again in **1848** and **1849** by Radde (230 pages) and included an introduction by Hering. It was again re-printed in **1860** as the 4th American Edition.

1846: *ORGANON DE HAHNEMANN OU EXPOSIÇÃO DAS DOUTRINAS HOMOEOPATHICAS* :
Samuel Hahnemann, MD
Typ. Nictheroyense de Rego e Comp., Niteroi (Rio de Janeiro); 121 pages.
First Brazilian edition. Translated by João Vicente Martins.

1849: *ORGANON OF MEDICINE*: Samuel Hahnemann, MD
Headland, London; 339 pages.
Translated from the 5th German edition by Robert Ellis Dudgeon, MD. It was revised in **1893** and has become, until recently the "standard" to which all others are compared. It was reprinted by Boericke and Tafel in **1901** (304 pages), as the 2nd edition in **1906**, again in **1911** and **1935**, and again, as the 10th American, in **1944** and **1950**.

1855: *TRADADO TEÓRICO PRACTICO DE HOMEOPATIA O SEA ORGANON DEL ARTE DE CURAR:*
Samuel Hahnemann, MD
Imprenta Chilena, Santiago, Chile; 489 pages.
First Chilean edition. Translated by Dr. Benito Garcia Fernandez. This was a single volume which also contained a translation of Hering's *Domestic Physician*.

1865: *ORGANON DER HEILKUNST:* Samuel Hahnemann, MD
Lutze, Köthen, Germany; 356 pages
This edition, edited by Arthur Lutze, purported to be the 6th edition, but, "It was alleged that Dr. Lutze took liberties with the original text, and sought to show that Hahnemann favored the

practice of alternation." It was discredited by most homœopaths.

Since Hahnemann's death in 1843 there had been discussion about the release of the 6th edition of the Organon. It was not a secret that a 6th edition had been in preparation. Dr. Süss-Hahnemann (a grandson of Hahnemann, and at the time a physician in London) claimed to have a manuscript of the 6th edition, although Melanie Hahnemann said that the ONLY manuscript was in her possession. The Süss-Hahnemann manuscript was used by Dr. Lutze as the basis of an edition that contained a revised Paragraph 274 that Lutze contended was written by Hahnemann and had been intended for the 5th edition but was withdrawn. The paragraph in question deals with the acceptance of the use of two remedies in alternation when a single remedy can not be found. The book was declared by the German homœopathic community (in the April 10, 1865 issue of the AHZ) to be "spurious and apocryphal." Madam Hahnemann asked the publisher not to sell it, and it was, effectively, removed from the market.

1876: *ORGANON OF THE ART OF HEALING*: Samuel Hahnemann, MD
Boericke and Tafel; 244 pages.
Translated from the 5th German by Conrad Wesselhoeft, MD. This re-translation and publication was undertaken for two reasons: There were inaccuracies in the prior English translation and the printing plates for the 4th American edition were destroyed. "This has had a very extensive sale." It was reprinted as late as **1917**.

It was said that this translation was the "favorite edition of the Transcendentalists."

1889: *THE ORGANON*: Samuel Hahnemann, MD
Journal of Homœopathics, New York.
Translated by Bernhardt Fincke, MD. This was to be done in parts, but the journal in which it appeared was discontinued after two issues, and the full translation was never published. Pieces were again published in *The Homœopathician* in 1916, but the journal ceased publication after the death of Kent, and the serialization ended. The manuscript, in Fincke's hand, is in the Library at the National Center for Homeopathy in Alexandria, VA. The manuscript has recently been transcribed and should be available, probably on the web, in late 2002.

The transcriber wrote to me: "I get the feeling that Sam knew more than he wrote. This manuscript kind of puts you into that point where you can almost feel his mind pondering over the information — like pushing a pancake around your plate to soak up the syrup— which is totally different to anything I've come across so far."

1889: *THE ORGANON OF RATIONAL HEALING*: Samuel Hahnemann, MD
(unpublished); translated by M. W. VanDenburg, MD
An announcement appeared in the March 1889 *Medical Advance* that Dr. VanDenburg will be retranslating the *Organon*. The article said it would restore the footnotes to the bottom of the page (instead of putting them at the end of the text as Wesselhoeft had done), have marginal headings for each of the sections, use type difference to mark comparative differences in text values, and include "…some brief, and I trust not too audacious nor self-confident notes."
As far as can be determined, this volume was never published.

1896: *A COMPEND OF THE PRINCIPLES OF HOMŒOPATHY*: William Boericke, MD
Boericke and Runyon, San Francisco, CA; 160 pages.
This book contain an appendix written by Samuel Lilienthal, MD, consisting of a "Catechism on Samuel Hahnemann's *Organon*." In this work Lilienthal reduced each aphorism to "simple language and especially written for the student."

c. 1900: *ORGANON DEL ARTE DE CURAR*: Samuel Hahnemann, MD
First Mexican edition translated into Spanish by Drs. Segura and Pesado. A second Mexican edition, was published in **1910**, translated by Dr. Higinio G. Perez (310 pages). A third edition, translated by Dr. Rafael Romero from the Boericke 6th edition was published in Meridia, Yucatan, **1927**.

1913: *THE ORGANON OF RATIONAL HEALING*: Samuel Hahnemann, MD ✱
J. M. Dent, London; 200 pages.
A translation of the 1st edition by Charles Wheeler, MD. This appeared as an "Everyman's Edition" and contained several other writings of Hahnemann including "Aesclepius in the Balance."

1921: *ORGANON DER HEILKUNST*: Samuel Hahnemann, MD
Schwabe, Leipzig; 347 pages.
The first publication of the 6th edition, edited by Richard Haehl, MD.

1922: *THE ORGANON OF MEDICINE*: Samuel Hahnemann, MD ✱ ✔
Boericke and Tafel; 314 pages.
The 6th edition. Not a full re-translation. William Boericke began with the 5th edition (the Dudgeon 1893 revision), and simply corrected it where Hahnemann had made changes. The philosophical questions raised by the differences found between the fifth and sixth edition are too complex to be detailed here. Nevertheless, Hahnemann made a number of changes and proposed a new method of remedy preparation and administration (the fifty millesimal potencies). The method was unknown to the great practitioners (Hering, Kent, etc.) who followed in his steps. The book was re-published in **1935**.

1925: *HAHNEMANN'S ORGANON OF THE ART OF HEALING RESTATED*: C. A. Baldwin, MD
Baldwin, Peru, Indiana; 52 pages.
A small pamphlet (3.5" x 5.5") with an outline of each aphorism. "The Organon is a monument of such nobility and dignity that to mutilate it is, in the opinion of some admirers, a sacrilege, an unforgivable vandalism. But if I can, by bringing you this fragment, induce you to visit the monument, and there dedicate yourself to the noble art for which it stands, I will feel that this desecration is justified."

1967: *ORGANON DE LA MEDICINA:* Samuel Hahnemann, MD
Editiones Marite, (Buenos Aires); unknown pages.
First Argentine edition. Based upon the Romero translation from Mexico.

1970: *THE ORGANON OF MEDICINE*: Samuel Hahnemann, MD ✔
B. Jain; 224 pages.
A combination of the 5th edition by Dudgeon (the 1893 revision) with the 6th edition by Boericke. Essentially, one can see the changes that Hahnemann made to the text of the 5th. An appendix outlines all the changes made from the first edition on.

A valuable study guide. Of all the published editions, this remains my favorite, since it clearly shows the changes in Hahnemann's thinking as some paragraphs in the fifth edition were modified and others completely re-written. This edition offers both versions interposed ("This paragraph was completely rewritten in the sixth…").

1979: *THE ORGANON OF MEDICINE*: Samuel Hahnemann, MD
Haug Verlag; 304 pages.
Translated by Kurt Hochstetter, this unique volume contains the German with translations in English, French, and Spanish— all viewable on the same page. The German was directly from Haehl's translation, the English directly from the Boericke/Dudgeon translation.

1979: *THE HEALING ART OF HOMOEOPATHY; THE ORGANON OF SAMUEL HAHNEMANN*:
Edward Hamlyn
Beaconsfield; 110 pages.
"To free the text from the out-dated and often obscure language of existing English language versions, to give the book the hearing it clearly deserves…" An abstract of the *Organon*. 25 aphorisms are not included "because of their irrelevance to the modern purpose of the book."

1982: *THE ORGANON OF MEDICINE*: Samuel Hahnemann, MD ✔
Jeremy Tarcher; 270 pages.
The first "new" translation of the text. It was undertaken by Alain Naudé, and Peter Pendelton, and was checked and corrected by Jost Künzli in Switzerland. It does *not* contain the lengthy introduction offered by Hahnemann. The work was done from a microfilm of the 6th edition at the University of California. Unfortunately, the translators did not know that when the book was being microfilmed, some paragraphs that were pasted on pieces of paper into the original by Hahnemann were not folded out, and thus not recorded. This edition was reprinted by Cooper Publishing in Blaine, WA in **1994**.

1989: *ORGANON OF THE THERAPEUTIC ART*: Samuel Hahnemann, MD
Pyrinos Kosmos, Athens; 306 pages.
First Greek edition, translated by Dr. Georges Papaphilippou.

1991: *ORGANON RACIONÁLNÍ LÉÈBY:* Samuel Hahnemann, MD
Alternativa, Prague, Czech Republic. 233 pages
First Czech edition. Translated by Emilie Harantova.

1992: *ORGANON DER HEILKUNST*: Samuel Hahnemann, MD ✔
Haug Verlag; 327 pages.
The complete text of the 6th edition, in German, annotated by Josef M. Schmidt, MD. Dr. Schmidt was able to examine the original manuscript in California, and annotated a complete German transcription from the hand-written notations.

This is the most accurate version available, and introduces several mysteries into an already mysterious work: the annotations that were added to the manuscript of the 5th German edition appeared in FOUR different hands— Hahnemann's, the scribe Hahnemann used to record some of his material, Haehl's, and an unknown one— it is not Melanie's hand. Since Haehl brought the book to the USA by sea, perhaps, during the voyage, he re-transcribed some of the pages that were fragile. He never mentioned anything about this, and by the time people became interested enough to take notice of these discrepancies, Haehl had long since died.

1994: *THE ORGANON OF MEDICINE*: Samuel Hahnemann, MD
Homoeopress, Ltd. Haifa, Israel; 319 pages of text, 62 page introduction, 92 page index.
The text of the *Organon* interspersed with explanations and commentary by influential Israeli homœopath Joseph Reves.

Reves approaches the material from a mystical and philosophical viewpoint, often explaining concepts by illustrating them as "on the circle"— the conceptual model used by a number of homœopaths and also called "The Mappa Mundi." In this way, the work of Hahnemann is subjected to a theoretical overlay even more mystical than the Swedenborgian model we see used by Kent.

1995: *THE UNFOLDED ORGANON: A PRÉCIS OF HAHNEMANN'S SIXTH EDITION*: Peter Crockett ✔
Islington School of Homeopathy, UK; 107 pages.
The author has offered each aphorism "in a précis form containing the fundamental idea, while excluding verbosity and repetition." The work contains a thorough index of the text.

A good idea which was supplanted by the publication of the translation by O'Reilly just a year later that included a similar précis next to each aphorism and also contained a full index and glossary.

1996: *THE ORGANON OF THE MEDICAL ART*: Samuel Hahnemann, MD ✔
Birdcage Books, Redmond, WA; 407 pages.
The work is based on an interlinear translation from the original German done by Stephen Decker. The interlinear has an English word directly below the original German text; it is a literal

translation. Here is an interlinear translations of the beginning of the Preface to the 5th edition, with the original German above and the exact rendering below:

Die alte Medicin (Allöopathie),   um   Etwas   im Allgemeinen über dieselbe zu sagen,   setzt
The old Medicine (Allopathy), in order to something in   general   about the same to say, (pre)supposes

The second task in the translation consists of rendering these sentences into English, where the sentence follows, as much as possible, Hahnemann's sentence structure. The above example is translated as:

"The Old Medicine (Allopathy), generally speaking, presupposes..."

Wenda Brewster O'Reilly, working with Decker and his interlinear translation, further adapted each sentence into a modern grammatical structure, often changing the format to make it more readable. Long continuous paragraphs consisting of sentences separated by commas and semi-colons, have been made into smaller, more manageable, paragraphs. A full glossary describes some of the translation difficulties.

An amazingly readable work that brought the work alive for me. It should always be read with Dudgeon's translation close at hand to serve as a point of comparison. In many places, I like Dudgeon's "take" on the paragraph better than that found in this edition. The glossary at the end is invaluable and discusses some of the problems involved in translating German concepts into English.

In all, there have been over 110 different editions of the *Organon* published in 18 countries.

Principles

The Principles

As homœopathic practice grew, some practitioners began to write about their particular view of the Art and Science of homœopathy. This led to books about the application of the principles stated by Hahnemann in the *Organon*.

The books listed here fall into three categories:
• principles
• theory and methodology
• general writings (usually in shorter essays).

The last category is found in few books— generally collected from varying sources and assembled as "Lesser Writings."

The dividing line between the first two categories is nebulous. A book like Kent's *Philosophy* or Vithoulkas' *Science of Homeopathy* is a bit of both; philosophical material woven together with clinical explanations and applications.

The early books are truly wonderful and, sorry to say, rarely available, and often out of print. Written in a very different time, they make fascinating reading. The authors, and the readers, were products of an educational system in which one had read Plato and Ovid as a matter of course and any reference to their works was clearly understood in the larger conceptual context. The early books, like Joslin's *Principles*, or Granier's *Conferences*, were written at a time when the industrial revolution was in full swing, and steam power was a true wonder and a resource for building all sorts of fanciful analogies. Similarly the study of the vacuum was of endless interest. Electricity (aside from that available from voltaic cells) was unknown, although there was a surge of interest with the arrival of generated power in the early 1880s.

To fully appreciate these early words one not only has to be steeped in the language, but needs to understand the social systems and the politics of the time as well as the science. Many of the references will be lost to the modern reader because they are referring to people and incidents well-known at the time, but not often remembered even a decade later. We do not have the "cultural literacy" needed to completely understand many of the allusions used in these works. They form a fascinating record of that society and its thought processes.

Principles

1828: *THE CHRONIC DISEASES; THEIR PECULIAR NATURE AND THEIR HOMŒOPATHIC CURE*: Samuel Hahnemann, MD ✲ ✔
Die chronischen Krankheiten, ihre eigenthümliche Natur und homöopathische Heilung, Arnold, Dresden.
The basic concepts of the "miasms" are discussed in part one ("theoretical part") and 48 Anti-psoric remedies are discussed in part two. The "Theoretical Part" was reprinted by Boericke and Tafel as a separate edition in **1904**. See the entry in the Materia Medica section.

Although the Organon *was the first book to explain homœopathy, the first part of these volumes established the "miasmatic theory."*

1840: *THEORY AND PRACTICE OF HOMŒOPATHY*: I. G. Rosenstein, MD
Henkle and Logan, Louisville; 288 pages.
One of the first books printed that discussed homœopathy and its principles. The introduction contains three letters from doctors, one saying, "I have hitherto been unable to pursue the homœopathic system of medicine, not knowing the German language; but I am happy to learn, through Dr. Rosenstein, that he has commenced to writing a work upon the subject of homœopathy, in the English language, which I hope the profession will be liberal enough to read…"

Little is known of Rosenstein. He studied with Augustus Phillip Biegler in Albany, New York in 1838, then moved to Louisville, Kentucky, where he wrote the book. He moved to Canada in 1842. It was a most interesting work because it was really a first— written by someone far away from the homœopathic centers of Philadelphia or New York, and thus approaching the subject in an "open" and unbiased manner.

1850: *THE PRINCIPLES OF HOMŒOPATHY IN FIVE LECTURES*: Benjamin Franklin Joslin, MD ✻
Radde; 185 pages.
The title speaks for itself. A flowery, rambling essay about the inductive method and the principles of homœopathy. Joslin was converted to homœopathy when, as a test, he took a few doses of a 3c, kept track of what symptoms he felt, and then compared them to the materia medica of the remedy taken.

1852: *THE LESSER WRITINGS OF SAMUEL HAHNEMANN*: Samuel Hahnemann, MD ✻ ✔
Radde; 784 pages.
A collection of essays and letters, edited by Robert Ellis Dudgeon, MD. This contains a number of valuable essays, including his first major essay that defined homœopathy "Essay on a New Curative Principle for Ascertaining the Curative Power of Drugs" (1796) and many others, including: "Cure and Prevention of Scarlet Fever" (1801); "Aesclepius in the Balance" (1805); "Medicine of Experience" (1805); "Contrasts of the Old and New Schools of Medicine" (1825).

The first book to pull together all of Hahnemann's other writings. It is still in print and remains the primary source for studying the development of Hahnemann's thought.

1854: *LECTURES ON THE THEORY AND PRACTICE OF HOMŒOPATHY*: Robert Ellis Dudgeon, MD ✻ ✔
Henry Turner; 565 pages.
A record of the lectures Dudgeon delivered to the Hahnemann Hospital School in London, 1852-53.

This book is invaluable. Unfortunately, the original was small in size and in typeface, and the Indian reproductions are difficult to read because of poor copying and printing. However, it is well worth the effort to go through it. It gives a record of thought by one of the best writers in the field, and from a time less than ten years after Hahnemann's death. It is the unvarnished beginning.

1857: *MEDICAL REFORM: BEING AN EXAMINATION INTO THE PREVAILING SYSTEMS OF MEDICINE*: Samuel Cockburn, MD
 Rademacher and Sheek; 180 pages.

1859: *CONFERENCES UPON HOMŒOPATHY*: Dr. Michel Granier
Leath and Ross; 425 pages.
First published in France in 1858. Translated by H. E. Wilkinson and C. A. C. Clark. A series of lectures about homœopathy delivered by Dr. Granier of Nimes. A contemporary review said it was "the best exposition and defense of homœopathy we have ever met."

This is one of those magnificent books that, despite its age and dated examples, deserves to be read by a wider audience. Coming to print just 13 years after Hahnemann's death it shows clearly the arguments posited against the system— the same which we still see 142 years later.

1865: *ON HIGH POTENCIES AND HOMŒOPATHICS*: Bernhardt Fincke, MD ✻
A. J. Tafel; 131 pages.
 "With an appendix containing Hahnemann's original views and rules on homœopathic dose, chronologically arranged."
Although the question of "high" potencies had been a subject of ongoing discussion in the homœopathic journals, this book was the first to explore the various methodologies of preparing remedies (straight centesimal, Korsakoff method, dry grafting, and fluxion potencies) and to discuss them on the basis of cured clinical cases.

A very early work that attempted to explore the value of high potencies by clinical use. The majority of the cases are not of very high quality. The book contains an appendix consisting of drawings that appear to be "geometric proofs" with explanations as to the possible action of the remedies. I have looked at them a number of times and they remain a complete mystery, althought they undoubtedly made sense to Dr. Fincke.

1870: TEXTBOOK OF HOMŒOPATHY: Eduard von Grauvogl, MD
Halsey; 739 pages.
Translated by George Shipman. Shipman was asked by the author, a homœopath in Nürnberg, to translate the work. The work was sold by prior subscription, i.e., the books were sold in advance of the printing. The printing plates were lost in the Chicago Fire of 1871. There was no demand for a second edition. Issued with a signed photograph of the author in front, it remains one of the rarer volumes in homœopathy. It has never been reprinted. Saying that "Homœopathy is a system of therapeutics resting upon the foundation of all the natural sciences," the book is truly a "textbook" that begins with anatomy and physiology, discusses the latest (at the time) understanding of the cellular work of Virchow, and establishes a model of how homœopathy relates to the other sciences. Since, "some of the empiric data [of homœopathy] still lacked foundation according to natural laws," the author attempted to remedy this by using examples seen in cases to "elucidate medical logic." The author introduces his ideas of the three constitutions: oxygenoid, hydrogenoid, and carbo nitrogenoid. When Hering read the book, he commented, "At last we have a thinker."

Keeping Hering's comment in mind, it is unfortunate that this work, through its lack of re-printing, is virtually unknown. It is, one must be warned, intensely written and not "light reading." To fully understand what the author is thinking about, one must have a good foundation in the history of medicine, cellular theory, and the concepts developed by Virchow.

1874: ON THE UNIVERSALITY OF THE HOMŒOPATHIC LAW OF CURE: Charles Neidhard, MD ✔
Boericke and Tafel; 34 pages.
A lecture given to the students at Hahnemann Medical College in 1872 which was an expanded version of the lecture he delivered to the Rhode Island Homœopathic Society in 1851— the first public lecture on the subject heard in that state.
As the title suggests, the author attempts to show that homœopathic law is universal, which prompted a critique in the *British Journal of Homœopathy* to say: "It is rather an example of perverted ingenuity to attempt to trace the working of homœopathic law in the department of morals, politics, education, agriculture, chemistry, and physics. Of course, far-fetched analogies may be found everywhere and even among the most unlike things, but the discovery of such analogies belongs more to the art of the poet than to that of the physician... we fancy his ingenuity in this essay is rather misplaced, and we must express a decided preference for his contributions to practical medicine, of which he has furnished us with many brilliant specimens."

1874: THE SCIENCE OF HOMŒOPATHY: Charles Julius Hempel, MD
Boericke and Tafel; 177 pages.
"A Critical and Synthetic Exposition of the Doctrines on the Homœopathic School." A second edition was printed in 1876.

A strange mix of Swedenborg and von Grauvogl!

1877: HOMŒOPATHY, THE SCIENCE OF THERAPEUTICS: Carroll Dunham, MD ✻ ✔
Francis Hart and Co., NY; 529 pages.
A collection of papers by Dunham, published posthumously. Although there are some papers on materia medica and direct therapeutics, the majority of the book concerns homœopathic philosophy and its practical application.
"More than one-half of this volume is devoted to a careful analysis of various drug provings... We urge the thoughtful and the studious to obtain the book, which they will esteem as second only to the *Organon* in its philosophy and learning."— *The American Homœopathist*

1880: *THE GROUNDS OF A HOMŒOPATH'S FAITH*: Samuel A. Jones, MD
Boericke and Tafel; 92 pages.
Three lectures that were delivered to the matriculates of the Department of Medicine and Surgery at Ann Arbor. They are: 1. The Law of Similars; its claims to be a science in that it enables Prevision; 2. The Single Remedy— a Necessity of Science; 3. The Minimum dose— an inevitable sequence.

Jones is a brilliant writer and thinker with a caustic wit and pen. Although his language usage appears as "flowery" as others of the period, somehow, he gets to the point in a more direct fashion and his digressions are easily followed. A classic work by one of the best.

1888: *FIFTY REASONS FOR BEING A HOMŒOPATH*: James Compton Burnett, MD ✔
Homœopathic Publishing Company; 175 pages.
"Over almonds and raisins" at a dinner party, Burnett met Dr. T. A. K. who got him so heated that "I lost my temper— and did not find it again that evening." Burnett told Dr. T. A. K. that he could give him 50 reasons for being a homœopath, to which the Doctor replied, "I have never heard one good reason yet." This book is the collection of those 50 reasons that Burnett posted to Dr. T. A. K.

A magnificently written book, with much food for thought. Burnett at his acerbic best.

1888: *SIMILIA SIMILIBUS CURANTUR? ADDRESSED TO THE MEDICAL PROFESSION*:
Charles S. Mack, MD
Otis Clapp; 32 pages.
A rambling essay about the application of the similar principle to disease.

1894: *THE TRUTH ABOUT HOMŒOPATHY*: William H. Holcombe, MD
Boericke and Tafel; 43 pages.
An allopathic doctor won a prize in Philadelphia for his anti-homœopathic essay "Modern Homœopathy: Its Absurdities and Inconsistencies." This small volume is a reply to that essay. It was found in Holcombe's papers, ready to send to the printer, after Holcombe died.

1894: *SEMI CENTENNIAL SECTION ON MATERIA MEDICA AND THERAPEUTICS*
AIH; 110 pages.
Edited by Frank Kraft, MD. This is a series of replies by some of the great homœopaths and teachers in response to questions pertaining to the teaching of Materia Medica, Therapeutics, and Homœopathic Philosophy. Among those replying are H. C. Allen, Thomas Skinner, and Willis A. Dewey.

1896: *DEFENSE OF THE ORGANON: Hahnemann's Defence of The Organon of Rational Medicine and of His Previous Homœopathic Works Against The Attacks of Professor Hecker*: Samuel Hahnemann, MD
Boericke and Tafel; 130 pages.
Translated by Robert Ellis Dudgeon, MD. This work was written in 1811, ostensibly by Hahnemann's son Friedrich in reply to a newspaper attack on the *Organon* by a prominent professor. Dudgeon, commenting that the letter "has hardly excited the amount of interest it merits," says that the writing is "evidently the work of the much more competent father."

A rare volume.

1896: *A COMPEND OF THE PRINCIPLES OF HOMEOPATHY*: William Boericke, MD ✔
Boericke and Runyon, SF; 160 pages.
An exposition of the fundamental principles of homœopathy. Includes an appendix by Lilienthal of a synopsis of the *Organon*.

A crystal clear, concise work. At the end of each chapter is a "for further study, read..." and lists articles from the current journals to read that pertain to the chapter.

1897: *THE SCIENTIFIC BASIS OF MEDICINE*: Isaac W. Heysinger , MD
Boericke and Tafel; 122 pages.
"The revolt from ignorance, which is called heresy of one age, becomes the reform of the next, and the established order of the third."

The author also wrote a book called The Source and Mode of Solar Energy Throughout the Universe. The book here is a rambling dialogue filled with allusion and digressions— typical of the writing of the time.

1900: *LECTURES ON HOMŒOPATHIC PHILOSOPHY*: James Tyler Kent, MD ✱ ✔
Examiner Printing House, Lancaster, PA; 290 pages.
Transcriptions of the lectures Kent gave to his classes in the study of the *Organon*. Although the year of the lectures is uncertain it was probably between 1896 (when Kent began to introduce Swedenborg concepts into his lectures) and 1899— the last year he taught the course at the Post Graduate School in Philadelphia. The first edition contained a "Homœopathic Catechism" written by Julia Loos, MD, consisting of 100 questions about the *Organon*. "It is deemed that anyone who can fully and comprehensively respond to this list of queries has a good working knowledge of the principles of Homœopathy and their application."
In **1917**, Ehrhart and Karl issued "The Memorial Edition" with a photograph of Kent as a frontispiece and several eulogies for Kent. The edition was re-printed several times. A 5th edition was printed in **1954**.

A "guidebook" to the 5th edition of the Organon as seen by Kent through his Swedenborgian filters. Because most of the teachers up to the present day were strongly influenced by the pupils of Kent, the models presented by Kent that discuss homœopathy with the Swedenborg overlay have formed the "whole cloth" of the homœopathic garment with little critical discussion comparing the work of Hahnemann (what **was** *said) and the work of Kent (what he* says *Hahnemann said).*

1904: *A PHILOSOPHY OF THERAPEUTICS*: Eldridge C. Price, MD
Nunn, Baltimore; 336 pages.
Price taught at the Southern Homœopathic Medical College in Baltimore. "The foundation of which rests upon the two postulates: first that it is the human organism that is the active factor in the healing of the sick, not the drugs, and second, that there are two therapeutic laws." (similia and contraria).

1908: *BÖNNINGHAUSEN'S LESSER WRITINGS*: C. von Bönninghausen ✔
Boericke and Tafel; 348 pages.
Compiled from German writings by T. L. Bradford, and translated by L. H. Tafel.
The first English translation of Bönninghausen's other writings. "The whole, with its many clinical cases, forms a good work for all who want to get down to a solid homœopathic foundation, for, in a sense, it is one of our homœopathic foundation stones."

Bönninghausen died in 1864 and left a large number of writings, all in German. It has been said that Hahnemann was the theoretician, but Bönninghausen was the practitioner. His writings were always informative and filled with exceptional insights into the practice of homœopathy. Although a few of his writings escaped the net cast by Bradford, the majority are represented in this volume.

1908: *THE CHRONIC MIASMS: PSORA AND PSEUDO PSORA*: James Henry Allen, MD ✔
Private; 286 pages.

1908: *THE CHRONIC MIASMS: SYCOSIS:* James Henry Allen, MD ✔
Private; 426 pages.

A very in-depth discussion of the theoretical side of the miasms by J. H. Allen, who taught the subject in Chicago at the Hering College. Allen wrote a third volume on Syphilis, but died before it was published. It was to be serialized in one of the Journals, but only one piece ever saw publication.

1909: *THE SCIENTIFIC REASONABLENESS OF HOMŒOPATHY*: Royal S. Copeland, MD
Copeland, 57 pages.
Published by the *Chironian*, it is a series of essays speaking to the title of the volume.

Copeland had just finished his term as AIH President, and was soon to settle in New York to assume the position of Dean of the NY Homœopathic Medical College. Eventually he became the Health Commissioner of New York City and later New York State Senator. These series of lectures show him clearly as someone who is, on one hand, committed to homœopathy, and on the other hand, not possessing a very deep understanding of it.

1910: *THE AGNOSTIC IN MEDICINE*: James William Ward, MD
The Murdock Press, San Francisco, CA; 21 pages.
The Presidential Address by Ward to the AIH on June 11, 1910. "The agnostic… sees only natural causes and natural results, and seeks to induce man to give up gazing into the void and empty space, that he may give his entire attention to the real world in which he lives."

A flowery and meandering discourse on the importance of homœopathy and it's development as seen through its philosophical antecedents through history.

1914: *THE CASE FOR HOMŒOPATHY*: Charles E. Wheeler, MD ✔
British Homœopathic Association; 99 pages.
Second edition in **1923**. Third edition with Frank Bodman in **1932**.

Wheeler (1868-1947) was one of the stalwart British homœopaths who linked the 19th and 20th centuries. He was a member of the "Cooper Club" with Clarke and Skinner after the death of Burnett and Cooper. When Wheeler talked, everyone listened. In his obituary, his death was said to be "the most grievous loss of this generation."

1923: *THE TREND OF MODERN MEDICINE*: John Weir, MD
John Bale and Sons., London; 23 pages.
A lecture which outlined many of the ways that modern medicine has used homœopathic ideas and principles.

1924: *THE VALUE AND LIMITATIONS OF HOMŒOPATHY*: James C. Wood, MD
Central Journal of Homœopathy, Cleveland, OH; 63 pages.

An essay that unfortunately shows the lack of this surgeon's homœopathic understanding.

1924: *THE GENIUS OF HOMŒOPATHY*: Stuart N. Close, MD ✔
Boericke and Tafel; 280 pages.
A series of lectures delivered at the New York Homœopathic Medical College. Close was a student of P. P. Wells and Bernhardt Fincke. This book is one of the clearest statements about the philosophical basis of homœopathic study ever compiled.

When talking of reading about homœopathic principles, this is my book of choice. It does not contain the Swedenborgian undertone that Kent brings to the subject. It is written with extreme clarity.

1925: *THE PRINCIPLES AND SCOPE OF HOMŒOPATHY*: James William Ward, MD
Private, San Francisco, CA; 72 pages.
Six lectures delivered March and April 1925 to the University of California Training School for Nurses. These were extemporaneous lectures that were "stenographically transcribed."

Six succinct lectures about homœopathy, starting with a brief biography of Hahnemann, and moving quickly into the philosophical issues of homœopathy and its practice. It was privately printed by Ward and distributed to his friends. It deserves wider recognition.

1925: *WHAT SHALL BE OUR ATTITUDE TOWARD HOMŒOPATHY?*: Dr. August Bier ✔
Boericke and Tafel from the *Homœopathic Recorder*, December 1925; 38 pages.
Translated by P. J. R. Schmahl, MD.
A lecture delivered by Dr. Bier in Berlin. Claiming that the Law of Similars is simply a branch of medical therapeutics, he appealed for the reconciliation of the allopathic and homœopathic schools, and the end of "sectarian" medicine.

In the paper, Bier suggested that there be an "understanding" with the "scientific homœopaths" and that "… if we tolerate the honest fanatics among their ranks then homœopathy will be enabled to shake off its objectionable entourage." This was not taken kindly by those in the International Hahnemannian Association, who saw Bier's work as little but appeasement and a justification as to why homœopathy should be subsumed by the allopaths.

1926: *NEW REMEDIES; Clinical Cases, Lesser Writings, Aphorisms, and Precepts*: James Tyler Kent, MD ✔
Ehrhart and Karl; 698 pages.
Compiled 10 years after Kent's death by W. W. Sherwood, MD, these writings were condensed from letters, published articles, and lectures. Although there is materia medica of 29 remedies, the majority of the work concerns the philosophy and application of homœopathy.

Although this work contains most of Kent's published work, there are a few pieces missing. There does not seem to be any order in which the pieces appear, and the index is incomplete. The book contains a number of "Aphorisms" attributed to Kent. It is a valuable book to further understand the thinking of this great homœopath, and has many treasures buried within— including an explanation of how he arrived at the 30, 200, 1M, 10M series and the meaning of the different type styles in the rubrics found in his Repertory. *The book was, however, superseded by the publication of a revised work by K-H. Gypser in 1987.*

1927: *CONSTITUTIONAL MEDICINE WITH ESPECIAL REFERENCE TO THE THREE CONSTITUTIONS OF VON GRAUVOGL*: John Henry Clarke, MD ✔
Homœopathic Publishing Company; 182 pages.

A fascinating essay and probably the best way to learn about Von Grauvogl's ideas.

1929: *A COMPEND OF THE PRINCIPLES OF HOMŒOPATHY FOR STUDENTS OF MEDICINE*: Garth Boericke, MD ✔
Boericke and Tafel; 178 pages.
"A modern textbook." These were the lectures that Garth Boericke gave to the students at Hahnemann Medical College in Philadelphia.

1931: *PHYSICS OF HIGH DILUTIONS*: Guy Beckley Stearns, MD
Homœopathic Recorder, June 1931; 22 pages.
An exploration into the possible mechanism behind the action of the high dilutions. See the entry under 1942.

1932: *THE HOMEOPATHIC PRINCIPLE IN THERAPEUTICS*: Thomas Hodge McGavack, MD ✔
Boericke and Tafel; 204 pages.
"The teachers of homœopathy, those who have to establish the homœopathic viewpoint in students trained to think entirely on the gross material plane, will especially welcome this compendium"— Garth Boericke's Introduction.

McGavack was the Head of the Homœopathy Department at the University of California Medical School, in San Francisco. The work is an attempt to show how homœopathy fits in to the model of modern medical research, and the laboratory standpoint. When discussing the effectiveness of ultra-molecular dilutions, he mentions the works of Kolisko who found activity in the 30x dilution.

I would hazard a guess that the book was not carefully edited. There is a chapter "Schools of Thot in Medicine" that had me going to the dictionary to look up "thot" since it is not only used at the head of each page, but in the subheading, "The Homœopathic School of Thot." Could it be a word and meaning I did not know? Is there another god in the Egyptian pantheon that has to do with medicine? Alas, there is no such word, and we are faced with a grand spelling error in the index, the chapter head, one subhead, and six page headings.
To further compound the errors in the book, the page numbers in the index cease to be accurate after chapter two.

1936: *THE PRINCIPLES AND ART OF CURE BY HOMŒOPATHY*: Herbert A. Roberts, MD ✔
Homœopathic Publishing Company; 285 pages.
Roberts, obviously influenced by Stuart Close and other members of the International Hahnemannian Association, wrote this text covering the principles and practice of homœopathy. The 1942 edition contains information about the "atomic theory" and relating homœopathy to some of the newer discoveries in "modern" medicine.

Although many have hailed this book as the text to use, I find the writing a bit stilted and not as clear as the earlier work of Close. Somehow, Close is timeless, and this work seems dated.

1936: *A STUDY OF THE SIMILE IN MEDICINE*: Linn J. Boyd, MD
Boericke and Tafel; 421 pages.
A scholarly discussion of the simile in medicine, through the period of Hahnemann, followed by the more "recent developments," largely through German sources: The Arndt-Schultz law, the work of Augustus Bier, etc.

Boyd had taught at The University of Michigan at Ann Arbor and was, according to John Renner, MD, driven out by the Hahnemannians because he was experimenting upon animals. Boyd went on to the New York Homœopathic Medica College, where he became Professor of Medicine and Head of The Department of Medicine, Pharmacology and Homœopathic Therapeutics. He stayed on at New York Medical College into the 1950s and was a noted pharmacologist.

1942: *A NEW SYNTHESIS*: Guy Beckley Stearns, MD and Edgar D. Evia
Foundation for Homœopathic Research, New York; 127 pages.
Divided into three sections: 1. The Physical Basis of Homœopathy (what a potency is and the possible physics of how it stores/transmits information); 2. A New Synthesis (the biology of living matter and its response to the environment); 3. Things to Do (experiments, Boyd's emanometer, and the use of autonomic reflex testing).

A brilliant synthesis of disparate material. Stearns was the first to suggest that the autonomic nervous system will react to a remedy. He measured this through both pulse testing and pupilary reaction, both of which are described in the book. Those who have tried these techniques swear by them. This work (as of this writing) has not been reprinted, although it has been quoted as a primary source by many working on the physics of high dilutions.

c. 1955: *HOMŒOPATHY: HUMAN MEDICINE*: Dr. Leon Vannier
Homœopathic Publishing Co.; 234 pages.
An exposition about "constitution" and "typology," with an explanation of Nebel's three constitutional types: Carbonic, Phosphoric, and Fluoric.

1967: *PRINCIPLES AND PRACTICE OF HOMŒOPATHY VOLUME 1*: M. L. Dhawale ✔
Karatak Publishing, Bombay: 638 pages.
An in-depth discussion of homœopathic philosophy and repertorization, derived from a series of courses taught for the Homœopathic Post-Graduate Association in Bombay.

A very in-depth and well presented study. The philosophy behind the repertories is explained and emphasized as to why one would be used in preference to another.

1977: *A BRIEF STUDY COURSE IN HOMEOPATHY*: Elizabeth Wright-Hubbard, MD ✔
Formur; 102 pages.
Prepared by Alain Naudé from a number of papers left by Dr. Hubbard, this small work remains a concise description of the theory and practice of homœopathy.

1978: *THE SCIENCE OF HOMŒOPATHY*: George Vithoulkas ✔
Athens School of Homeopathic Medicine; 373 pages.
The first "modern text." The author, with major structural help by Bill Gray, MD, pulls together the work of Hahnemann and the work of Kent. The homœopathy presented is derivative of the thinking of Kent and presents it in the light of "high potency" classical thinkers. It was *the* book that served as the introduction to homœopathy for many professionals and shaped the thinking of a whole generation of prescribers. Reprinted in **1980** by Grove Press.

Until this book, the only "modern" text was Roberts' Principles and Art of Cure. *Vithoulkas' text served as an introduction to many of the newer homœopaths world-wide. It covered the whole range from the "philosophical" to the practical. But it was all seen through Vithoulkas' modeling, and subsequent generations were taught about the "stacking cones" of the "mental, emotional, and physical" and have been introduced to Vithoulkas' concept of "freedom" as a criteria in "health." It is important to understand that although many of these ideas had their root in the work of Hering and Hahnemann, the "spin" is decidedly Kentian, with a more modern layer of spirituality applied to that. It grew out of the times of the late 60s and early 70s where many were looking for spiritual gurus in a world that had seemingly lost itself. The book spoke very directly to those of that generation. As useful as the book is, one should remember that this is homœopathy through Vithoulkas' filters — NOT those of Hahnemann.*

1980: *PSYCHE AND SUBSTANCE: Essays on Homœopathy in the light of Jungian Psychology*:
Edward Whitmont, MD ✔
North Atlantic Books; 190 pages.
A series of essays by a Jungian trained homœopath, about symbolic ways of seeing homœopathic remedies through the archetypal images of the remedy sources. All but two of the essays appeared in the *Homœopathic Recorder* between 1948 and 1955. The thinking presented in this book served as the base for one of the leading edge of modern homœopathy. A 2nd edition, of 238 pages, was printed in **1991**.

1980: *NOTES ON THE MIASMS OR HAHNEMANN'S CHRONIC DISEASES:*
Dr. Proceso Sanchez Ortega ✔
National Homoeopathic Pharmacy, New Delhi; 295 Pages
Originally published in **1977** as *Apuntes sobre los Miasmas o Enfermedades Crónicas de Hahnemann*. Primera edición. Biblioteca de Homeopatía de México A.C. México D.F.
The English edition was published under the supervision of Diwan Harish Chand. This book is an in-depth look at miasmatic analysis of cases.

According to Dana Ullman, the English translation was paid for by Don Gerrard, who also put up the first money to start the IFPH which later became the International Foundation for Hmeopathy.

1982: *INTRODUCTION TO HOMŒOPATHIC PRESCRIBING*: S. M. Gunavante ✔
B. Jain; 300 pages.
An in-depth review of homœopathic principles and practice, with many references to past works of the masters. The 4th edition in 1990 (335 pages) was revised and expanded with the inclusion of a number of repertory exercises and a brief materia medica of nine remedies.

Gunavante is a "lay-person" who developed a deep interest in homœopathy. The book contains a few errors (Radium brom. is not *an imponderable!), but, generally, it is a well-researched and documented exposition of homœopathic principles and practice. Each chapter ends with a short "self-test" and suggestions as to which books to consult for more information. Many authors are quoted throughout, and the appendices include a listing of books to read at various levels of expertise, as well as remedy suggestions for "specifics" and "causations." This is not a well known book and has a great amount of information buried within its pages.*

1986: *THE HANDBOOK OF HOMEOPATHY; ITS PRINCIPLES AND PRACTICE*: Gerhard Köhler, MD ✔
Thorsens; 240 pages.
Published in Germany in 1983 as *Lehrbuch der Homöopathie*. Translated by A. R. Meuss. A complete exposition on the principles and practice of homœopathy.

Although it contains a few errors (it gives the date of Kent's Repertory as 1877 instead of 1897, and has a very confused statement on the meaning of the repertory gradings) and has some advice that many homœopaths would certainly not agree with (i.e., the symptom in the patient must match the grade in the repertory; if the patient shows a symptom strongly, it must be in Bold type in the repertory), the book is, generally, very thorough in its explanations and definitions of homœopathic practice.

1987: *KENT'S MINOR WRITINGS ON HOMŒOPATHY*: James Tyler Kent, MD
Haug Verlag, Heidelberg; 766 pages.
Edited by Klaus-Henning Gypser, MD, this is a scholarly revision of Kent's "Lesser Writings." This book contains *only* those pieces directly attributable to Kent (i.e., signed by him), and arranged in chronological order of publication. The editor of the previous work, W. W. Sherwood, had split some of the cases away from the articles which had contained them. This volume places it all back together.

The ultimate "Kent Reader." A fascinating study of how Kent developed his ideas, since his thinking can be traced through the chronological order of publication. Original sources for all the material are noted. It contains several articles that were missed by Sherwood in his 1926 work. It does NOT contain the "Aphorisms" since they were only attributed to Kent but never appeared under his signature. Similarly it does not contain the editorial from The Homœopathician *in which Kent supposedly discussed prescribing upon pathology, since the editorial in question did not appear under Kent's name, and was probably written by co-editor Julia Loos.*

1991: *A NEW MODEL OF HEALTH AND DISEASE*: George Vithoulkas ✔
North Atlantic Books and Health and Habitat; 205 pages.
"The book is written with a threefold objective in mind: 1. To show that established medicine has failed in its mission to prevent and cure disease… 2. To present a new model of health and disease as a new paradigm for the science of medicine… 3. To point out that such therapeutic systems exist and are available today…"

Although the author apologizes for his "polemic or prejudiced manner" in asserting that all the modern diseases (AIDS, cancer, immune diseases) are caused by the use of modern drug therapies, the book tends to alienate all but the "true believer." I was reading the book on a plane, and in the seat next to me was a physician who was interested in the title. I let him look at the book, and he was both offended at the assertion of blame and mystified by it. No matter what its intent, the book is preaching to the converted and is not offered in a manner that would encourage those of the "medical establishment" to read further.

1991: *THE SPIRIT OF HOMEOPATHY*: Rajan Sankaran ✔
Homeopathic Medical Publishers, Mumbai; 328 pages.
The book is divided into five sections: Philosophy, The Mind, Casetaking, Finding the Remedy, and Materia Medica. Sankaran introduces his idea of "situational materia medica" which postulates that disease originates from traumatic situations in which the person adopts a behavior to help with the situation, but the behavior continues after the trauma is past, and this results in sickness— which is an inappropriate response of mind or body. This state of mind and body is maintained by what Sankaran terms the central disturbance. The core of the central disturbance is the basic delusion (the imaginary situation to which the organism reacts) and it is this central disturbance that has to be perceived and then cured.

The first book written by Rajan Sankaran, the son of P. Sankaran, a great Indian homœopath.

1991: *A GUIDE TO THE METHODOLOGIES OF HOMEOPATHY*: Ian Watson ✔
Cutting Edge Publications, Cumbria, UK; 166 pages.
Definitions and explanations of the varying methodological approaches found in homœopathy— "essence" prescribing, unicist, pluralist, complexisist, etc.

1991: *TREATISE ON HOMEOPATHIC MEDICINE*: Francisco Eizayaga, MD
Ediciones Marcel, Buenos Aires; 315 Pages.
First published in Argentina in **1972**. A complete overview of homœopathy by the great Argentinian homœopath.

Eizayaga taught extensively in the USA in the mid 1980s. His analytical approach and his use of daily dosing with lower potencies, was a great contrast to the "single dose and wait" that was the fashion among "essence" prescribers. This book explains his methodology and his reasons for looking at homœopathy in his unique manner. Although a masterful work, the translation leaves a lot to be desired— the book suffers from a "choppy" style and awkward constructions. In a time when homœopathy was becoming more metaphysical and psychological in its approach, this book is a clear statement of the opposite side of the coin.

1992: *TYPOLOGY IN HOMŒOPATHY*: Dr. Leon Vannier ✔
Beaconsfield; 176 pages.
Originally published in France in **1955** as *La Typologie et Ses Applications Thérapeutiques Les Tempéraments, Prototypes et Métatypes*. Translated by Marianne Harling, FFHom.
"Typology" is the classification of human beings according to their physical and psychological characteristics. The author starts with Nebel's three constitutional types and develops them through the temperaments of Greco-Roman mythology. "These planetary beings are considered prototypes of human psycho-physio-pathological behavior and are described at length..." Illustrated with paintings, statuary, and composite models, the author describes the eight "Prototypes," the 13 "Metatypes," and the six "Earth types," along with the diseases to which they are prone and the homœopathic remedies to which they best respond.

A beautiful example of a speculative and synthetic structure being placed over the homœopathic model— everything that Hahnemann cautioned against.

1993: *24 CHAPTERS ON HOMEOPATHY*: Joseph Reves ✔
Homœopress Ltd., Haifa, Israel; 256 pages.
"In 24 chapters we have done our best to bring the reader the principles and way of homœopathic thought."

Joseph Reves practices and teaches in Israel. His approach to homœopathy is heavily Kentian with a major metaphysical overlay. The book is not very easy going, but that might be the nature of the translation. It is about as dense as Hahnemann's Organon— *read a paragraph at a time... then think a lot.*

1993: *THE ALCHEMY OF HEALING*: Edward Whitmont, MD ✔
North Atlantic Books; 240 pages.
Said one reviewer, "This makes for a writing style that resists easy passage." Whitmont discusses the nature of the healer's self and roles with regard to himself/herself and to the patient, and he clarifies these relationships by the use of an archetypal analysis of those interactive roles.
Whitmont summarizes contemporary developments in different fields of knowledge, and the result is a summary of such areas as the new physics, the Gaia hypothesis, and Jungian studies. Homœopathy comes and goes through the work. It is *not* about homœopathy but is a work written by a Jungian analyst who understands the principles of homœopathy and pays his respect to them.

1994: *THE SUBSTANCE OF HOMEOPATHY*: Rajan Sankaran ✔
Homeopathic Medical Publishers, Mumbai; 303 pages.
In this book, which builds on Sankaran's previous work, the author offers an expanded theory of the miasms, along with other typologies, mostly those of the mineral remedies, using the periodic table as a way to deduce "themes" in the remedies. The first third of the book concerns itself with a delusion-based interpretation of the theory of miasms intended for diagnostic use, and a system of classification by delusion for the purpose of finding the simillimum.
The rest of the book introduces the concepts of the differences between the remedies from the different kingdoms (animal, vegetable, and mineral) and how one can use the behaviors (and "situation") of the patient to point the way to the kingdom in which the remedy for the case exists.

These two works (The Spirit *and* The Substance) *by Sankaran have become the popular "cutting-edge" of homœopathy, and have led to more and more speculative musings about the remedies needed in the case— the information gleaned not as much from the case but by the synthetic overlay of the kingdom analysis and the perception of the core delusion. The path is fraught with danger, especially in the hands of those with little grounding in the materia medica, who see these methods as an easy way to find remedies. As "essence" prescribing was the password in 1980s, the "core delusion" and "kingdom analysis" became the "hot ticket" in the 1990s.*

1995: *HOMEOPATHY RENEWED*: Rudolph Verspoor and Patricia Smith ✔
Private printing, Ottawa, CANADA; 133 pages.
An erudite exposition of the conceptual structure of "Sequential Therapy" as first outlined by Swiss physician, Jean Elminger, MD.

Although Verspoor's ideas are backed up along the way by quotes from a number of homœopathic "greats," the book tends to be "soft" around the edges and fails to give a detailed picture of the subject. The case that is presented at the end as an example of "sequential prescribing" leaves large gaps in the possible interpretation of of the symptoms. We are asked to believe that the original remedy was properly prescribed (and failed) when little of the case is shown to the reader.

1998: *CROSSROADS TO CURE: THE HOMEOPATH'S GUIDE TO THE SECOND PRESCRIPTION*: Nicola Henriques ✔
Totality Press, Saffron Walden, UK; 165 pages.
The author has collected all the writings from the "greats" about the "second prescription" and assembled it in a logical order.

1999: *THE HERSCU LETTER*: Paul Herscu ND ✔
New England School of Homeopathy, Amherst, MA; 16 pages.
A bi-monthly "lesson" in homeopathy. Essentially, lessons in the principles of homeopathy, illustrated by examples from practice.

Not really a book, but by now it is read regularly by over 700 people, and so becomes an influential source of information. Each edition discusses a single issue of principle, gives an example of how it is seen in practice, and gives a short assignment— the answers to which are answered in the next edition.
At some point it would be a delight to see them all bound into a book. It would provide our current homeopaths with a volume which has a depth of thinking not seen since Dudgeon's Theory and Practice *over 150 years ago.*

1999: *HAHNEMANN REVISITED: A TEXTBOOK OF CLASSICAL HOMEOPATHY FOR THE PROFESSIONAL*; Luc De Schepper, MD ✔
Full of Life Publishing, Santa Fe, NM; 573 pages.
An in-depth text designed to guide the experienced professional. There is a chapter on the use of LM potencies.

A bit too prescriptive or dogmatic for my tastes. The author has a tendency to say, "this is the way," rather than

to place it in the context of his personal experience which would say, "this is the way it has been in MY practice." Nevertheless, a lot of useful information is presented. As the title says, it is for the experienced, practicing homœopath.

1999: HOMEOPATHY RE-EXAMINED: BEYOND THE CLASSICAL PARADIGM: Rudolph Verspoor and Stephen Decker ✔
Hahnemann Center for Heilkunst, Gloucester, Canada; 400 pages.
An exposition of homœopathy in light of the Organon and a careful analysis of what is contained therein.

This book is bound to upset many. There has not been a solid book discussing the Organon *in depth since Kent's Lectures in 1900. All other "philosophy" books worked from Kent or the unspoken assumptions that were passed through generations. This is the first new look at the meaning of Hahnemann's seminal work without the filters of the past. It is not light reading— but, then again, neither is the* Organon. *It loses cohesion every so often, but it is a must read for anyone interested in the practice of homœopathy beyond simple "first-aid" depth. The book poses a lot of questions around the interpretation of Hahnemann's work. The interpretations of the* Organon *are derived from the unpublished inter-linear translation done by Decker. Keep in mind that Verspoor is an advocate of "sequential therapy" and has, seemingly, "read into" many of Hahnemann's words a justification for that practice. The ideas presented, however, are thought provoking and deserve to be opened up for debate after all these years. But as Kent should be read in the light of his Swedenborg overlay, the authors of this work bring to it their own "overlay" that is never mentioned.*

2000: *THE SYSTEM OF HOMEOPATHY*: Rajan Sankaran ✔
Homeopathic Medical Publishers, Mumbai ; 494 pages.
Sankaran briefly introduces his first twenty-five case histories, presents about fifty pages outlining his "system," and follows with another ten cases. He clarifies his thoughts on miasm and kingdom classification in an appendix. There is a final summary by Dr. Bill Gray.

Sankaran is adamant that no theorizing or speculating must enter into case analysis, and yet he uses intangibles such as patterns in speech, dreams and life events as hard data— and it certainly looks *like theorizing and speculation. The book would make little sense without his other two works, and he refers readers to his materia medica,* The Soul of Remedies, *for a better understanding of the prescription.*
Says one reviewer: "This book is like a window into a gifted mind finding the fullness of his delusions. Much is borrowed from homœopathy and much is invented. All the references to 'my system' and 'my concepts' etc. seem like egotistical aberrations, for while Sankaran offers valuable insights into many aspects of the work, the original writings are readily available and much more rationally laid out by Hahnemann and his closest followers. There is a continual drifting between fragments of rational, established methods of practice and his own somewhat irrational twists of theory. With each step, he takes you a little further into his imaginative thinking that demands organization, hence everything dissolves into themes and stages that are somehow supposed to represent a system. The 'System' is finally a mass of generalizations that need to be carefully sifted as to their worthiness. Instead of being called 'The System of Homeopathy' a better title would be 'An Interpretive Approach to Medicine based on Homeopathy.'"

Materia Medica

The Homœopathic Materia Medica

The first need of a practitioner, after a good text on homœopathic principles, is a materia medica— a list of the medical materials that the practitioner will be using. The homœopathic materia medica is quite different from that of its allopathic counterpart, in that it is not only a listing of the chemical makeup of the material and its possible uses, but, most importantly, it is a detailed listing of the symptomatic response of a healthy person under controlled circumstances (proving) to the medicinal influence. Hahnemann, as he constructed the first materia medica used the *de capite ad calcem* (from head to foot) that had been in general use in medicine. At first, he started with the symptoms of the head moving down through the body ending with "sleep" and "moral symptoms." In his later work he began with the symptoms of the mind and the senses and then moved down the body to end with sleep and fever.

As other provings were done and more information was gathered, the Hahnemannian schema began to be the standard layout used. Hering, writing in 1867, commented that the schema makes the most sense when it is considered in light of the "laws of cure"— the symptoms are listed from above to below, and from inside to outside with the skin being last.

As practitioners gained experience in the use of the remedies they began to uncover problems in the interactions of various remedies— which remedies followed each other, which ones would antidote others, etc. As the importance of the conditions of aggravation and amelioration were recognized, a separate category of those conditions which were considered to be of the "general" nature were included in the materia medica of the remedy. The next series of books that were published reflected these new experiences. These new materia medica added this new material to the Hahnemannian schema.

As further experience was gained, other materia medicae became more than mere lists of provings; they became accounts of personal experiences with the remedies. Some authors, like Teste, began to group the remedies into similar categories. Others began to put the information together using clinical information as the schema, where the "disease" is defined and the ways in which each homœopathic remedy relates to it is outlined.

Each materia medica that was written after Hahnemann's work (with the exception of other provings) is essentially a record of personal experiences with the remedies that Hahnemann outlined or of remedies that were added through new provings. The more provings that were done, the larger grew the materia medicæ. Hering commented, "Who would object to a library because it is too large? If you have good catalogs, you always have a better chance of finding what you are looking for than in a small one."

There are a number of ways in which materia medica can be presented:
• Straight from the proving, in the words of the prover, as in Hughes' *Cyclopedia*. Hahnemann arranged these records in the "above to below" schema, and that is generally followed through most materia medica documentation.
• Experiential recording, often of clinical data gleaned by the practitioner in the use of the remedy.
• A free narrative about the remedy, where the above information is woven into a "word picture" of the characteristics of the remedy. These were often derived from lectures delivered by teachers like Dunham, Farrington, etc.
• Regional materia medica: in which the remedies are limited only to those that are found to relate to a specific region (mind, lungs, back, etc.). In this category, those that are pure materia medica are rare. Most regional materia medica have their primary interest in therapeutics and, therefore, are considered in this work as therapeutic texts.
• Comparative materia medica: in which remedies which have similar actions are compared and referenced to their modalities, as the work of Gross.

All of these presentations can be mixed and matched into other categories.

Once the remedy has been used with success, it becomes difficult to discuss the remedy without giving clinical examples of its use. Because of this, the distinction between pure materia medica and therapeutics grows rather fuzzy.

The Heritage of Homœopathic Literature

For our purposes, if the book "reads" as a materia medica, then it will be placed into that category.

Once the materia medica is written, there is always the desire to make it accessible by compiling an index. Many of the books presented in the listing here include a "clinical index" which is simply a listing of conditions cross referenced with a list of remedies that might be helpful. If one uses the clinical index one is always referred back to the materia medica for the final selection.

The other kind of index is a "repertory." A clinical index is very different from a "repertory" since it does not involve itself with the uniqueness of the remedy as seen through the modalities. The clinical index will simply say "Sore throat." The repertory will break the symptom (sore throat) into its components: worse at night, worse when swallowing, stitching on the left side, etc.

For our purposes here, I have chosen to separate those books which are materia medica with a clinical index from those which are a combined materia medica and repertory in one.

Those books which discuss therapeutics as their main focus are listed under "Therapeutics" and those books that are primarily repertories are listed in the "Repertory" section.

Materia Medica (provings, experiential/clinical, narrative)

1805: *FRAGMENTA DE VIRIBUS MEDICAMENTORUM POSITIVIS SIVE IN SANO CORPORE HUMANO OBSERVATIS*: Samuel Hahnemann, MD
Sumtu Joan, Ambros. Barthii, Leipzig; 713 pages.
The first materia medica by Hahnemann contained the proving information of 27 remedies in the first part (269 pages) and a 470 page repertory in alphabetical order in the second part. The first part, edited by Frederick Foster Hervey Quin, MD in England, was re-published there as a 214 page book (again in Latin) in **1834**.

1811-1821: *THE MATERIA MEDICA PURA*: Samuel Hahnemann, MD ✱ ✔
Reine Arzneimittellehre, Arnold, Dresden. Vol. 1, **1811**, Vol. 2, **1816**, Vol. 3, **1816**, Vol. 4 , **1818**, Vol. 5, **1819**, Vol. 6, **1821**. 53 remedies.
The second edition (in six volumes) was published between **1822-1827**. The third edition (in two volumes) was published between **1830-1833**. Of the 53 remedies, 15 were found to be of an antipsoric nature and were included, in expanded form, in *The Chronic Diseases*. The first English translation was done by Charles Hempel, and published by William Radde in **1846**. R. E. Dudgeon did a translation that was published by the Hahnemann Publishing House (London) in **1880**.

1828-1830: *THE CHRONIC DISEASES; THEIR PECULIAR NATURE AND THEIR HOMŒOPATHIC CURE*: Samuel Hahnemann, MD ✱ ✔
Die chronischen Krankheiten, ihre eigenthümliche Natur und homöopathische Heilung, Arnold, Dresden.
Vol. 1, **1828**, Vol. 2, **1828**, Vol. 3, **1828**, Vol. 4, **1830**.
The first English edition was by Geddes M. Scott, MD of Glasgow, Scotland in **1842**. It was translated from the **1832** French edition. In **1845**, William Radde published a translation made by Hempel from the German. Because of complaints of poor translation and missing symptoms in the Hempel translation, a further translation (of 1600 pages), direct from the German, was made by Louis Tafel in **1896**, and published by Boericke and Tafel. It is this massive volume that is currently available from Indian booksellers.
The basic concepts of the "miasms" are discussed in part one (theoretical part) and 48 Anti-psoric remedies are discussed in part two. The "Theoretical Part" was reprinted by Boericke and Tafel as a separate edition in **1904**.

1836: *JAHR'S MANUAL OF HOMŒOPATHIC MEDICINE*: Georg Heinrich Gottlieb Jahr
Academical Bookstore; 419 pages.
Translated and edited by Constantine Hering, MD. (This book was first published in France in **1834** under the title: *Manuel d' Medicine Homeopathique.*)
This 1836 volume, published under the auspices of the North American Academy of the Homeopathic Healing Art at Allentown, PA, was the first homœopathic materia medica published in English in the USA. The first part was the Materia Medica, "Symptomology." The book was used as the base for an edition published by William Radde in **1841**. It was edited and amended by Amos Gerald Hull, MD, a pupil of Hans Burch Gram, and one of the earliest converts to homœopathy. This translation is structured as a list of remedies with their outstanding physical characteristics. A repertory was included in the second volume. This edition was known as *HULL'S JAHR.*
In **1861** the book was revised and edited by Frederick Snelling, MD. This two volume update was divided into symptomology (vol.1) and repertory (vol.2). It was published by Radde. In **1879**, Boericke and Tafel republished the Snelling revision of the Materia Medica, and republished the Repertory in **1884**.

1838: *THE PATHOGENIC EFFECTS OF SOME OF THE PRINCIPAL HOMŒOPATHIC REMEDIES*:
Harris Dunsford, MD
Balliere, London; 276 pages.
This was compiled mostly from the works of Bönninghausen and Jahr. It presents 50 remedies in the Hahnemann schema. It might be the first book in the English language on materia medica.

1841: *PRACTICAL OBSERVATIONS ON SOME OF THE CHIEF HOMŒOPATHIC REMEDIES:*
Franz Hartmann, MD.
J. Dobson; 171 pages.
Translated by A. Howard Okie. A second volume was published in **1846** by William Radde.

1843: *MANUAL OF HOMŒOPATHIC MATERIA MEDICA*: Alphons Noack, MD and
Carl Friedrich G. Trinks, MD
Handbuch der homöopathischen Arzneimittellehre. Schumann, Leipzig;
Volume I (*Aconitum* to *Kreosotum*) 1010 pages.
Said the *British Journal of Homœopathy* at the time: "An extremely important & useful work... contains the provings of all medicines which have appeared up to the date of its publication, slightly abridged it is true, but only to avoid repetition, without omitting any characteristic symptom."
The final work was issued in two volumes in **1847**, with Volume II (*Lactuca* to *Zingiber*) having 1570 pages. Although the work is often quoted in other materia medicae, a full English translation was never done.

Schumann had asked Noack to complete a handbook of materia medica. Noack asked Trinks for his contributions. Because of lack of time, Trinks gave Noack his notes. Noack completed the first volume up till Kali hydroiodicum, then left Leipzig and moved to Lyons. The first edition of the first volume was postponed. Schumann asked Trinks to complete the work. He accepted the task (with the help of Clotar Müller). It was written to compete with Jahr's "Symptomen-Codex" which was selling well.

1846: *THE TRANSACTIONS OF THE AMERICAN INSTITUTE OF HOMŒOPATHY*
Charles Rademacher, Philadelphia; 299 pages.
The minutes of the first meeting of the AIH comprise the first ten pages. The next 243 pages contain the text of ten provings (*Fluoric acid, Oxalic acid, Elaterium, Eupatorium perfoliatum, Podophyllum,* etc.), and the final 46 pages is a brief repertory of the remedies discussed.

1846: *ADDITIONS TO THE MATERIA MEDICA PURA:* Ernst Stapf, MD.
Radde; 292 pages.
Translated by Hempel. The proving of 12 remedies (*Clematis, Coffea, Crocus, Juniperus, Ranunculus bulbosus, Ranunculus scleratus, Rhododendron, Sabadilla, Senega, Teucrium, Valariana, Vitex agnus castus*)

1852: *FLORA HOMŒOPATHICA:* Edward Hamilton, MD ✔
Balliere; 523 pages.
Illustrations and descriptions of 66 medicinal plants used as homœopathic remedies. Both a botany book and a materia medica, it has information about the symptomology of poisonings, and records of cases where the plant was successfully used, as well as a description of the homœopathic uses. The original book contained magnificent hand-colored illustrations. The book was reprinted by the Faculty of Homeopathy in **1981**, as a limited edition. It has subsequently been reprinted in India.

1853: *THE HOMEOPATHIC MATERIA MEDICA, ARRANGED SYSTEMATICALLY AND PRACTICALLY:* Alphonse Teste, MD ✔
Rademacher and Sheek; 634 pages.
Translated from the French by Charles Hempel. This book is arranged, as the author says, "systematically and practically." The remedies are grouped into twenty sets that Teste found to be related. Each set has a listing of common characteristics and then similar remedies are differentiated. For example, the first set is *Arnica*, with the sub-headings under it as *Led., Crot-t., Ferr-mag., Rhus-t., Spig.*

1853: *PROVINGS OF THE PRINCIPAL ANIMAL AND VEGETABLE POISONS OF THE BRAZILIAN EMPIRE*: Benoit Mure, MD
Radde; 220 pages.
Mure, a French merchant in the last stages of consumption, read the *Organon* and went to Count Des Guidi in Lyons for treatment. After being cured, he enrolled at Montpellier and became a physician. He started practice in Malta in 1836. It was said, "Dr. Mure in his proselytizing ardor was no stickler for professional etiquette." He worked in Palermo, then in Paris with Jahr. He went to Rio de Janeiro in 1840 and started the first homœopathic school in Brazil. He returned to France in 1847. He practiced in Egypt and the Sudan in 1851. He was the first to suggest low potencies are for acute conditions and high potencies are for chronic conditions.
The book contains provings of 38 remedies including: *Crotalus cascavella, Elaps corallinus, Pediculus capitis, Mimosa humilis, Mancinella, Hura, Lepidium, Plumbago littoralis, Paullinia pinnata, Amphisoboena, Jacaranda,* and *Aristolohcia milhones*, and *Spiggurus martini* (the porcupine) among others. The book was originally published in French. It was reprinted in Brazil in **1999** as *PATHOGENESIA BRASILEIRA*.

A rare work with beautiful line illustrations of each of the remedy sources.

1853: *HOMŒOPATHIC PROVINGS:* James W. Metcalf, MD
Radde; 417 pages.
Originally issued as a supplement to the *North American Homeopathic Journal*, the book contains the provings of 14 remedies.

1854: *KEY TO THE MATERIA MEDICA OR COMPARATIVE PHARMACODYNAMICS*: Adolph Lippe, MD
Henry Duffield, Philadelphia; 142 pages.
An early work from a great prescriber. "Being aware that this work— a first effort of the kind— will admit of improvement, I shall very gladly and thankfully receive suggestions from any source as to imperfections that may exist, and corrections tending to make it more useful."
Certainly, a "work in progress." The author presents a series of characteristic symptoms of remedies (starting with the polychrests) in the left column, and remedies that have similar symptoms or bear comparing, are listed opposite each symptom in the right column.

1859: *A NEW AND COMPREHENSIVE SYSTEM OF MATERIA MEDICA AND THERAPEUTICS:*
Charles Hempel, MD
Radde; 1202 pages.
"Arranged upon a Physiologico-Pathological Basis, for the use of Practitioners and Students of Medicine." Revised and Enlarged (as two volumes) in **1865**, and again (edited by H. R. Arndt) in **1880**. The second volume is a materia medica.

1859: *HOMŒOPATHIC MATERIA MEDICA*: Martin Freligh, MD
Charles T. Hurlburt; 201 pages.
"Being a Summary of the Curative Action of the Principal Remedial Agents employed in Homœopathic Practice." A compilation from the works of Hahnemann, Jahr, Hull, Teste, etc.

1862: *A MONOGRAPH ON GELSEMIUM:* Edwin M. Hale, MD
E. A. Lodge; 56 pages.
Incorporated into Hale's later work.

1864: *NEW REMEDIES; THEIR PATHOGENIC EFFECTS AND THERAPEUTIC APPLICATIONS IN PRACTICE:* Edwin M. Hale, MD ✔
E. A. Lodge; 448 pages.
Called simply "New Remedies," this was the first of many editions. The book was a record of provings of 44 indigenous remedies (*Gelsemium, Cimicifuga, Podophyllum, Collinsonia*, etc.) and clinical cases in which the remedy was successfully used. Realizing that much of the work was simply "suggestive or theoretical deductions," the author acknowledges that as experience is gathered in the use of the remedies, the "necessity for these suggestions and theoretical deductions will be done away with."
The work was enlarged in a second edition of 1144 pages in **1867** titled: *THE MATERIA MEDICA OF THE NEW REMEDIES; THEIR BOTANICAL DESCRIPTION, MEDICAL HISTORY, PATHOGENIC EFFECTS AND THERAPEUTIC APPLICATION IN PRACTICE.* By **1873**, 80 new remedies were added, and included were only characteristic symptoms, without the provings and descriptions of the remedy. In the 4th edition in **1875**, called *THE MATERIA MEDICA AND SPECIAL THERAPEUTICS OF THE NEW REMEDIES*, the author "at the behest of the profession" re-introduced the material he took out of the 2nd edition to prepare the 3rd. The 4th edition was offered in two volumes: "Symptomology "and "Therapeutics." The Symptomology volume was a materia medica derived from the provings— a listing of symptoms set out in the Hahnemann schema. The "Therapeutics" volume presented the history and botanical description of the remedy and cured cases using the remedy. The information in the second volume was based on the lectures Hale gave at the Hahnemann Medical College of Chicago during 1873-74. A 5th edition was published by Boericke and Tafel in **1897**.

The first and second editions are the most "pure," having the reports of the poisonings and provings, with little further commentary. By the time the 3rd edition was done, the actual reports were replaced with characteristic symptoms. The first edition is difficult to find, although I have seen a number of second editions for sale through the years. The second edition also contained some beautiful line drawings of the plants. The two volume fourth edition is the one that has currently been reprinted.

1866: *TEXTBOOK OF MATERIA MEDICA*: Adolph Lippe, MD ✔
A. J. Tafel; 714 pages.
Lippe was one of Hering's earliest pupils. The book uses Hahnemann's schema, and lists the characteristics and most prominent symptoms of each remedy. It was originally published in five parts.

Lippe is considered by many to be one of the finest Hahnemannian homœopaths ever, and his symptomatology in this book is very reliable. This book formed the base for Hering's Condensed Materia Medica *which started as an interleaved copy of Lippe's work, with Hering's additions.*

1867: *A MANUAL OF PHARMACODYNAMICS*: Richard Hughes, MD ✲ ✔
Leath and Ross and Henry Turner; 560 pages.
A transcription of the lectures on materia medica delivered to his classes in London. Although much of the material in the book concerns the pharmacological action of the remedies, Hughes' scholarship is flawless. He says this work is "in no way a substitute for the materia medica. It is, rather, a guide and companion to it." The back of the book has a remedy index with clinical indications listed. The book was issued by William Radde in **1868**, and had its 5th edition in the UK in **1886**.

George Royal relates that he was told by his preceptor to study Hering's Condensed Materia Medica, *but he couldn't make head nor tail of it. He then met Erastus Case who said, "That foolish man! Why did he not give you Hughes'* Pharmacodynamics *first? Get that and read it through. Then you can appreciate Hering."*

Although Kent considered Hughes a "skunk" for his emphasis on the pathological symptoms and advocacy of substantial doses, the book by Hughes is one of the best essays in the basics of homœopathic materia medica. However it should be kept in mind that Hughes was concerned with the pathological symptoms seen in the provings and many of our most "characteristic symptoms" we find in discussing remedies today will not be found in Hughes' work. Many of them developed through clinical symptoms after this work was published, and many Hughes would disregard because they are not in the provings.

Said Dr. Fornias in the April 1888 issue of The Medical Advance: *"It is a book written in elegant, forcible English, well adapted to inveigle or induce our old–school friends to look into the subject… it contains information well to know, but I pity the Homœopathist who goes into the sick–chamber provided only with the limited knowledge of symtomatology which can be obtained from this book."*

Says H. C. Allen, of the book, "It teaches us how to practice Allopathy with homœopathic remedies. Nothing more. The prescriber is taught to guess both at the pathology of the disease and the pathological action of the remedy, but he can never make an accurate Homœopathic prescription if he follows its teaching. Is it to not be wondered at that 'our old–school friends' are often disappointed?"

1869: *CHARACTERISTIC MATERIA MEDICA:* William Burt, MD ✔
A. J. Tafel; 460 pages.
Burt was one of the major provers of the "new remedies." Saying that the book was "not offered as a substitute for materia medica," the author condensed the experiences of Guernsey, Hering, and others into a materia medica of the characteristic symptoms, always referred back to the source. The book was reprinted by Gross and Delbridge in **1880** as *Physiological Materia Medica*, and again in **1888** as the 4th edition with 1109 pages.

1869: *EPITOME OF HOMŒOPATHIC MEDICINES:* William L. Breyfogle, MD
Boericke and Tafel; 383 pages.
Reprinted **1872, 1879, 1891.** The leading symptoms are listed with comparisons, followed by a short statement about the "curative range" of the remedy.

1873: *MATERIA MEDICA VOL. 1*: Constantine Hering, MD
Boericke and Tafel; 706 pages.
Originally published as a supplement to the *American Journal of Homeopathic Materia Medica*, it contained monographs of 16 remedies. Further volumes were never published.

1874: *THE ENCYCLOPÆDIA OF PURE MATERIA MEDICA; A RECORD OF THE POSITIVE EFFECTS OF DRUGS UPON THE HEALTHY HUMAN ORGANISM:* Timothy Field Allen, MD (10 volumes) ✔
Boericke and Tafel; 10 volumes.
This massive work was listed in the Hahnemann schema. It is an almost complete record of all provings and poisonings recorded to that date. Each symptom is referenced as to the prover, the dosage which elicited the symptom, and the source of the information. Allen credits Hughes, Dunham, Hering, and Lippe with helping him compile the information. The volumes were issued over a five year period: vol. 1 (*Abies* to *Atropin*) **1874**; vol. 2 (*Aurum* to *Carduus*): **1875**; vol. 3 (*Carlsbad* to *Cubeba*): **1876**; vols. 4 (*Cundurango* to *Hydrocotyle*), 5 (*Hydroc.acid* to *Lycopersicum*), 6 (*Lycopodium* to *Niccolum*): **1877**; vols. 7 (*Nicotinum* to *Plumbago*), 8 (*Plumbum* to *Serpentaria*): **1878**; vols. 9 (*Silica* to *Thuja*), 10 (*Tilia* to *Zizia*): **1879**.
In **1881** Allen published *A CRITICAL REVISION OF THE ENCYCLOPÆDIA OF PURE MATERIA MEDICA*. A reprint from the *North American Journal of Homeopathy* of 16 pages, this small work is, essentially, an errata for his larger work. It covers revisions to remedies from *Agaricus* to *Carbo veg*. No further work was done.
In a small four-page printing with no date, Allen gives the number of the symptoms that have been clinically verified by Dunham.

A classic work, considered an essential reference in the serious practitioner's library. However, at the time of its publication a review in the December 1879 Homœopathic Times, *described the work as "Dr. Allen's gigantic and most discredible fiasco." The review described the work as a "…mass of trash, of wild vagaries, of symptoms which seem to have been gathered at random from every language under heaven, from every insane asylum in the land, and from nurseries where fond mothers take seriously to heart the symptoms and sayings of their young offspring. Mixed with all this trash, the trained searcher may possibly find the real gems of our therapeutics, for they are there; but they are often so covered with what is perfectly worthless, that a special training is necessary to evolve them from the surrounding rubbish." It seems that Allen himself claimed responsibility for all the translations from the German, but in the reviewer's perusal of the* Nux vomica *chapter, several gross translation errors were found. For example, a literal translation of Hahnemann reads: "She regards the present pain as intolerable." while Allen translated it as: "The usual pain seems intolerable." Hahnemann says: "After midnight, very violent palpitations, with extreme anxiety which* impels *him to* suicide." *Which Allen translates as: "Extreme anxiety with violent palpitation which impels him to suicide."*

Says the reviewer: "…if we find a simple translation, from so important writer as Hahnemann, full of errors, what reliance can be placed on any of the editor's work?"

This review, although unsigned, was probably written by Egbert Guernsey, one of the editors of the Journal. It places into question the accuracy of a book which has been thought by many to be one of the primary sources of materia medica.

1877: *CONDENSED MATERIA MEDICA*: Constantine Hering, MD ✱ ✔
Boericke and Tafel; 870 pages.
This was an early work which lead to Hering's authoritative *Guiding Symptoms*. It was prepared with the help of two of his students, Augustus Korndoerfer and Ernest A. Farrington. It was dedicated to Charles Raue, his pupil and assistant. A 2nd edition was issued in **1879**; a 3rd, edited by Ernest A. Farrington, was issued in **1884**, and a 4th in **1894**.

1878: *AN ELEMENTARY TEXTBOOK OF MATERIA MEDICA:* Allen Corson Cowperthwaite, MD ✔
Duncan Brothers; 399 pages.
Cowperthwaite taught at the Hahnemann Medical College in Chicago. This book begins with a general analysis of each remedy, characteristic symptoms, and also includes therapeutic and clinical indices. A second edition was published in **1882**. A third edition was published by Gross and Delbridge in **1885**, a 4th in **1887**, a 5th in **1890**, a 6th (834 pages) in **1891**, and a 10th (with 894 pages) by Boericke and Tafel in **1909**.

1878: *CLINICAL THERAPEUTICS:* Temple Hoyne, MD ✔
Duncan Brothers; 602 pages.
Although titled "Therapeutics" this book is presented as materia medica, using the symptomatology of the remedy as a framework. It is interspersed with clinical cases gleaned from the literature, which serve to illustrate the remedies. A second volume of 643 pages was published in **1880**. "During the last four or five years, I have been repeatedly asked by the students of Hahnemann Medical College to publish my lectures in book form, in order that they, as well as their preceptors, might be able to make frequent reference to them."

1878: *LECTURES ON MATERIA MEDICA:* Carroll Dunham, MD ✔
Francis Hart and Co., New York; 828 pages in two volumes.
Dunham, a student under Bönninghausen, held the position of Chair of Materia Medica at New York Homœopathic Medical College. Dunham died in 1876 at the age of 49. The notes from his lectures were compiled by his students and published two years after his death. Said Samuel A. Jones, "His lectures are not today in such shape as he would have given them to the world; they are to us as though we had stolen into the classroom unseen and overheard him talking to the boys." A second edition was published by Boericke and Tafel in **1880**.

Kent, in 1899, wrote that he hoped the Dunham College of Chicago would "…teach materia medica as Dunham taught it."

1878: *NATRUM MURIATICUM AS A TEST OF THE DOCTRINE OF DRUG DYNAMIZATION:* James Compton Burnett, MD ✔
Gould; 84 pages.

The first of many books by this prolific writer. Along with his next work (Gold, below), the materia medica presented is seen through provings and through clinical cures.

1879: *GOLD AS A REMEDY IN DISEASE:* James Compton Burnett, MD ✔
Homœopathic Publishing Co.; 156 pages.

Burnett's proving of Gold is worth reading!

1879: *THE GUIDING SYMPTOMS OF THE MATERIA MEDICA:* Constantine Hering, MD ✔
J. M. Stoddart (vol. 1-4), The Estate of C. Hering (vols. 5-10).
1879 marked the release of the first volume, *Abies* to *Amoracea sativa*. The second volume, *Arnica* to *Bromium*, was released in **1880** shortly before Hering's death. The subsequent volumes were completed by his students Raue, Knerr, and Mohr. They were as follows: vol. 3 (*Bryonia* to *Chamomilla*): **1881**; vol. 4 (*Chelidonium* to *Cubeba*): **1884**; vol. 5 (*Cundurango* to *Helonias*): **1887**; vol. 6 (*Hepar* to *Lachesis*), 7 (*Lachnanthes* to *Natrum muriaticum*): **1888**; vol. 8 (*Natrum phos.* to *Pulsatilla*): **1889**; vol. 9 (*Ranunculus bulbosa* to *Stannum*): **1890**; vol. 10 (*Staphisagria* to *Zizia*): **1891**.

Sadly, the book was not completed by Hering, (who died during proof-reading Cainca *in Volume 3) but by his pupils, and thus contains innumerable questionable judgments about remedy and symptom grading. Says Kent: "The first two volumes were very good, but after the dear old man was taken from us the rest of the work was not up to standard and is full of foolish things. Though it is the best reference book of the present day, it is far from the perfect work needed." The information is a grand record of confirmed symptoms seen in over 50 years of practice. It is, with all its faults, an invaluable resource to the homœopathic practitioner and should be one of the first "larger" purchases when one is looking for a very complete materia medica.*

1879: *THE INCOMPATIBLE REMEDIES:* Charles Mohr, MD
Boericke and Tafel; 9 pages.
A paper presented to the Homeopathic Medical Society of Philadelphia. The author discusses the concept of "incompatible," gives some case examples from practice, and presents a list of remedy relationships.

1882: *MATERIA MEDICA MEMORIZER:* Andrew Leight Monroe, MD ✔
J. P. Morton, Lexington, KY; 50 pages.
Contains the keynotes of 44 remedies set to verse, where the first letter of each line spells out the name of a remedy.

A condition of veins, when well understood
Recalls it whenever its use would do good;
Namely *"stasis"* and *"extravasation"* of blood
It this may be used after *trauma* or *strain*
Convulsions, **C**ontusions or **C**ough with sore pain,
And Typhus' bad breath and Petechial stain.

1885: *A CYCLOPEDIA OF DRUG PATHOGENESY* (4 volumes): Richard Hughes, MD and Jabez P. Dake, MD, editors. ✔
Published jointly by the British Homœopathic Society and the American Institute of Homœopathy. The four volumes contain records of all provings done to date. Hughes believed that Allen's *Encyclopedia* had several faults, among them poor translations of the provings and admitting all published provings without checking their veracity. This latter issue was quite touchy since several years

earlier a German physician, C. W. Fickel, had published (to enhance his reputation) several provings that were pure inventions. He had published under several pseudonyms as well and his work was often quoted by opponents of the homœopathic system.
This work was assembled by a committee including Drysdale, Dudgeon, and Pope in the UK, and Conrad Wesselhoeft, E. A. Farrington, and H. R. Arndt in the USA.

As usual, with the work by Hughes, the scholarship is outstanding. If you have questions about symptoms in Allen's 10 volumes, a check of these four volumes might resolve doubts. But in the process, Hughes, ever the advocate of the physiological dose, eliminated all provings that were done with the higher potencies, thus eliminating much useful information.

1887: *A CLINICAL MATERIA MEDICA:* Ernest A. Farrington, MD ✻ ✔
Sherman & Co.; 752 pages.
Farrington, a protégé of Hering, died at the early age of 38 in 1885. This edition was edited by Lilienthal and is comprised of Farrington's lectures to his class at Hahnemann Medical College in Philadelphia that were "reported phonographically."
The material is presented in "family" order. A lecture on Spiders— The Arachnida; A lecture on the Compositae (*Arnica, Artemisia, Millefolium*, etc.); the Umbelliferæ; The acids; The Ammonium preparations, etc. In the 72 transcribed lectures, he discusses the topic and then compares the remedies to others— a comparative materia medica. The lecture on Halogens includes a part about *Spongia*— as it is rich in iodine and shares many symptoms of that group. A second edition was published by Hahnemann Printing House in **1890**.

With the current trend to looking at the "families" of remedies, it is interesting to reexamine this work and see that there is not much new, but a lot to be re-discovered.

1888: *SALIENT MATERIA MEDICA AND THERAPEUTICS:* Charles Luther Cleveland, MD ✔
Boericke; 171 pages.
191 remedies. The last 30 pages are a clinical index. "A practical, simple, and salient work is desired by many… how well I have succeeded will be quickly determined."
The same format is followed for all the remedies: 1. Temperament 2. Location and Nature 3. Objective [symptoms] 4. Causal 5. General characteristics 6. Aggravations 7. Ameliorations 8. Therapeutic range 9. Administration [dosage suggestions].

1888: *A MATERIA MEDICA CONTAINING PROVINGS AND CLINICAL VERIFICATIONS OF NOSODES AND MORBIFIC PRODUCTS:* Samuel Swan, MD
Pusey & Co., New York; 121 pages.
38 pages are provings of *Saccarum lactis*, the rest are provings of *Lac caninum*. Others volumes were planned, but "demand did not show a long-felt want" and no more provings were published.

1889: *HANDBOOK OF MATERIA MEDICA AND HOMŒOPATHIC THERAPEUTICS:*
Timothy Field Allen, MD ✻ ✔
Boericke; Quarto size, 1165 pages.
Originally sold by subscription only. An immense work, primarily derived from his *Encyclopædia* and his clinical notes. Hahnemann's schema is followed and is interspersed with clinical notes. It is of interest to note that most of the remedies proved by Mure have been deleted because "scarcely any have been found valuable."

That last sentence is very interesting! A perusal of some current (last 30 years) literature finds a fair number of cases of remedies proved by Mure and found in his 1853 book—Hura, Mancinella, Elaps, and Crotalus cascavella. Could it be that the symptomatology elicited in the provings was not observed in patients until "modern times"?

1892: *A PRIMER OF MATERIA MEDICA:* Timothy Field Allen, MD ✔
Boericke and Tafel; 408 pages.
"The characteristic features of the most important drugs" designed to "give the 'gist' of each drug rather than its symptomology."

1894: *POCKET CHARACTERISTICS*: Timothy Field Allen, MD
Privately printed by Allen; 150 pages.
A small (approx. 3" x 5") quiz compend that presents a single symptom per page, with the corresponding remedy name on the reverse side of the page.

A rare little volume. On front: "Eructations tasting of the ingesta."; *On reverse:* Antimonium Crudum

1894: *ESSENTIALS OF MATERIA MEDICA:* Willis A. Dewey, MD ✔
Boericke and Tafel; 294 pages.
A brief "Quiz Compend" that contains questions like: "What are the urinary symptoms of *Sepia*? How does *Causticum* compare?" followed by a detailed answer. Dewey taught materia medica at the University of Michigan at Ann Arbor, Michigan, and *this* was what he expected his students to know at the end of four years. There was a 4th edition in **1908**, and a 5th edition (372 pages) in **1926**. It was translated into French, German, and Portuguese.

This is a magnificent quiz compend, and puts into perspective the education that is now offered compared to that in the "golden age of homœopathy." Kent cautioned that "memorizers have no perception," but if one can absorb what is in this book it would provide an incomparable knowledge of basic homœopathic materia medica.

1894: *PROVINGS AND CLINICAL OBSERVATIONS WITH HIGH POTENCIES*: Malcolm Macfarlan, MD ✔
The Homœopathic Physician, Philadelphia, PA; 150 pages.
"My object has been to collate a few reliable symptoms, not as many as possible. What is written is, to the best of my knowledge, true, and was worked out originally for my own guidance and information. It is now given for what it may be worth to the profession." The information is culled from 25 years of practice. The provings were done with high potencies— from 200 up and most were made by Fincke. "The Medicines were given in water as a rule. Patients never knew they were making provings of medicines… Symptoms generally occurred on the third day. The provers, in many cases, had local ailments, fractures, injuries, etc., which did not interfere much with their general health or complicate medicinal symptoms." The work was published in *The Homœopathic Physician* (1892-1894), and then printed as a book.

Truly a wonderful collection. Having had Macfarlan's original hand-written notes in my possession, I saw the great care that went into this work. This work is rare and deserves to be better known by the profession.

1895: *PATHOGENIC MATERIA MEDICA:* Medical Investigation Club of Baltimore, MD
Boericke and Tafel; 347 pages.
A synthesis of Hughes' *Cyclopedia of Drug Pathogenesy* with the information listed as: proving remarks; sphere of action; symptomatology (in the Hahnemann schema); therapeutic applications.

1897: *NOTES ON MATERIA MEDICA LECTURES:* W. W. Winans, MD
Burnett Printing, Rochester, NY; 190 pages.
The sophomore and junior year notes from lectures at the Hahnemann Medical College in Philadelphia, during the 1896 and 1897 sessions. For each remedy, the notes of the sophomore year are presented first, followed by those of the junior year.

It is instructive to see how little pure materia medica was being taught at that time and how the allopathic uses and dosage forms of the remedies were stressed.

1898: *SAW PALMETTO:* Edwin B. Hale, MD
Boericke and Tafel; 96 pages.
A monograph on *Sabal serrulata*.

1898: *KEYNOTES TO THE MATERIA MEDICA:* Henry Clay Allen, MD ✱ ✔
Boericke and Tafel; 179 pages.
A small pocket book which keynotes the symptoms of 188 remedies. "To master that which is guiding and characteristic." This materia medica offers a section on remedy relationship and remedies that "follow well." A second edition which came out within a year of the first was expanded to 318 pages.
A 6th edition was printed in **1931**. It was printed by Boericke and Tafel into the 1950s.

1899: *LEADERS IN THERAPEUTICS:* E. B. Nash, MD ✱ ✔
Boericke and Tafel; 381 pages.
Nash covers over 200 remedies in the order he thinks of them ("to follow the bent of my inclinations, or, as it is sometimes expressed, the moving of the spirit"), *not* in alphabetical sequence. This book gives some interesting insights into the thought processes of one of the great old homœopaths. The 6th edition was published in **1946**. "Dr. Nash awoke one morning and found himself famous— as soon as this book was known— and the binder could scarcely keep up with the demand, and a second edition was soon called for… It is safe to say that no one is disappointed with this book, and it is a fascinating read from cover to cover."

A delightful volume which is very readable and filled with personal experiences and tid-bits from a grand prescriber. One of my favorite books, filled with useful hints and insights. Said one reviewer, "I will guarantee that no physician, be he homœopath, eclectic, regular, or what not, can read [this book] and not be a better physician."

1900: *A DICTIONARY OF PRACTICAL MATERIA MEDICA:* John Henry Clarke, MD ✱ ✔
Homeopathic Publishing Co.; 3 volumes.
A pulling together of Allen's *Encyclopedia*, Hering's *Guiding Symptoms*, and Hale's *New Remedies*. The clinical uses of the remedies are discussed, cases are given as examples of use, and then the remedy symptoms are listed using the Hahnemann schema. When some felt that the work was too long, Clarke replied: "My work is a *DICTIONARY* and I have never found a dictionary that explained too many words."
The first volume was issued in 1900. Volumes 2 and 3 were completed in **1902**.

If one needed just a single materia medica, this set might serve the purpose. Although the materia medica in the Hahnemann Schema is of use, the real "gold" of this work is found in the narrative that precedes the listing, where stories of the remedies are related, snippets from Burnett, Skinner, and Cooper are found, and unique characteristics of the remedy under discussion are presented.

1900: *NEW, OLD, AND FORGOTTEN REMEDIES:* Edward Pollock Anshutz ✔
Boericke and Tafel; 386 pages.
A collection of essays gleaned from homœopathic literature, encompassing 117 remedies. "Many of the drugs we recognize as nuggets, which, although have not received the stamp of the official assayer, possess an indisputable value which gives them currency." A 2nd edition, greatly enlarged to 608 pages, was published in **1917**.

A fascinating view into some smaller remedies, culled from literature to which most have no access. The making of Mullein oil, and the story behind the proving of Blatta are worth the price of the book.

1901: *MATERIA MEDICA:* William Boericke, MD ✱ ✔
Boericke and Runyon; 572 pages.
A 2nd edition by Homeopathic Publishing Co. in **1903**; 3rd edition by Boericke and Runyon in **1906** which contained a repertory by William's brother Oscar. The 9th edition was published in **1927**

and is still in print. This book has been compared to "trying to build a small house with many large rooms." Over a thousand remedies are mentioned. Although the polychrests are covered in less detail than in other *Materia Medica*, many other remedies are mentioned that are found only in larger works such as Clarke's *Dictionary*. Boericke wrote of choosing the specific font used in the book because of its visual clarity. The last printing with the original plates was done in the early 1980s, and the plates were showing their age, and there were places where the printing was unclear. When Boericke and Tafel chose to reissue the book in **1990**, they changed the type style.

I am sorry that this volume is no longer available with the black leatherette cover and the gold-edged, bible paper pages. It has (when in that form) eased my way while traveling through airports, as people avoided me, thinking they were to be evangelical targets!

1901: *A MANUAL OF HOMŒOPATHIC MATERIA MEDICA*: J. C. Fahnestock, MD
Published by the Author, Piqua, Ohio; 264 pages, interleaved.
Outlines of prominent features of 118 remedies with "specific action or 'elective affinity' included."

The author was a Hahnemannian homœopath who was not a member of the IHA.

1901: *ABC MANUAL OF MATERIA MEDICA:* George Hardy Clark, MD
Boericke and Tafel; 197 pages.
"Physiological effects of medicinal substances upon man is the safest and most useful guide to their selection in diseased states." An elaboration of the characteristics, toxic symptoms, doses used, and therapeutic uses. A step away from basic provings. A second edition, enlarged to 301 pages, was published in **1905**.

1901: *CHARACTERISTICS OF MATERIA MEDICA:* M. E. Douglas, MD
Boericke and Runyon; 974 pages.
"Many new drugs have been introduced… the aim of the author is to collect these… into practical and convenient shape for handy reference." A materia medica gleaned from many sources and verified by the author over 20 years of practice. Includes a 33 page clinical index. *The Medical Advance* said,
 "…the characteristic symptomatology of many remedies that they never before heard of, and which can be found in no other work, and for which they will thank the indefatigable author."

1904: *THE MNEMONIC SIMILIAD*: Stacy Jones, MD
Boericke and Tafel; 350 pages.
"I have endeavored to introduce a scheme for aiding the memory in grasping and retaining in mind *groups* of remedies having a general indication in *common*. To what extent I have succeeded must be determined by a fair trial, made by those who may feel disposed to test it… I beg the pardon of all the Muses of pathetic and sentimental song for introducing upon the rhythmic stage my plain domestic Muse, whose cognomen is USE. She is, indeed, plain and simple, but withal a most sincere and honest dame."
The author uses three devices: indication of letters, personification of remedies, and versification.

BROMINE (Brother; Broker)
Bromine,— We to thee assign,
Place with sponge and iodine,
As in goitre, hoarseness or croup,
Or a chest catarrhal group…

In the last 50 or so pages, the author develops "mnemonic sentences" with advice to refer back to the versification. For "Absence of Mind" he offers: "Who? Agnus, who is away on the coast of India, with the *hopeless* Nun of St. Para."

Surely one of the strangest exercises in the range of materia medica!

1905: *LECTURES ON MATERIA MEDICA:* James Tyler Kent, MD ✽ ✔
Boericke and Tafel; 965 pages.
Transcribed by his students from the lectures he presented at his Post-graduate School of Homœopathics in Philadelphia. It is reported that he stood with his interleaved and annotated copy of Hering's *Guiding Symptoms* on the lectern, and talked about the remedy, presenting symptoms from the book, and subjective reports from his own practice.
The transcribed lectures are sometimes seen in archives as a bound collection of typewritten pages. The National Center for Homeopathy has a unique series of his lectures that are hand-written, and while some are nearly identical to the material in the book, others are substantially different. A 2nd edition was printed in **1911**, a 3rd edition in **1923**, a 4th edition in **1932** and reprinted in **1956**.
In **1991**, Jay Yasgur and Chris Ellithorp published *THE DUNHAM LECTURES*— an additional series of lectures on materia medica that Kent delivered as a guest lecturer at the Dunham College in Chicago in 1899.

A valuable series of lectures which should be placed in historical perspective— this material is NOT primary materia medica. It is filtered through Kent and often filtered through Hering before him. The material is wonderful to read and contains many valuable therapeutic hints. Unfortunately, too many use this book as a primary source of materia medica. It isn't.

1906: *MANUAL OF MATERIA MEDICA, THERAPEUTICS, AND PHARMACOLOGY:*
A. L. Blackwood, MD ✔
Boericke and Tafel; 711 pages.
Pages 53-632 are a materia medica; pages 633-692 are a clinical index. Second edition in **1923**.

Often referred to as a "Dispensatory of the Homœopathic School."

1906: *TEST DRUG PROVING:* The O. O. & L. Society
O. O. & L. Society, Boston; 665 pages.
A reproving of *Belladonna* conducted by the Ophthalmological, Otological, and Laryngological Society in Baltimore.

A very involved re-proving of a grand old remedy. Despite all the efforts at being precise, exact, and as "scientific" as they understood at the time, the book contains nothing new in understanding the pathogenesis of Belladonna.

1907: *THE LIBRARY OF HOMŒOPATHIC CLASSICS, Volume I:* P. W. Shedd, editor
Journal Publishing Co., New York; 384 pages.
Published as a supplement to the *NORTH AMERICAN JOURNAL OF HOMŒOPATHY*. It contained articles by Hering, Dahlke, Kent, Neidhard, etc. This seems to be the only volume published.
"…will include everything of value in homœopathic materia medica as published in archives and journals in all languages of the homœopathic school from its inception to the present day."

1907: *SULPHUR AND COMPARISONS:* E. B. Nash, MD ✔
Boericke and Tafel; 159 pages.
"One remedy well studied is better than several not half understood." The characteristics of *Sulphur*, and comparisons and differentiations to other remedies.

1910: *THE MATERIA MEDICA OF THE NOSODES:* Henry Clay Allen, MD ✔
Boericke and Tafel; 583 pages.
This book covers 42 remedies and includes the provings done in 1897 of potentized *X-Ray* by Bernhardt Fincke. Published posthumously.

Although one step removed from the primary sources, it is still one of the best sources for information on the nosodes.

1911: *PATHOGENIC MATERIA MEDICA*: Elizabeth Enz, MD
Burton Publishing Co., Kansas City, MO; 367 pages.
A brief materia medica in which the pathological features of the remedies are outlined. The first heading (after a description of the source) is about "which centers are altered" (i.e., respiratory, mucous membranes, etc.) and is followed by a description of the pathology of those alterations.

The first materia medica (and perhaps any other homœopathic text) written by a woman.

1915: *GUNPOWDER AS A WAR REMEDY:* John Henry Clarke, MD ✔
Homeopathic Publishing Co.; 31 pages.
A small pamphlet. Black gunpowder is a mixture of Sulphur, Carbon, Potassium nitrate (*Kali-nit*). Farmers, it was said, often sprinkled it in sandwiches or took it as teaspoonful doses mixed with hot water to prevent infection. Clarke credits Rev. Roland Upcher (who wrote about it in 1911) with pointing out its virtues to him.

A wonderfully useful little work.

1919: *AN INTRODUCTION TO THE PRINCIPLES AND PRACTICE OF HOMŒOPATHY:*
Charles E. Wheeler, MD ✔
British Homœopathic Association, London; 308 pages.
The first 19 pages discuss general homœopathic philosophy as it relates to the single dose, and the administration of the remedy. The rest of the book is narrative materia medica. The 3rd edition was printed in **1948**.

1924: *700 RED-LINE SYMPTOMS:* J. W. Hutchinson, MD ✔
Ehrhart and Karl; 38 pages.
A short listing of the most characteristic symptoms derived from the work of Cowperthwaite. Originally compiled by the class of 1897 at the Chicago Homeopathic Medical College.

1928: *RADIUM:* William H. Diffenbach, MD
Reprinted from the *Homeopathic Recorder* 1928; 52 pages.
A history of *Radium bromide.* and a re-proving, including some objective laboratory tests.

1930: *MATERIA MEDICA IN VERSE:* V. M. Kulkarni
Roy and Co., Calcutta; 279 pages.
Presented to students at the Bombay Homeopathic Medical College. 150 remedies summarized in verse, with separate sections for Generals, Mind, Head, Eye, etc.

Our Aconite has full domain
O'er inflammations with much pain.
Congestions all which come with great dread
and hemorrhages of blood red…

1935: *TEXTBOOK OF MATERIA MEDICA:* Otto Leeser, MD ✔
Boericke and Tafel; 927 pages. Translated from the German by Linn Boyd.
Prepared for Leeser's post-graduate course at the Stuttgart Homeopathic Hospital 1926, 1928, and 1930. "How well I succeed will be determined by the reception…" An in-depth review of the mineral remedies "in conformity with scientific chemistry," and its known effects both as poisonings and through provings.

In light of the work done by Jan Scholten, attempting to find links between families of remedies according to their periodic table placement, it is amazing to look at this book, see the diagrams of the periodic table, and read work that was moving toward the ideas of Scholten— some 60 years earlier (and Hering had suggested similar work even earlier!)

1936: *CONCISE PICTURES OF DRUGS PERSONALLY PROVEN:* Donald Macfarlan, MD
Published by the author, Philadelphia, PA; 51 pages.
11 remedies proven over a period of 20 years.

1936: *KEY TO HOMEOPATHIC MATERIA MEDICA:* Alfred Pulford, MD and Dayton Pulford, MD ✔
Published by the authors, Toledo, OH; 136 pages.
"A start in the right direction." The authors stress that this is *not* a materia medica but, rather, just a key to it. 25 remedies are presented. Each remedy has a short sentence for "Identification," a longer paragraph of "Essential" information, followed by a clinical use comment section.

1939: *MATERIA MEDICA CARDS:* Garth Boericke, MD
Boericke and Tafel; 25 cards.
Keynotes of the remedy on one side, with the remedy name on the reverse side.

I have seen only three of these sets. They were developed by Dr. Boericke as a "quiz compend" for his students at Hahnemann Medical College in Philadelphia.

1942: *HOMEOPATHIC DRUG PICTURES:* Margaret L. Tyler, MD ✔
Homeopathic Publishing Co.; 868 pages.
125 remedies covered in a narrative style. Many quotes appear from other authors. Reprinted through present day. So many other sources are quoted, that it is almost a "Reader's Digest" of materia medica.

Her flowing, narrative style makes this an exceptionally readable book, and a great book for the neophyte. Of course, one should look at her writing with a view to the historical perspective; when she says of a remedy type, "look out the window you can see this type in the street," please remember she is talking about the mid- 1930s in London and not the present day in San Francisco!

1944: *THE HOMEOPATHIC MATERIA MEDICA AND HOW IT SHOULD BE STUDIED:*
Noel Puddephatt
Health Science Press; 32 pages.
13 remedies with the symptoms outlined in the Hahnemann schema.

Puddephatt was one of the grand "lay-homœopaths" in England. He eventually moved to South Africa where he taught a number of other practitioners among them Sheilagh Creasy and George Vithoulkas.

1944: *MATERIA MEDICA OF GRAPHIC DRUG PICTURES:* Alfred Pulford, MD and
Dayton Pulford, MD ✔
Published by the authors, Toledo, OH; 318 pages.
In a magnificent five-page introduction, the authors explain that provings consist of both the symptoms generated by the remedy on the prover, and the symptoms that are idiosyncratic to the prover and not necessarily *of* the remedy. The former are reliable symptoms, the latter are of interest but not as reliable. The book presents "graphic pictures" of the reliable proving symptoms in a brief narrative, followed by some clinical uses and experiences which are only "suggestive."

Says Vermeulen: "Whoever takes the trouble to wade through the chaos of commas and semi-colons used by Pulford to further the cause of codification and grammatical correctness will be regularly rewarded by real pearls of wisdom."

1944: *DRUGS OF HINDOOSTAN:* Sarat Chandra Ghose, MD ✔
Original publisher unknown; 342 pages.
The author knew many of the older homœopaths, Boger, Kent, Clarke, etc. The book contains 131 remedies that were originally used in India. Claiming there is nothing original in the work he says, "I do not possess the acumen or intelligence of a Hale…" The book contains 50 remedies. It was republished in **1984** by the Hahnemann Publishing Co., Calcutta.

1947: *MASTER KEY TO HOMŒOPATHIC MATERIA MEDICA*: K. C. Bhanja, MD ✔
Gilbert, Darjeeling, India; 504 pages.
Materia medica drawn from Hahnemann, Hering, Dunham, and other great homœopaths. Each remedy is by "general guiding symptoms," "marked features," and "other leading indications" with comparisons.

Those that have seen the book consider it as one of their favorites.

1949: *SONG OF SYMPTOMS:* Patersimilias
True Health Publishing, London; 151 pages.
71 remedies. Written by a member of the Faculty of Homeopathy, who preferred to remain anonymous, the left page presents the keynotes of the remedy in question, and the right page contains a poetic verse about the remedy and visual illustrations of the characteristics. The book was re-issued by Health Science Press in **1974**.

The author of this amusing short tome was Dr. Percival Henry Sharp and the illustrations were by J. A. Browne. It is a real classic, and deserves to be in print.

1951: *A PHYSICIAN'S POSY:* Dorothy Shepherd, MD ✔
Health Science Press; 291 pages.
21 remedies discussed in a narrative style, based on the author's experience.

Shepherd, who studied at the Hering Medical College in Chicago in 1906, presents a very "chatty" narrative, making it eminently "readable" and a great value for the beginner.

1958: *THE CARCINOSIN DRUG PICTURE:* Donald Foubister, MD ✔
Unknown publisher; 18 pages.
A small pamphlet with information about this little-written-about remedy. It was updated in **1967**. Further information appears in Foubister's *TUTORIALS ON HOMEOPATHY* published by Beaconsfield in **1989**, a year after Foubister's death.

1971: *MATERIA MEDICA OF NEW REMEDIES:* O. A. Julian, MD ✔
Matière Médicale d'Homéothérapie, Librairie Le François, édit. Paris 1971.
Translated from the French, this book has the results of limited provings of over 100 remedies including many derived from modern pharmacological substances: penicillin, sulfanilamide, etc. Translated into English in **1979**, and published by Beaconsfield Press (UK); 625 pages.

This book, along with the other two by the same author, becomes a fertile field from which to gather information about many nosodes, isodes, and sarcodes.

1972: *SYSTEMATIC MATERIA MEDICA*: Dr. Kailash Narain Mathur ✔
B. Jain; 1034 pages.
Discusses 200 remedies. The author expresses concern that homœopathy is disappearing because the materia medica is not "interesting and instructive to the new generation." The materia medica is presented in a "systematic way so that a new generation of homœopaths who do not have much time to go through all old materia medica may derive maximum benefit…" The source of each remedy and its provers are listed, along with a brief section of comparative remedies. The major information is presented in a grid of three columns headed: complaints and characteristics, generalities and modalities, and causes and diseases.

1974: *THE PEOPLE OF THE MATERIA MEDICA WORLD:* Frederica E. Gladwin, MD ✔
National Homeopathic Pharmacy , New Delhi; 164 pages.
Written in 1921 for Pierre Schmidt, her favorite pupil, this book was finally published 52 years later at the urging of Diwan Harish Chand. Gladwin, an early pupil of Kent, presents 25 distinct remedies and many comparisons in a series of delightful stories which bring the remedy characteristics into

a clear focus. *Calcarea phos* is discussed as being the child resulting from the marriage of Mr. Phosphorus to Miss Calcarea. There is a delightful chapter called "Afternoon at the Crocuses."

A very informal materia medica written by one of Kent's pupils. Although there are many generalizations expressed through the array of characters, it makes delightful reading and can serve to fix the characteristics of the remedies in one's memory.

1976: *SIGNPOSTS TO THE HOMEOPATHIC REMEDIES:* Noel Puddephatt and Marjorie Kincaid Smith
Bockberg, Devon, UK; 132 pages.
A narrative of a drive through "homœopathic" country. "The people who inhabit the town of *APIS* exhibit, when ill, curious characteristics…" 72 remedies are discussed, of which 16 were completed by Puddephatt before his death and the rest by his associate.

1977: *MATERIA MEDICA OF HOMEOPATHIC REMEDIES:* Dr. S. R. Phatak ✔
IBPS, Bombay; 630 pages.
A brief materia medica derived primarily from the works of Boger, with additions. "He [Boger] has given clues in his *Synoptic Key* for compiling such books. With my poor intellect and limited knowledge of homœopathy, I have tried to fulfill his wish. How far I am successful in my attempt, only time will show." Republished in the UK in **1988**.

While most practitioners in the USA who wanted a small "pocket manual" often chose the Boericke work, many in the UK preferred the Phatak work. In a comparison between them one may find Phatak to be a bit more readable. Those who have used it say that the summaries he presents of the remedies contain useful details that are not found in Boericke's.

1980: *ESSENTIALS OF HOMEOPATHIC MATERIA MEDICA:* Jacques Jouanny, MD
Editions Boiron; 454 pages.
The author suggests that in learning the materia medica "one finds oneself hopelessly lost in the thick and thorny copse of pathogenesis and unable to distinguish anything clear…" His work is an attempt to "learn, in the first stage, that which is essential." He presents the pathogenic action, typology, characteristic symptoms, and the principal clinical indications of the remedies.

Written in 1980, when focus on the mental symptoms was gaining popularity in the "Vithoulkas/Kentian camp," the author suggested that the only mental symptoms that should be considered in any case were the ones that were produced "experimentally" — that is, seen in the provings themselves.

1983: *ESSENTIAL THEORY GUIDE TO MATERIA MEDICA:* Subatra Kumar Banerjea, BMS ✔
World Homeopathic Links; 328 pages.
49 remedies. A quiz compend with questions and answers.

1984: *SYNOPTIC MEMORIZER:* Subatra Kumar Banerjea, BMS ✔
World Homeopathic Links; 184 pages.
"To write a new materia medica is a greatest absurdity… it can only be delineated in a new approach and illustration…" The first part of the book defines the characteristics of the remedy by the name:
A= ailments from
P= pains
I= incontinence of urine
S= sensitivity
This is followed by a fuller exposition of the characteristics of the remedy. The book also contains a listing of peculiar and uncommon symptoms, and finishes with a comparative materia medica.

One more work that attempts to find a system to help commit the characteristics of a remedy to memory. Like others works of this nature, the method is unique to the author and may or may not be useful to the reader. Personally I found this method idiosyncratic and not useful.

1985: *THE MATERIA MEDICA OF THE HUMAN MIND:* Dr. M. L. Agrawal ✔
Pankaj Publications; 358 pages.
The first effort made to inverse the repertory and extract the information as materia medica. The extractions were gleaned from the "Mind" section of Kent's *Repertory*. An 8th edition was published in **1996**.

This idea, painstakingly done by hand, was made much easier with the advent of the computer repertories. See the 1995 extraction by Heli O. Retzek.

1986: *SCORPION:* Jeremy Sherr, FSHom ✔
Society of Homœopaths, UK; 60 pages.
A proving. re-printed in **1990**. The first of many provings conducted and supervised by Sherr.

1986: *PORTRAITS OF HOMEOPATHIC MEDICINES VOL. I:* Catherine R. Coulter ✔
North Atlantic Books; 422 pages.
The first of a series. Greatly influenced by the "portraits" and work of Edward Whitmont, this first volume contains a narrative discussion, based upon historical literature and cases seen in her own years of practice. Nine remedies are discussed: *Phosphorus, Calcarea carbonica, Lycopodium, Sepia, Sulphur, Pulsatilla, Arsenicum, Lachesis,* and *Natrum muriaticum.*

The first new look at materia medica since Pulford's work in the 1940s. Although the author is quick to stress that the entire pathogenesis of the case should be studied, these "pictures" present the remedies as "essences" that could easily be used as the main filter for the case rather than as a filter at the end to narrow the choice of remedy. The wish to prescribe on "essence" is very seductive, and the urge to do so should be carefully moderated by references to the primary materia medica (as the author does regularly). That said, this, and her subsequent books, are especially readable, and have proven to be of use in the practices of many homœopaths.

1986: *CHARACTERISTICS OF THE HOMEOPATHIC MATERIA MEDICA:* Horst Barthel, MD
Berg am Starnberger See; 478 pages.
The book defines 12 ways in which remedies may be "characteristic" and then presents those characteristics for 115 remedies.
Using *Phosphorus* as an example, here are the 12 ways a symptom may be "characteristic":
1. The symptom is peculiar in itself: "long narrow stool."
2. The symptom is peculiar through the modality: "mania for work before menses."
3. The symptom is peculiar through its localization: "cold knees at night."
4. The symptom is peculiar through sensations: "anus feels open."
5. The symptom is peculiar through extension: "coryza extends to the chest."
6. The symptom is peculiar through beginning, progression, and end: "pain increases and decreases with the sun."
7. The symptom is peculiar through contrary symptoms: "lack of vital heat, but heat aggravates."
8. The symptom is peculiar through its periodicity: "headaches every 7th day."
9. The symptom is peculiar through alternating symptoms: "weeping alternating with laughter."
10. The symptom is peculiar through sequences: "bloody vomiting following suppressed menses."
11. The symptom is peculiar through vicarious symptoms: "vicarious epistaxis."
12. The symptom is peculiar through the absence of expected symptom: "increased sexual desire without erections."

1987: *STUDIES OF HOMEOPATHIC REMEDIES:* Douglas Gibson, MD ✔
Beaconsfield; 538 pages.
An assembled collection of materia medica lectures presented by Gibson to the Faculty of Homeopathy from 1963-1977. Over 100 remedies are covered in a concise, narrative style.

1988: *ESSENCES OF MATERIA MEDICA*: George Vithoulkas ✔
Jain; 213 pages. 53 remedies.
In the late 1970s George Vithoulkas taught a number of seminars in the USA. After the first seminar at Esalen in 1979, Bill Gray transcribed George's class notes and distributed them to class members. The following year, those who took the course received the "essence" class notes from the year before. Those who took the class the third year received the notes from the second year as well. The attendees were asked to sign an agreement promising not to copy or distribute the material. It was very clear that Vithoulkas felt that these were not ready for publication and that he didn't want them to be distributed. By the fourth year of the course someone (who shall remain nameless) receiving the notes copied them and distributed them to friends. These became the "Stolen Essences."
In **1988**, the "essences" were finally edited by Vithoulkas, and given to Jain to publish. They are, by agreement, *not* available for sale in the USA.

I remember seeing a copy of the "class notes" that belonged to Dr. Karl Robinson, one of those attending the first Esalen course. They were, obviously, unfinished ideas. Sentences trailing off, and uncompleted thoughts. It looked as if they had been typed on several different machines (which they were!) and not well photocopied.

1988: *PORTRAITS OF HOMEOPATHIC MEDICINES VOL. II:* Catherine R. Coulter ✔
North Atlantic Books; 422 pages.
The second volume, containing *Nux vomica, Silica, Ignatia,* a discussion of the Nosodes (*Psorinum, Medorrhinum, Syphilinum, Tuberculinum,* and *Carcinosin*), and a comparative materia medica of *Staphisagria* in "Indignation."

1990: *SYNTHETIC MATERIA MEDICA OF THE MIND*: Dr. Hari Singh
Smriti Publishing, New Delhi; 483 pages.
The computer repertory program of Kent's *Repertory*, *MacRepertory*, was used to create a listing of the rubric headings of the mind symptoms of 485 remedies, highlighting those rubrics which are unique to that remedy.

1991: *LACHESIS; METAPHOR AS MEDICINE:* Greg Bedayn, RSHom (NA)
Hahnemann College of Homeopathy, Oakland, CA; 44 pages.
Contains an English translation of the article, published in French, of Hering's account of his first encounter with *Lachesis* and the subsequent proving he did.

A valuable work which was subsequently reproduced in the journal Simillimum. *We find that during the proving of Lachesis, Hering did* not *become comatose, nor was his wife present to take notes— as the story goes that we read in Clarke. Another myth bites the dust!*

1991: *THE HOMEOPATHIC TREATMENT OF CHILDREN:* Paul Herscu, ND ✔
North Atlantic Books; 374 pages.
A discussion of eight remedies (*Calcarea, Lycopodium, Medorrhinum, Natrum muriaticum, Phosphorus, Pulsatilla, Sulphur, Tuberculinum*) and how they relate to the treatment of children. Each chapter contains a very full narrative of the remedy based on many years of clinical cases, notes about the presentation of the remedy in relation to infants, an outline of the salient points of the remedy, and a listing of confirmatory symptoms.

A very clear and concise book, based upon the author's extensive practice. Very reliable information.

1992: *THE SYNOPTIC MATERIA MEDICA:* Frans Vermeulen ✔
Merlijn Publishers; 414 pages.
"Originally compiled as a remedy summary for the Finnish and Irish Schools of Homœopathy, this materia medica soon grew into a book from which, I hope, others may also benefit."

Saying how difficult it was to compose a cohesive picture of a remedy from the fragmentary and often contradictory information in most materia medicae, the author summarized the remedies "in such a way that the mental picture (M), the generalities (G), and the physical symptoms (P) are clear to the reader." The exposition of 194 remedies is followed by a listing of rubrics derived from VanZandvoort's *Complete Repertory*. Each entry has space for "Notes" at the end, encouraging users to add their own information.

The work has gone through six editions, all unchanged from the original. A seventh edition, revised and enlarged, is due in December 2001.

1992: *PROVING OF HYDROGEN:* Jeremy Sherr, FSHom ✔
Dynamis; 180 pages.

1992: *MATERIA MEDICA VIVA VOLUME 1:* George Vithoulkas ✔
Health and Habitat, Mill Valley, CA; 267 pages.
Claiming he has "little to add" to the volumes of existing literature, the author presents information gleaned from homœopathic literature and enhanced with his own experience. Each entry presents information about pharmacy and toxicology, physiological action, essential features, general symptoms and keynotes, and cured cases from *other* authors, if any were found in a literature search. No cases from his own practice are given, as that will be the subject of another book. The first volume contained *Abelmoschus* to *Ambrosia*.
VOLUME 2 was published in **1995** by Hahnemann Book Publishers in London, and contained *Ammoniacum gummi* to *Argentum nitricum*, in pages 247-528.
VOLUME 3 was published in **1995** by Hahnemann Book Publishers in London, and contained *Arnica* to *Avena sativa*, in pages 529-788.
VOLUME 4 was published in **1997** by the International Academy of Classical Homeopathy in Greece, and contained *Baccilinum* to *Benzoic acid*, in pages 789-1004.
VOLUME 5 was published in **1997** by the International Academy of Classical Homeopathy in Greece, and contained *Berberis vulgaris* to *Butyric Acid*, in pages 1005-1229.
VOLUME 6 was published in **1997** by the International Academy of Classical Homeopathy in Greece, and contained *Cactus grandiflorus* to *Calcarea silicata* in pages 1231-1445.
VOLUME 7 was published in **1997** by the International Academy of Classical Homeopathy in Greece, and contained *Calendula* to *Carcinosin* in pages 1447-1656.

1993: *METAPHORIC NATURALISM:* Greg Bedayn, RSHom (NA)
Published by the author, Layfayette, CA; 61 pages.
A collection of essays, several published previously in homeopathic journals. An interesting and speculative view into four remedies: *Lachesis, Bufo, Agaricus, Tarentula*.

I loved the view of Agaricus— the red cap mushroom with the white spots (which grows, among other places, in Siberia)— leading to the descriptions of old St. Nick (red suit, white spots), driving his reindeer (who love Agaricus) across the sky in a mushroom induced hallucination.

1993: *HOMEOPATHY AND MINERALS:* Jan Scholten ✔
Stiching Alonnissos; 295 pages.
An exploration of the mineral remedies, and the "themes" related to the groupings (i.e., the natrums, the kaliums, the carbonicums). The author develops a synthetic understanding of the remedies and uses these concepts to predict the curative possibilities of unknown remedies.

1993: *THE PROVING OF CHOCOLATE:* Jeremy Sherr, FSHom ✔
Dynamis; 195 pages.

Yum yum! An interesting proving of a most addictive substance. The proving has led to several reported cases where the remedy proved curative. Too bad the cover wasn't edible!

1993: *THE DESKTOP GUIDE TO KEYNOTES AND CONFIRMATORY SYMPTOMS:*
Roger Morrison, MD ✔
Hahnemann Clinic Publishing; 440 pages.
A concise reference for confirmatory symptoms. The information is derived mostly from the author's practice and includes no remedies "which I have only very little experience or only theoretical knowledge." Asking, "Does our profession really need this text?", the author answers it by saying he conceived the book from his own "desire to have at my desk exactly the book I was contemplating writing."

Considered by many to be an ideal desktop reference.

1994: *CORE ELEMENTS OF THE MATERIA MEDICA OF THE MIND:* Ananda Zaren
Ulrich Burgdorf, Germany; Volume 1: 254 pages; Volume 2: 318 pages.
The materia medica as seen through the author's concept of "the wound, the wall, the mask." The first volume contains her experiences with *Calcarea phosphorica, Cannabis indica, Causticum, Hyoscyamus, Medorrhinum, Silica*. The second volume contains *Anacardium, Calcarea carbonica, Natrum carbonicum, Sulphur, Thuja*.

1994: *THE PROVING OF LAC HUMANUM:* Jacquelyn Houghton and Elisabeth Halahan ✔
Private printing; 52 pages.
The proving of human breast-milk.

1994: *COMPREHENSIVE HOMEOPATHIC MATERIA MEDICA OF THE MIND*: Dr. H. L. Chitkara
Jain; 692 pages.
A listing of symptoms derived primarily from the *Synthetic Repertory* of Barthel and Klunker.

1994: *THE MAD HATTER'S TEA PARTY*: Melissa Assilem ✔
Helios Pharmacy, Tunbridge Wells, UK; 78 pages.
A loose narrative materia medica about the history and use of four remedies: *Thea, Coffea, Saccharum officinalis*, and *Lac humanum*.

1995: *LOTUS MATERIA MEDICA:* Robin Murphy, ND ✔
Lotus Star Academy, Pagosa Springs, CO; 1876 pages.
Contains the history, folklore, planetary signs, and therapeutic uses of 1200 remedies. Condensed from many other sources. Includes spagyric uses— where the leftover from the tincture process, after the liquid is extracted, is burned to an ash, triturated, and re-introduced to the preparation. Re-issued as the *HOMEOPATHIC REMEDY GUIDE* in **2000**.

1995: *HOMEOPATHIC PSYCHOLOGY*: Philip Bailey, MD
North Atlantic Books; 418 pages.
"Personality profiles of the major constitutional remedies." Written by an Australian psychotherapist who studied with Vithoulkas. The author discusses how 34 basic remedies act on a psychological level, and describes why people needing certain remedies behave the way they do.

This book is another work that suggests people can be easily identified as one of many polychrest states by their outward appearance and behavior. While it does contain one therapist's insights into extreme mental states of illness it can be looked at as "new age pop-psychology" with a homœopathic flavor. The author openly disparages the "older repertories" in favor of his unsystematic office impressions, and his routine dosing of every patient with a 10M potency frequently has no effect, which would indicate to some that he is probably giving either the wrong remedy or the wrong potency. Said one reviewer, "The book inadvertently serves as a much better psychological study of Philip Bailey than it does of humanity at large."
It is not a book for beginners who lack the experience and depth of knowledge necessary to evaluate the material. Many of the author's generalizations can be questioned. For example, he says that in his experience in England, North America and Australia, about one-third of all the people are in need of the Natrum series of remedies.

1995: *1001 SMALL REMEDIES*: Frederik Schroyens, MD ✔
Homeopathic Publishing; 1504 pages.
An extraction from the *Synthesis Repertory* of the symptoms of one thousand (and one) lesser known remedies.

1995: *THE COMPLETE MATERIA MEDICA OF THE MIND:* Heli O. Retzek, MD ✔
IRHIS; 1932 pages.
Nicknamed "the brick" because of its size and weight (7.5 pounds/ 3.36kg), this volume is an extraction of material found in the *Complete Repertory*, and placed into remedy order. The rubrics (symptoms) and the author of the source of each remedy are given.

1996: *STRAMONIUM:* Paul Herscu, ND ✔
New England School of Homeopathy, Amherst, MA; 220 pages.
A discussion of *Stramonium* with an emphasis on comparative materia medica and the introduction of his "cycles and segments" concept. Also discussed is his concept of "Map of Hierarchy."

1996: *THE ELEMENTS OF HOMŒOPATHY:* Dr. Pichiah Sankaran, edited by Rajan Sankaran ✔
Homœopathic Medical Publishers; 430 pages vol. 1, 310 pages volume 2.
Two volumes of compiled writings by a prolific author and master homœopath. Volume 1, Part II contains a narrative materia medica on 51 remedies and an essay on the Bowel Nosodes. See "Other Books."

1996: *HOMEOPATHY AND THE ELEMENTS:* Jan Scholten ✔
Stitching Alonnissos; 880 pages.
A continuation of the ideas begun in *Homeopathy and the Minerals*. This volume explores relationships between the elements and the structure of the periodic table. The elements are discussed in terms of "series" (the relationship of the remedies in the lines across the table) and the "stages" (the relationship of the remedies in the rows from the top to the bottom of the table). As with his previous book, the author develops a synthetic understanding of the relationships between the elements, extrapolating from what we know of the elements already in our materia medica, and using these concepts to predict the curative possibilities of unknown remedies. Case examples from the author's and other's practices are given.

A "cutting edge" of homœopathy, the information is interesting, yet much of the materia medica is synthetic and, therefore, theoretical. It should be approached with caution. Not for the novice homœopath or one without experience.

1996: *AMBRA GRISEA: ROAD TO HOMEOPATHIC PRACTICE, VOL. I:* Michael Thompson, FSHom. ✔
Doghaus Publishing, Northampton, UK; 40 pages.
An "inside out" materia medica, beginning with 9 cases that have responded to the remedy, and then developing the materia medica as reflected in the cases. It includes many quotes about the remedy from authors of the past, and includes an essay about sperm whale hunting and the nature of ambergris.

1996: *THE SYNOPTIC MATERIA MEDICA, VOL. II:* Frans Vermeulen ✔
Merlijn Publishers; 909 pages. second edition revised and enlarged: August **1998**: 979 pages.
The first edition is nominated by a Roman II, the second uses a Latin 2. A continuation of the first volume, it includes 342 remedies that are less well known than those in the first volume.

1997: *PHARMACOLOGY AND HOMEOPATHIC MATERIA MEDICA*: Jacques Jouanny, MD, Denis Demarque, MD, Bernard Poitevin, MD ✔
Editions Boiron; 417 pages.
A materia medica of 300 remedies, with information about the origins, general action, characteristic signs, corresponding etiologies, and clinical indications of each.

"French flavored" said a brief review, meaning much stress is laid on the pathological symptoms provoked in the proving.

1997: *THE SOUL OF REMEDIES:* Rajan Sankaran ✔
Homeopathic Medical Publishers; 286 pages.
The author speaks about the "dangers inherent in the undertaking" of writing a book about remedies, specifically the danger of a "beginner in the field to become fixed on these remedy pictures" and forget the larger pictures of the remedies discussed. 100 remedies are presented in a narrative style, followed by a listing of useful rubrics. Much of the information has been condensed from the author's other books.

1994: *CONCORDANT MATERIA MEDICA:* Frans Vermeulen ✔
Merlijn; 1018 pages.
The second edition, enlarged with Hering's *Guiding Symptoms*, was published in **1997**; 1686 pages. The third edition [millennium edition] released in late 2000 has some minor revisions and substitutions. 847 remedies. The author started with the full text of Boericke's *Materia Medica* and then checked it against over a half-dozen other works. Essentially, it is a "filled out" Boericke.

Probably the most valuable of the newer materia medica (along with The Synoptic 1 and 2)— since it has taken everything from most of the other books, sorted it, and eliminated all the duplications. Nevertheless, the individual books from which the author gleaned his information offer an indescribable "something" that is not present when all the works are condensed under a single cover.

1997: *PROVING OF BAMBOO:* Bernd Schuster ✔
Verlag fur Homöopathie, Weilberg, Germany; 237 pages.

1997: *DYNAMIC PROVINGS:* Jeremy Sherr, FSHom ✔
Dynamis; 442 pages.
Edited by Melanie Grimes. Provings of *Adamas*, *Scorpion*, *Brassica*, *Germanium*, *Eagle*, *Indium*, and *Neon*.

A series of well conducted provings, following the methodology discussed in his book . See "Other Books."

1997: *PROVING OF GRANITE, MARBLE, LIMESTONE:* Nuala Eising ✔
Burren School, Galway, Ireland; 91 pages.
Subsequent work by the author included a proving of *Ignis Alcoholis* (Fire) and *Succinum* (amber).

1997: *PROVING OF OZONE:* Anne Schadde ✔
Alethea Books, Seattle, WA; 150 pages.

1997: *PROVING OF TUNGSTEN:* Annette Bond ✔
North West College of Homeopathy, Manchester; 78 pages.

1998: *MATERIA POETICA:* Sylvia Seroussi Chatroux, MD ✔
Poetica Press, Ashland, OR; 103 pages.
"Written to entertain with the intention that the personality and essence of the remedy comes to life for the reader." This book contains descriptive verses for 101 remedies.

A beautifully produced little volume. It makes an ideal gift for the homœopath in your life. And the verses are beautifully constructed as well.

1998: *PROVINGS:* Rajan Sankaran ✔
Homeopathic Medical Publishers; 247 pages.
Provings of 11 remedies including *Black Mamba*, *Coca Cola*, *Lac Caprinum* (goat milk), and *Polystyrene*.

Poor examples of proving methodology. The Coca-Cola proving was done at a seminar over two days, and all those present were asked to record their symptoms, whether they had taken the remedy or not.

In the proving of Crotalus cascavella, *12 provers participated, one was given placebo. That person's symptoms were recorded in the proving record but were also entered into the "rubrics"— although the symptoms were not the result of ingesting the substance. This is poor methodology, and has led to even more absurd proving methodologies as seen though the increase in "dream provings" or "seminar provings" where any and all symptoms reported by those present are entered into the record— even symptoms that were experienced before the substance was ingested. Provings are the backbone of homœopathic methodology. If the symptoms of everyone present are seen as part of the proving, whether or not they have taken the substance, what can be the ultimate value— except to degrade the idea of provings?*

1998: *PORTRAITS OF HOMEOPATHIC MEDICINES VOL. III:* Catherine R. Coulter ✔
Quality Medical Publishers; 338 pages.
The third of the series containing remedies *Aurum*, *Thuja*, and *Graphites*. Also included is a comparative materia medica of clairvoyance, generosity, and suspicion, as well as the comparative materia medica of indifference, which had been released as a supplement to Volume II (1989).

1998: *THE SPIRIT OF HOMEOPATHIC MEDICINES:* Didier Grandgeorge, MD ✔
North Atlantic Books; 221 pages.
Subtitled, "essential insights into 300 remedies," the book consists of a narrative description of each remedy, followed by "Observations"— examples of cases seen in the author's practice.

A delightful book to read, filled with puns, double meanings, and quality homœopathic prescribing.

1998: *ANIMAL MINDS, HUMAN VOICES:* Nancy Herrick, PA ✔
Hahnemann Clinic Publishing; 407 pages.
Provings of eight "animal" remedies: *Sanguis soricis* (Rat blood), *Lac loxodonta africana* (elephant milk), *Lac leoninum* (lion milk), *Lac lupinum* (wolf milk), *Lac delphinum* (dolphin milk), *Maiasaura lapidea* (fossilized dinosaur bone), *Limenitis bredowii* (butterfly), *Lac equinum* (horse milk).

Right on the leading edge of the "new homœopathy," the author presents much information outside of the provings based upon anthropomorphic speculations, and draws conclusions about "themes" that often stretch rational thought processes. If the information was kept separate— "this is factual, this is speculative"— the book would be quite different, but by linking it all together, it is hard to get an impartial picture of the remedies under discussion. The methodology of the provings themselves are "looser" than the ideal.

1999: *RHYMING REMEDIES:* Sally Yamini ✔
Wolfin Publishing, Dallas, TX; 117 pages.
A brief and basic materia medica in verse, each consisting of two verses of four lines.

1999: *PROVING OF COLA NITIDA:* Bernd Schuster ✔
Verlag fur Homöopathie, Weilberg, Germany; 305 pages.

2000: *NATURE AND HUMAN PERSONALITY:* Catherine R. Coulter ✔
Quality Medical Publishers; 210 pages.
A condensation of the earlier volumes with 12 remedies described and useful charts detailing modalities and ameliorations aggravations.

The Materia Medica (comparative)

1867: *DR. H GROSS' COMPARATIVE MATERIA MEDICA:* Edited by Constantine Hering, MD ✱ ✔
Boericke; 520 pages.
A book of differential comparisons. Remedies which share similar characteristics are placed side

by side on a page. At the bottom of each page there is a comparison of the conditions of aggravation and amelioration. The remedies are arranged alphabetically. In the introduction Gross mentions that he paid no attention to the "remedy groupings" suggested by Teste.

This work contains a preface by Hering. Hering's major works were all compilations of symptoms based on his practice. He wrote very little about the actual practice of homœopathy, so when we find anything written by Hering, it pays to read it because it never fails to offer insights and excellent advice. His writing was always direct and to the point. His commentaries here offer insights into the nature of "similarities" and the ways one might use remedy comparisons in one's daily practice.

1874: *SUPPLEMENT TO GROSS' COMPARATIVE MATERIA MEDICA:* Ernest Albert Farrington, MD ✔
Published as an appendix to the *American Journal of Homœopathics*; 152 pages.
It was re-published by *The Journal of Homœopathics* in **1901** and again in **1936** by Saltzer, in India, who added many of Farrington's "therapeutic hints" from his other works.

1911: *PLAIN TALKS ON MATERIA MEDICA:* Willard Ide Pierce, MD ✔
Boericke and Tafel; 792 pages.
A book for "inducing the student to get the repertory habit," this is a comparative materia medica arranged by symptom. The first part is called "comparisons" and is almost a repertory. The second part (from p. 217 on) is the materia medica, based upon lectures presented by the author at the New York Homœopathic Medical College, 1898-1908.
Said one reviewer, "It is the best thing since Farrington's *Clinical Materia Medica* appeared."
The value of the book is not apparent upon first inspection. It takes using to appreciate. The book contains numbers in brackets (after some symptoms in the materia medica) that seem to be confusing— but if they are followed, treasures await. For example, under the first drug considered, *Abies nigra*, reference is made to the classical symptom, "sensation of an undigested hard-boiled egg in the stomach (179)."
Turn to page 179 of the "comparisons" and there are seven other drugs with almost the same sensation:
Argentum nitricum: Sensation of a stone with ineffectual efforts to eructate.
Bismuth: Eructations with burning pains with a feeling of a load or hard lump in the stomach.
Bryonia: Food seems to lie like a lump or load in the stomach, with sensitiveness of the epigastric region to touch.
Gelsemium: No thirst; either a sensation of emptiness or weakness in the stomach, or a feeling of a heavy load lying there.
Kali carb: bloating, sour eructations, heartburn and a feeling of a lump in the pit of the stomach
Nux m: dyspepsia, distress appearing while the patient is eating, feeling as if the food formed hard lumps, with soreness of the stomach.
Nux v: Pain in epigastrium as from a stone, in the morning or immediately after eating.

The materia medica section gives very good information about the sources of the remedy, the preparation of it, and details of the provings.

This is certainly one of the "buried treasures." I am sure that many have picked it up and not understood, from a quick glance, the value of the work. It deserves to be better utilized.

1941: *THE STUDY OF REMEDIES BY COMPARISON:* Herbert A. Roberts, MD ✔
Published by the author, Darby, CT; 90 pages.
Quarto sized. Based on the post-graduate lectures at the American Foundation for Homeopathy course from 1933-37. A number of charts comparing a range of related remedies. The first grouping is *Aconite, Belladonna, Hyoscyamus*, and *Stramonium*. Another is *Sepia, Murex, Iodine*, and *Spongia tosta*. There are two series of comparisons of the snake remedies, and one series on the spider remedies.

Still in print, this is a rarely referenced book that contains an extraordinary amount of useful information. When I showed my copy to a practicing homœopath (who had never seen the work) she was amazed that nowhere in her years of training had this book been mentioned.

1989: *PORTRAITS OF INDIFFERENCE:* Catherine R. Coulter
North Atlantic Books; 49 pages.
A brief comparative materia medica.

1989: *COMPARATIVE MATERIA MEDICA:* Eugenio Candegabe, MD ✔
Published as *Materia Medica Comparada* in Argentina, it was translated and republished in **1997** by Beaconsfield; 330 pages.
Seven major remedies are discussed in a narrative style, with comparisons to 37 other remedies. There is emphasis placed on the mental symptoms.

Materia Medica (regional)

1890: *THE RUBRICAL AND REGIONAL TEXTBOOK OF THE HOMEOPATHIC MATERIA MEDICA, WITH SECTIONS ON URINE AND THE URINARY ORGANS:* William Gentry, MD ✔
Hahnemann Publishing House; 240 pages.
Encompassing 372 remedies, only symptoms relating to the urinary organs are listed. The author says that this is the first of a possible series, just to show what can be done with this kind of arrangement. No further books were produced.

Shortly after this book was written, the author underwent a religious conversion, abandoned homœopathy, and became a "hands on" faith healer who wrote that all others were charlatans and that "I alone can speak to you in the name of Jesus Christ."

1895: *REGIONAL AND COMPARATIVE MATERIA MEDICA:* John Malcom, MD and Oscar Moss, MD
Malcom and Moss, Chicago, IL; 919 pages.
260 remedies. An interesting way of looking at the materia medica. The sections are divided into regions, following the Hahnemannian schema, and the symptoms of that region are listed for each remedy, in the alphabetical order of the remedy. So under the heading "Eyes" is found each remedy and the eye symptoms known for it. After the materia medica section, there is repertory of what has just been covered, and this is followed by the next section, "Ears," etc. The materia medica section also includes clinical hints and often gives suggestions of potency.
The work was updated by a 76-page supplement in **1899**, published by The News Company. This small volume has a similar arrangement covering 412 remedies. When combined with the earlier work, 460 remedies are discussed.

What comes around, comes around. In the German edition of the "Symptomen Codex," Jahr presented a materia medica in the same way— a fact either not known by the authors, or not acknowledged. A review of the book appeared in the Medical Advance of June 1895, v.33, number 6, p. 402, where the reviewer said, "We find this the most helpful materia medica in our office and refer to it more oftener than all the others combined… it is simply astonishing in its completeness… almost every important symptom to be found in the Guiding Symptoms *or Hahnemann's* Materia Medica *may be found in this work…"*
This work, which was held so highly at the time, has never been re-published.

1901: *REGIONAL LEADERS:* E. B. Nash, MD ✔
Boericke and Tafel; 282 pages.
A regional quiz compend. The symptoms are printed at the outside of the pages, while the indicated remedy is printed in the page gutter. The original books came with a strip of aluminum (with the book's name printed on it) that could be used to cover the "answers."

Another magnificent quiz compend.

c. 1944 : *DIGESTIVE DRUGS*: Douglas Borland, MD ✔
British Homœopathic Association; 96 pages.
Based on lectures presented at the London Homœopathic Hospital in 1940.

Materia Medica
(including a repertory)

1834: *MANUAL OF HOMEOPATHIC MEDICINE*: George Heinrich Gottlieb Jahr
Published in France under the title: *Manuel 'des Médicaments Homoeopathiques.*
The materia medica was published in **1836** under the auspices of the North American Academy of the Homeopathic Healing Art at Allentown, PA. The repertory was published in **1838**.
Published as two volumes by William Radde in **1841**, it was edited and amended by Amos Gerald Hull, MD, and thus known simply as *HULL'S JAHR*. It consists of the materia medica in the first part and a repertory in the second part.
In **1861** the book was revised and edited by Frederick Snelling, MD, and published by Radde. In **1879**, Boericke and Tafel republished the Snelling revision of the *Materia Medica*, and republished the *Repertory* in **1884**.

1887: *KEYNOTES TO THE MATERIA MEDICA:* Henry N. Guernsey, MD ✱ ✔
Boericke; 267 pages.
This small volume was compiled by Guernsey from his personal experiences. It was based upon two previous works: a nine-page article "The Key-Note System" published in the *Hahnemann Monthly* (1868), and *Notes on Lectures on Materia Medica*, published by W. P. Kildare in 1873. The book was compiled by Joseph C. Guernsey, H. N. Guernsey's son. It was based upon lectures H. N. Guernsey gave at Hahnemann Medical College (PA) from 1871-73, and published posthumously. Pages 1-178 are the materia medica; pages 179-243 are the repertory.

1888: *THE TWELVE TISSUE REMEDIES*: William A. Boericke, MD and Willis A. Dewey, MD ✱ ✔
Boericke and Tafel; 303 pages.
In 1858, German pathologist Rudolph Virchow published a paper entitled "Cellular Pathology." In that paper he postulated that disease results from pathological changes of healthy body cells. In 1873, a German physician, Schüssler, wrote a paper concerning the "Biochemic Theory of Disease." His observations were influenced by Virchow and led him to conclude that healthy cells in the body have a balanced amount of mineral components, and that the lack of the proper balance of minerals can lead to diseased states. He isolated twelve salts (actually 11 salts and the mineral silica) that could be used to re-establish health in diseased states. At the time, this was seen as being in step with the advances of science. His article was translated by Constantine Hering who suggested that further investigations (provings) be conducted of the remedies Schüssler suggested. Although Dr. Schüssler denied all connections with homœopathy and insisted that his system was based upon physiologico-chemical processes in the body, his 12 remedies were embraced by the homœopathic community. This book by Boericke and Dewey stands as the most complete work on the subject of the 12 remedies. It must be remembered that they were not writing about the 12 remedies from the view of Schüssler, but were trying to bring the 12 remedies into the mainstream of homœopathic practice. In the introduction, the authors state:
"Whatever opposition there may be in our ranks to Schüssler's methods, because it is not pure homœopathic practice, would speedily disappear if all critics could join in proving and confirming these valuable remedies, introduced first to American Homœopathy by our own Hering, who surely could not be accused of fathering and furthering anything absolutely mongrel and detrimental to the best interests of our school.
"We do not sympathize with the attempts of Schüssler and few others to look upon the Tissue Salts as being sufficient for all purposes— provings alone can verify this. For the present, we think, with

Dr. J. C. Morgan, that Schüssler throws away a great and necessary compliment to his Materia Medica in discarding all organic drugs, as Bellad., Hyos., Acon., etc. which really make the Tissue Remedies more valuable, acting as the opposite blade of the scissors..."

The repertory, by the fact that it is only a repertory of 12 remedies, is very slim. The book stands as the best work done on the Cell Salts as seen from the homœopathic perspective.

1892: *COMPENDIUM OF MATERIA MEDICA, THERAPEUTICS, AND REPERTORY OF THE DIGESTIVE SYSTEM:* Arkell McMichael, MD
Boericke and Tafel; 359 pages.
A folio-sized book. Section I deals with the stomach and digestion. It comprises a Materia Medica that is arranged in columns across two pages. The remedy is in the first column, and the other columns contain the details of symptoms of the stomach, appetite and thirst, taste and tongue, concomitants, mouth and teeth, nausea and vomiting, eructations and flatulence, and clinical indications. This is followed by a repertory. Section II repeats the arrangement, but deals with stool, rectum, anus, etc.

1906: *HOMEOPATHIC MATERIA MEDICA COMPRISING THE CHARACTERISTIC AND GUIDING SYMPTOMS OF THE REMEDIES*: William Boericke, MD and Oscar Boericke, MD ✔
Boericke and Runyon; 572 pages.
This was the 3rd edition of the *MATERIA MEDICA* and was the first to contain a repertory written by William's brother Oscar. The 9th edition was published in **1927** and is still in print.

Perhaps the best known and most widely used of the Materia Medica/Repertory combinations, although most buy it for the materia medica and pay scant attention to the repertory. This lack of attention could be because the repertory is set out in a manner somewhat similar to the ideas of Bönninghausen, where stress is placed on the location and the modalities. It is so different from Kent's work that most people look at it and pass it by. Nevertheless it is a serviceable repertory if the time is taken to acquaint oneself with its use.

1915: *THE SYNOPTIC KEY:* Cyrus Maxwell Boger, MD ✻ ✔
Printed by the author, Parkersburg, WV; 224 pages.
A brief repertory/materia medica combination. Only 323 remedies are covered. The repertory section is divided into four categories:
a) the periods of aggravation (times)
b) conditions of aggravation and amelioration
c) generalities (sensations and general conditions)
d) regional repertory (parts of the body affected)
Although it is not as "full" as the Boericke book (in terms of remedies covered), many practitioners find it an ideal reference book at the bedside.
Many people have bought the book, but few read the introduction which outlines Boger's ideas about how to "order" the case, and explains that the materia medica of each remedy is presented in *that* "order." Once *this* is understood, and time is spent concentrating on the details of the case-taking (as Boger explains it), the book takes on a new level of usefulness.

Boger is one whose entire being oozed the ability to abstract, condense, and then condense further. His writing, likewise, is condensed and abstracted, and one can easily miss the depth of meaning because a paragraph is so short. Phatak described the need to have Boger's "intellect and acumen," and said the work is useful if "well understood." Thus said, this volume could serve as the only book one might need as a reference for general practice.

1916: *A STUDY ON MATERIA MEDICA*: Dr. N. M. Choudhuri ✻ ✔
Re-published by Jain in **1978**; 1085 pages.
A repertory was added to the book in **1929**. Choudhuri was the principal of the Bengal Allen Medical College in Calcutta, and had attended Hering Medical College in Chicago. He preceptored with P. C. Majumdar. The text is based on his lectures and includes many comparisons.

1920: *TEXTBOOK OF HOMEOPATHIC MATERIA MEDICA:* George Royal, MD
Boericke and Tafel; 391 pages.
Based on his lectures given to students at the State University of Iowa, Royal presents the material based upon his unique understanding of materia medica, which is derived from understanding the physiological systems of the body, and the affinity for the remedies to certain systems. Presented in a narrative style, the book contains a repertory that is divided into sections based upon the systems: Bones and Blood, Brain and Nerves, Mucous membranes, Glands and glandular organs, Muscles, Joints, etc.

The work of George Royal is vastly under-appreciated. This book (and his others) deserve careful reading. There are gems buried within.

1927: *MANUAL OF HOMŒOTHERAPEUTICS*: Edwin A. Neatby, MD and
Thomas George Stonham, MD ✔
John Bale, London; 1047 pages.
"This volume has been written in the hope that it may meet the need of two classes of readers—missionaries to foreign countries who have had a year's training in the elements of medicine and surgery and students and members of the medical profession inquiring into the subject of homœopathy." Contains a large materia medica with clinical indications. There is a "Clinical Index"— a clinical repertory and a repertory of aggravations and ameliorations.
The book was re-printed by Foxlee-Vaughn Publishers in Great Britain in **1987**. It is a re-print of the **1948** third edition, and contains a foreword by Sheilagh Creasy. It is presented in the original red binding.

1963: *HAHNEMANNIAN PROVINGS:* James H. Stephenson, MD ✔
Roy and Co.; 150 pages.
Contains provings of 37 remedies conducted between 1924 and 1959. 21 other remedies are mentioned that the author says do not meet Kent's criteria of having three provers. The literature sources of those remedies are given. A full repertory is appended, set out as Kent's with the understanding that these symptoms can be integrated into the Kent's *Repertory*.

Done with extreme detail and thoroughness by an IHA stalwart, this book was the prime reference source for information on provings of rare remedies, some of them isodes like Alloxan *and sarcodes, like* Cortisone *and* Pituitary.

1974: *INTRODUCTION TO HOMEOTHERAPEUTICS:* Wyrth Post Baker, MD, William W. Young, MD, Alan Neiswander, MD
American Foundation for Homeopathy; 262 pages.
This quarto sized paperback is a compilation of the materia medica from H. A. Farrington's *Course in Homeotherapeutics* and the Repertory from Boger's *Synoptic Key*.

This book was designed to be used as the text for the AFH beginning courses. At the time it was published, few books, other than the Boericke MateriaMedica, *were available.*

1981: *DICTIONARY OF MATERIA MEDICA:* O. A. Julian, MD ✔
Jain; 410 pages.
Originally published as *Dictionnaire de Matière Médicale Homéopathique*– Masson et Cie, édit. Paris, it was translated into English in 1984, but the translation leaves a lot to be desired. It discusses 131 remedies, many from his earlier work. It also contains a *Clinical Repertory* by P. Freche and M. Haffen.

Repertories

The Repertory

When I first became interested in homœopathy I heard that the local "natural health" store had a "homœopathy" section. Upon looking at the two shelves of books, I figured that the best book was the biggest. I pulled it out, and opened it up. It made less sense than a phone book. I placed it back on the shelf. That was my first encounter with the repertory.

Frederica Gladwin, who was one of those who worked with Kent on the preparation of his repertory recounted her first experience with a repertory. She says:

"Before me was the symptom, 'disposition to commit suicide by drowning.' Among the words following were 'Ant' and 'Bell.' They were words I knew but I was sorely puzzled to know what an ant and a bell had to do with drowning. A little further on I recognized 'Hell' and 'Puls' but they had left off the 'e' in the spelling of 'pulse'. I wondered, but had a vague idea that the pulse and hell might be some relation to 'wanting to drown oneself.' I tried to read more but found it no use. It was just words and words; most of them meaningless, so I gave up."

Why a repertory is needed

Within 40 years of the publication in 1810 of *The Organon*, the amount of material collected in the various *Materia Medicæ* had become virtually inaccessible without a system of cross referencing. Jahr, in his *Therapeutic Guide* mentioned the need to study the materia medica and realized what a monumental task it was. In his introduction he said, "At this time [1868] such a careful study of materia medica is unfortunately no longer possible to the beginner in Homœopathy."

When homœopathic practice was in its infancy there were few remedies to work with and thus there was not a lot of information to be cross referenced. As more and more remedies were introduced, the list of possible symptoms also grew. Therefore a method of systematically cross referencing symptoms and remedies became paramount.

Hahnemann made an attempt at constructing such a system, but it went unpublished. The task of putting together the first repertory that could be used in practice fell to Clemens Maria Franz von Bönninghausen, a lawyer who became interested in homœopathy through his own cure by the system. Bönninghausen's work was known and respected by Hahnemann.

Within a few years of the publication of Bönninghausen's repertory in 1832 it became obvious that this new tool was beginning to create problems. In a letter to Bönninghausen on Dec. 26, 1834, Hahnemann says:

"Even if the homœopathician perceives that the repertory is insufficient for finding the best remedy for every case of disease, nevertheless, they calm down when they have such an overview in their hands, and even believe with some probability to be able to dispense with sources [materia medica], and they don't buy them and use them."

Even at that time, 169 years ago, the concern was expressed that the people were using the repertory as a shortcut to find the remedy, without bothering to look further in the materia medica to more finely differentiate remedies.

In the introduction to his *Manual*, Jahr cautions against using the repertory "mechanically." Giving a case example, defined by a disease name, he goes through all the possible remedies for symptoms, narrowing to the single remedy, and says:

"From these examples the reader can perceive how perfectly impossible it is for him to do justice to homœopathy in contenting himself to turn over the leaves of the *Repertory* to establish the choice of a good medicament, and how perfectly indispensable to that result is a knowledge of the entire materia medica… Frequently great risk will be run of committing the most serious errors by searching mechanically for the symptoms of disease in the *Repertory*. If we wished we could multiply by the hundred the mistakes we have known through the mechanical use of the repertory; but it answers our ends to signalize them in a general manner, in order to prevent beginners, and especially those who only see a mechanical labor in the researches of the medicaments, from encountering the numerous shoals on which they can be wrecked."

The distinction between a Repertory and a Therapeutic Index

A "therapeutic index" (a book like Clarke's *Prescriber*) is very different than a "repertory." The therapeutic book is ordered by "disease name," while a repertory is ordered by the pathological phenomena; the symptoms. Looking under "throat, pain" in a therapeutic index will lead one to a series of remedy differentials: this remedy has these modalities, that remedy has those modalities, etc. The repertory, on the other hand, will break the symptom (throat, pain) into its components: worse at night, worse when swallowing, stitching on the left side, etc., and following each with possible remedies that have shown those symptoms in the proving or through lengthy clinical experience.

Repertory construction and its influence on the outcome

How does one take the mass of information from the materia medica and structure it into a repertory? The Hahnemannian schema (Mind, and then body from the top down)? Alphabetical? An order that might be useful in case taking? Each has its uses, and each author will view it differently.

The introduction to most of the individual repertories adequately discusses the reasoning and logic behind their structure. This work is not intended to delve deeper into the finer details.

Bönninghausen was a master of generalization. He could look at several symptoms in the provings, see the "thread" which ran through them, and summarize it in a single rubric. If the same modality (or sensation) occurred (in the proving) in different parts, and being clearly expressed in several provers, he called it a "red string symptom" and said that the remedy could cure that symptom in parts other than those it occurred in during the proving.

Seeing a "complete symptom" as having a location, a sensation, and a modality, his repertory was, essentially, built to ease the finding of those specifics. If a stitching [sensation] in the forehead [location], was aggravated by stooping, one has to look in three different parts of the repertory: Location, Sensation, Aggravation.

Kent, on the other hand, believed that the modality belonged to the part. So one would look for the single rubric under "Head, Pain, Stitching, Forehead, stooping."

One method looked at the general and moved to the specific, and the other looked at the specific and moved to the general. They are very different ways of approaching the subject.

C. M. Boger said during a meeting of the International Hahnemannian Association (Reported in the October 1932 *Homœopathic Recorder*, page 737):

"If you will read the preface in Jahr's *Handbook* and if you read the lexicon in German, you will see that Jahr's *Handbook* with its repertory and Bönninghausen's *Antipsorics* came out within two years of each other.

"It is an impossibility for two men to construct repertories practically identical in the rubrics within two years of each other. I can't prove this, but I take it that they have their common origins in the regional repertories, scattered through the lexicons.

"As Dr. Green said, repertories are generally a repetition of some previous one, or the result of combining two.

"As to the compilation of repertories, I think that every man should construct a repertory for himself, even if it is just a little one, not any larger than the one I have here in my pocket… Even if you haven't anything larger than this, construct it after your own ideas and then you will know where to find what you need, because every man's mind works a little differently from other minds… I am free to say I have never been able to follow *Kent* literally at all, but *Kent* less than *Bönninghausen*. I had Lee's *Repertory* long before *Kent's* was ever published and never could make a great use of it and when I got *Kent's* I didn't make so much more use of it, at that."

Said Dr. Alfred Pulford (at the same meeting):

"I bought seven copies of Kent's *Repertory* and I wouldn't be without it as an index. It is indispensable to us, but I never rely on prescribing on it. We have three repertories, *Kent*, *Bönninghausen*, and *Knerr*. *Kent* is the most readily available and the least, to me, reliable. *Bönninghausen* is less available, but more reliable. *Knerr* is the least of all available and the most reliable."

Said Dr. H. A. Roberts: "Repertories are tools, nothing else. It has been said in order to understand a repertory properly, you must know how to use that tool. I believe I have forty-three different repertories in my office…"

Royal E. S. Hayes, discussing the use of *Repertories* by Erastus Case, said:

"Apparently he used all repertories using one or another to some reason of his own, not accepting the belief that *Kent's* swallowed all the others. He dropped remarks to me about them at various times. Of *Gentry* he said, 'I use it sometimes, but you do not have to buy it.' Of *Lippe's*, 'It is very good, but not as complete as I would like.' Of *Jahr's*, 'You can find things in there that you can find nowhere else.' Of *Kent's*, 'I use it for my daily work.' Of *Bönninghausen's*, 'I use *Kent's* every day at my desk, but for hard chronic cases I always go to *Bönninghausen*.' Of the *Symptom Register*, 'Yes, you should have it. It is rather awkward to use. You have to get acquainted with it.' He also used the 'As If' repertory and chuckled about the things he found in it sometimes."

At the turn of the 19th century, there were a handful of people who were using the Bönninghausen *Repertory* with Cyrus M. Boger being the leading advocate. Since the major education in homœopathy was being done by Kent at his Post-graduate School in Philadelphia (and, after 1900, in Chicago), his pupils were those who were really using the method with diligence, and because of their influence in subsequent education, the Kent *Repertory* slowly became the standard.

By 1922, most of the homœopathic schools in the USA had closed. The American Foundation for Homeopathy took up the education of those handful who wished to learn at the post-graduate level. In 1931, two of the teachers treated the class to a "repertory duel"— Frederica Gladwin used the *Kent* book and Boger used *Bönninghausen*— to find the simillimum for a case. Boger finished about a minute earlier than Gladwin. Both came up with the same remedy.

Although still championed by H. A. Roberts and a number of his pupils, the Bönninghausen method ceased to be taught as the practitioners who understood it passed away, and the Kent's *Repertory* became the standard. The last course in the use of the *Bönninghausen Therapeutic Pocket Book* was offered by Dr. Allan Sutherland at the AFH School (now under the auspices of the National Center for Homeopathy) in 1979.

In 1886, George W. Winterburn authored a small (182 pages) *Pocket Repertory*. In the introduction he says:

"As a *memory refreshener* [my italics—JW] the repertory is of hourly service to the busy practitioner, and will enable him to select at the bedside, with certainty and confidence, the true drug-similar to the disease-condition before him."

And H. A. Roberts says, in 1932:

"There isn't a repertory on earth which has ever been made or ever will be made that will be the final analysis, but they are a great help in getting us down somewhere near the simillimum. Then, when you have come somewhere near the simillimum, go back to your materia medica, to your pharmacology, your provings and you can get results without hunting so far."

But the repertory is still a compilation. Rubrics have been copied from one another. Even with the *Kent* work we have no record of how Kent obtained some of the information included, and only vague ideas about his intent concerning various rubrics.

Although Bönninghausen stressed the need of the materia medica as the final arbiter in remedy selection, the way to get to the materia medica is often by way of the repertory— a book that is known to have inaccuracies and inconsistencies, where we often have no understanding why some remedies are in certain rubrics. Occasionally, we don't even know what certain rubrics mean. The repertory is an imperfect tool.

We should, above all else, recognize the repertory for what it is— a tool that helps us do the job— an index to remind and point us in the right direction. Hahnemann, in the introduction to *The Chronic Diseases*, said (in reference to repertories): "…these books are only intended to give light hints as to one or another remedy that might be selected, but they can never dispense him from making the research at the first fountain heads."

Buried in the pile of repertories are treasures that we have forgotten. Often the introductions by the authors are enlightening, and insightfully refreshing.

We should be aware that many of the "special" repertories (such as moon phases, and epilepsy —to name two) were published in journals such as the *Medical Advance* and the *Homœopathic Physician*, and have not been re-printed.

Although many of these old repertories have had their content incorporated into the newer, larger books, there is a piece other than the raw data which cannot be transferred— the conceptual framework of the structure that was the key to the wholeness of the work. The new books might be complete in their content but, because of their nature as a compilation, they often lack the individuality and "wholeness" that is found in the separate works.

It is a problem Kent faced when compiling his repertory over 100 years ago, and it a problem we still face. The compilations are useful, but the individual parts from which the compilation is derived should not be forgotten.

Repertories

1805: *FRAGMENTA DE VIRIBUS MEDICAMENTORUM POSITIVIS SIVE IN SANO CORPORE HUMANO OBSERVATIS*: Samuel Hahnemann, MD
Sumpter Joan Ambros Barthii, Leipzig; 713 pages.
The first materia medica by Hahnemann contained the proving information of 27 remedies in the first part (269 pages) and a 470 page repertory in alphabetical order in the second part.

1817: *THE SYMPTOM DICTIONARY*: Samuel Hahnemann, MD (handwritten)
Hahnemann made an attempt at constructing an index. The work is preserved in the archives at the Robert Bosch Institute in Stuttgart. It is a large folio volume in which he pasted symptoms that were obviously cut from his hand-written materia medica. Of the effort he wrote: "Only the dictionary (repertory) would give the seeker more information…" And again: "My repertory was an alphabetical record which could be of great services in looking up the necessary symptoms of medicine, if very complete and this perfection is not yet found in mine. It therefore remains unpublished."

1826: *SYSTEMATIC DESCRIPTION OF THE PURE EFFECTS OF REMEDIES (Systematische Darstellung der Reinen Arzneiwirkungen)*: Carl Georg Christian Hartlaub
Baumgärtner, Leipzig; 538 pages (volume I).
Produced by a student of Hahnemann, this was, according to Pierre Schmidt, the first printed repertory. .It was issues in six volumes, printed between 1826 and 1827.

1830: *SYSTEMATIC DESCRIPTION OF ANTIPSORIC REMEDIES (Systematische Darstellung der Antipsorische Arzneimittel)*: Georg Adolph Weber
Vieweg, Braunschweig; 536 pages.
A repertory of deteriorations and ameliorations in health, ranging fom head to toe, and ending with slepp and mental symptoms.

1831: *SYSTEMATIC PRESENTATION OF ALL HOMŒOPATHIC MEDICINES:* Ernst Ferdinand Rückert
Schumann, Leipzig; 1285 pages in three volumes.
Rückert hand-copied Hahnemann's massive dictionary, re-arranged it, and published it in three volumes. It was more of an ordering of the materia medica than a true repertory.

1832: *REPERTORY OF ANTIPSORIC MEDICINES (Systematisch-Alphabetisches Repertorium der Antipsorischen Arzneien)*: C. von Bönninghausen
Coppenrath, Münster; 256 pages.
A 2nd edition was published in **1833**. This work remained in German until Boger issued an English translation in **1900**.

1834: *JAHR'S MANUAL*: Georg Heinrich Gottlieb Jahr ✱
Schaub, Dusseldorf; 727 pages.
The book was a combination materia medica and *Repertory*, based upon the work of Hahnemann. It was first published in German. It included an Alphabetical Repertory (*Systematic Alphabetical Repertory*).

1835: *REPERTORY OF MEDICINES THAT ARE NOT ANTIPSORIC (Systematisch-Alphabetisches Repertorium der nicht-antipsorischen Arzneien)*: C. von Bönninghausen.
Coppenrath, Münster; 266 pages.
The work contained a Preface by Hahnemann. It was not translated into English until Boger did it in **1900**.

1838: *REPERTORY TO THE MANUAL:* edited by Constantine Hering, MD
Academical Book Store; 419 pages.
In 1838, Jahr's *Manual* was translated into English by Constantine Hering and published by the Academical Bookstore at Allentown, PA— the publishing division of his school. It was the first repertory in the English language. It was a much "purer" work than Jahr's original work— using only that which related to the symptoms experienced and not the disease states. In retrospect it was a milestone as it became the precursor to Kent's *Repertory* over 50 years later.

1838: *REPERTORIUM FÜR DIE HOMÖOPATHISCHE PRAXIS:* A. Joseph Fredericus Ruoff
Stuttgart; 256 pages.
This book was translated by A. Howard Okie, MD, and published by J. Dobson in **1840**. In the original German, this book referenced each symptom to the original source in the literature and included literature reference for cured cases. When Okie did the translation he deleted all the sources and reference, just leaving indications.

1841: *HULL'S JAHR; A NEW MANUAL OF HOMŒOPATHIC PRACTICE*: A. Gerald Hull, MD
William Radde; 2 volumes, 651/710 pages.
Re-translated, revised and edited by A. Gerald Hull. This *New Manual of Homœopathic Practice* became known simply as "Hull's Jahr" and was the most common repertory in use. It followed Jahr's later format. The first part is a materia medica, the second, the *Repertory*. Jahr, it seemed, tried to meet the students on the ground of their previous instruction and lead them into homœopathic thinking. Jahr began by listing remedies for diseases, then remedies for the symptoms of disease. Finally he listed the symptoms of the patient, general symptoms modified and lastly particular symptoms with their modifications. He emphasized that the symptoms of the patient were the most important. What he came up with was two repertories in one: a repertory of diseases and a repertory of the patient. Two type styles, regular and italic, were used, and they matched the type used by Hahnemann in the *Materia Medica Pura*. The first part, the diseases and the differentials, became the basis for Lilienthal's *Homœopathic Therapeutics*. It is said that Mary Baker Eddy, the founder of Christian Science, always carried two books with her: a Bible and Hull's *Jahr*.

1842: *PURE SYMPTOMATOLOGY OR SYNOPTIC PATTERN OF ALL THE MATERIA MEDICA PURA (Symptomatologie Homoeopathique ou Tableau Synoptique de Toute Matière Médicale Pure, a l'aide duquel se trouve immédiatement tout symptome ou groupe de symptomes cherché)*: P. J. Lafitte
Baillière, Paris; 974 pages.
Based mainly on the work of Hahnemann. Each heading is written in a string divided in columns: nature and sensation; accessory symptoms according to location, nature and sensation; causes, conditions according to place, time, schedules and circumstances; aggravations; improvements; ceasing.
Although the information is good, the layout takes up much space, making it difficult to visualize for purposes of repertorization.

1846: *THE THERAPEUTIC POCKET BOOK (For Homœopathic Physicians, to be Used at the Bedside of the Patient and in Studying the Materia Medica Pura) (Therapeutisches Tachenbuch)*: C. von Bönninghausen. ✱ ✔
Along with the German edition in **1846**, there was also an English edition (translated by Stapf), and a French edition.

Several other editions were printed: **1847**, translated by A. Howard Oke; Otis Clapp; 483 pages. **1847**, translated by Charles J. Hempel; William Radde; 504 pages. **1891**, edited by T. F. Allen, MD, Hahnemann Publishing House; 484 pages.

In 1846 Bönninghausen produced his *Therapeutic Pocket Book*. It served as the final synthesis for his ideas. Five type faces were used to indicate the manner in which the remedies were encountered in the provings: parentheses for those remedies which are doubtful; symptom seen in a proving (plain); symptom seen in several provings (italic); symptom seen in provings and verified as cured (lower case bold); symptom seen in provings and repeatedly verified (upper case bold). Several translations were made of this work over the years, the most recent being the revision by Gypser and Dimitriadis in 2000.

It is THIS book that most people see as "Bönninghausen" and it is this book that Kent talked about when he said he didn't understand the method of Bönninghausen. It was never well explained except through the teaching that took place through preceptorships. It was thought to be so valuable that Erastus Case, MD, copied one by hand when he could not find a copy for sale. It was more than a repertory— it was a method. Bönninghausen was not only a lawyer, he was a botanist and taxonomist. He saw things in large generalities, and used this ability to synthesize several rubrics into a generality— something Kent never quite understood. As the title implies, the book was also intended to be used in the reverse as well— as a guide to the study of the materia medica. With the recent revision in print, more people are beginning to understand and use the method with the book.

1850: *ALPHABETICAL REPERTORY OF THE SKIN SYMPTOMS*: G. H. G. Jahr
Radde; 515 pages.
Translated by Hempel. "…together with the Morbid Phenomena Observed in the Glandular, Osseous, Mucous, and Circulatory Systems arranged with Pathological Remarks on Diseases of the Skin."

1850: *PATHOGENIC CYCLOPEDIA*: Robert Ellis Dudgeon, MD
Samuel Highley, London; 591 pages.
Printed for the Hahnemann Society. Only one part was issued, "Symptoms of Mind, Disposition, and Head." A Therapeutic index more than a repertory. The first heading is "Symptoms relating to the Disposition" sub-head, "Unimpressionable Disposition." Each remedy is listed with the differential, e.g.,
Asarum: He is quite stupid in the head and has pleasure in nothing.
Berberis: Disposed to indifference, apathy.
Cannabis: Nothing pleases him, is indifferent to everything.

1851: *A POCKET MANUAL OR REPERTORY OF HOMŒOPATHIC MEDICINE*: Joel Bryant, MD ✔
William Radde; 352 pages.
A small manual that went through many printings. The design was threefold: "First— to furnish Physicians, especially beginners in homœopathic practice, with a convenient *Vade Mecum*, or work of ready reference, at the bedside of the patient. Secondly: to provide travelers, who are liable to attacks of illness where it is impossible to procure the services of a homœopathic physician, with a valuable *Medical Companion*. And lastly, to supply families, residing at a distance from any homœopathic physician, with a work which may be used by them as a *Family Physician* in *cases of emergency* and for the many *minor ills* that flesh is heir to."
Included descriptions of diseases as well as a section on poisons and antidotes.

The edition I have was printed by Boericke and Tafel almost 30 years later, in 1880. It was a very popular book— used by physicians, and as a "domestic manual" by laypersons.

1853: *JAHR AND POSSART'S NEW MANUAL OF HOMŒOPATHIC MATERIA MEDICA, ACCOMPANIED BY AN ALPHABETIC REPERTORY*: G. H. G. Jahr.
William Radde; 923 pages.
Translated by Hempel. Includes the *REPERTORIUM* by Possart, that was published that year in Germany.

1853: *THE COMPLETE REPERTORY*: Charles J. Hempel, MD
William Radde; 1159 pages.
Intended as the third volume of Jahr's *Symptomen-Codex*— a materia medica that Hempel translated in 1848. It includes a 58 page index.
"The classification of the symptoms which has been adopted in this work is more complete, and at the same time more simple and practical than anything of the kind published in any language. I scarcely need to remark that the perfection of such a work involves an immense deal of toil. I have devoted upwards of four years' steady labor to it, and the reader will not throw away his kindness by excusing any little omission which may have accidentally occurred in spite of my best efforts to avoid every cause of complaint.
"Kind reader, I ask your indulgence. Remember that it is an easy thing to criticize, but not so easy to achieve an immense work like the present. The mental concentration required to preserve the unity of the execution, would have exceeded my energies, if I had not been encouraged in the performance of my arduous task by the desire of being serviceable to our cause and its adherents, and supplying a want which has been sadly felt by thousands."

1854: *THE SIDES OF THE BODY AND DRUG AFFINITIES:* C. M. von Bönninghausen
Rademacher and Sheek; 28 pages.

1859: *REPERTORY OF THE HOMŒOPATHIC MATERIA MEDICA (CYPHER REPERTORY)*:
Robert Ellis Dudgeon, MD
Henry Turner, Manchester.
This book was published in several parts. It was then published in **1878** as two volumes bound as one.
"It is necessary to provide a mode by which one individual aspect may be found, but also to give the detail of the symptom.
"Jahr gave up the task as one of insurmountable difficulty. If only four points of view of each symptom are given, the number of repetitions would be so great that 48 volumes would be needed to hold it all… A system of symbols or cyphers has been devised by which a whole symptom may be expressed within the compass of little more than the abbreviations of the medicines ordinarily used in repertories. The abbreviations of the names of the medicines have, in the first place, all been reduced to 3 letters. All symptoms which are common to several organs are represented by the letters of the alphabet in Roman type, the symbolical value of the letter being the same throughout the book, e.g., 'a' appearance, 'b' coldness, 'n' hemorrhage. 'a' with a superscript 'b' is 'bright, sparkling' (subgroup under 'a' appearance). Aspects peculiar to each chapter are given letters in Roman or old English letters, and they only apply to that chapter." In the chapter "Teeth and Gums," Phosphorus is listed as "continued tearing and boring in one molar tooth, worse by touch and chewing." This appears in the Cypher as:

$$\text{Mo. Pho. I}^{ch}.\text{V}^3.\text{VI}^4.11\text{-}60.$$

A special committee was set up to create this work by the Hahnemann Publishing Society — first suggested in 1853. It was compiled by a number of people, primarily Drs. Drysdale and Dudgeon, with help from Drs. Atkin, Black, Irvine, Kerr, Madden, Russell, Craig, Stokes, Hayward, and Raynor.
A section of the listing under "Indifference—Concomitants" appears like this:

$r^1p.$ *Heat of hands.*—ver^b.𝔥.æ^a.n.
$rv.$ *Paralysis of limbs.*—con.𝔨.4.
$\phi.$ *Sleepiness.*—alo.—crn.—mgn.
　 𝔥.—rs-r.—til.𝔥^c.
$\chi^1.$ *Chilliness.*—k-cl.𝔨.m.5.
$\omega^2.$ *Debility.*—ag-n.𝔨.ω^8—rum^b.α^1.
$\omega^8.$ *Trembling.*—ag-n^2.𝔨.ω^2.

Boger described the book as "pure gold" but it was very difficult to use because it was, essentially, written in an almost indecipherable code.

1861: *HULL'S JAHR:* revised and edited by Frederick Snelling, MD
William Radde; This two volume update was divided into a 1204 page symptomology (vol.1) and an 804 page repertory (vol.2).
Boericke and Tafel reprinted Part 1 in **1879**, and Part 2 in **1884**.

1868: *REPERTORY OF THE NEW REMEDIES*: Temple Hoyne, MD
Luyties and Co. St. Louis; 70 pages.
"Classification of a Few of the New Remedies, according to the Parts of the Body acted upon, after the plan of Bönninghausen." First printed in the *Western Homœopathic Observer*, Volume 4.
The "New Remedies" were those that did not appear in Hahnemann's original works. They were, generally, native to the USA and included Iris versicolor, Hydrastis canadensis, Phytolacca decandra, Gelsemium sempervirens, and others.

1869: *A REPERTORY OF THE SYMPTOMS OF THE EYES AND HEAD*: Edward William Berridge, MD
Published as a supplement in the *Hahnemannian Monthly*, Feb. 1869 to December 1871. 220 pages.

1872: *REPERTORY OF LEUCORRHOEA*: Alvin Matthew Cushing, MD ✔
T. P. Nichols, Boston; 70 pages.

1873: *COMPLETE REPERTORY TO THE HOMŒOPATHIC MATERIA MEDICA/ DISEASES OF THE EYES*: Edward William Berridge, MD ✔
Alfred Heath, London; 321 pages.
Only the "Eye" section was ever completed. "A perfect repertory should contain a reference to every symptom of the materia medica under every rubric where it can possibly be looked for. To effect this, I have divided each chapter of the repertory into two sections: I— the symptoms themselves; and II— their conditions (Including concomitants)."
In a footnote:
"It is often difficult or impossible to decide from the provings alone what symptoms are really connected with each other… whereas if a group of symptoms are cured homœopathically, there can be no doubt of the necessary connection of its constituent elements."
"With regard to the abbreviation of the [remedy] names… I have adopted a uniform and scientific method of ciphering, as it is quite time that such absurd names as Hepar Sulfuris… be discarded… The cyphers of the simple haloid salts are the same as their chemical symbols; the —*ate* salts are cyphered by adding — *a*; the —*ite* salts by adding —*i*... Thus:
Na= sodium
Na.s.- sulfide of sodium
Na.sa= sulphate of sodium
Na.si= sulphite of sodium
The book has 1171 remedies listed.

1875: *ANALYTICAL THERAPEUTICS*: Constantine Hering, MD ✱ ✔
Boericke and Tafel; 352 pages.
Hering's first and only attempt at a repertory. Re-issued in **1881** as *Analytical Repertory of the Symptoms of the Mind*. "The arrangement as well as the style of printing, has the one object especially in view, viz.: to make it as easy as possible for the eye, and through the eye, for the mind to find what is looked for."
"… while the materia medica requires a constant synthesis in the mind of the reader... the therapeutical work requires a constant analysis."
Hering cautions never to indiscriminately mix what symptoms have been produced by the drug with those symptoms reported as cured by the drug.
"Dr. Dunham, during his stay with Bönninghausen, was allowed to copy the author's own marks, corroborations and additions, which had been made from his practice, during more than ten years. Dr. Dunham, with his well-known liberality left his copy long enough in Philadelphia to be compared and carefully copied."

The book contains 48 chapters, in the Hahnemannian schema— from Mind and Disposition through Fever, and ending with "Stages of life" and "Relationship with other drugs". At about Chapter 40 Hering interspersed several chapters on Relation to Time, and Relation to Space— i.e., moving, standing, changing place, etc. Section 43 is called "Sensations Classified" and has a two page index.

He uses four signs based on Bönninghausen's four degrees:

| Observed on the healthy
|| Observed often and repeatedly
I   Applied successfully with the sick
II   Applied very often and repeatedly

A book filled with interesting information by the father of American homœopathy. It is somewhat confusing in the way it is laid out, thus keeping the gems within hidden. Hering's inclusion of categories such as "Relation to space" gives us an invaluable insight into what he looked for in a case. As previously mentioned, writing by Hering is rarely seen, so the lengthy introduction to this work is well worth reading and gives us a view into the thinking of one the grand minds in homœopathy.

1876: *REPERTORY OF NEW REMEDIES*: Charles Porter Hart, MD
Boericke and Tafel; 199 pages.
Based on the Materia Medica work of E. M. Hale, this repertory strives to bring these new remedies— *Cimicifuga, Gelsemium, Podophyllum, Iris versicolor*—into clinical practice.
"We urge upon every student and practitioner the importance of using the repertory in connection with the work upon which it is based. No repertory can give the symptoms in sufficient detail for practice. To attempt this, as is too often done, is to wrench it from its legitimate sphere; to bring its usefulness into discredit by repeated failures, and to pervert our noble calling, which under all circumstances requires the exercise of sound discrimination and judgment, and the scientific application of established principles. The most that can be expected of a repertory is, that it shall inform us where to find the symptom and at the same time give us a general idea of their character— the finer shades and mutual relations of the various symptoms can ofttimes be found only in the full text of the symptomatology."

1879: *REPERTORY TO THE MORE CHARACTERISTIC SYMPTOMS OF THE MATERIA MEDICA*: Constantine Lippe, MD ✔
Bedell Brothers, New York; 112 pages.
Constantine Lippe was the son of Adolph Lippe. He patterned this book after Hering's *Allentown Repertory* of 1838. He added sections from many others. The Hahnemann schema is followed and ends with a section called "Generalities" with which all previous sections are to be compared. One of the shortcomings of the book, mentioned by Julia M. Green, was that many of the rubrics have so few remedies listed that combining them could lead nowhere. Said Green, "The book needed to be enlarged; students could not find enough in it." When Kent began to compile his *Repertory*, he began by writing notes into his copy of Lippe's, and then interleaving pages with additional notes.
Ill health prevented Lippe from editing a 2nd edition. He gave his work to E. J. Lee of Philadelphia, who further refined it and published the Mind section in **1889**. Constantine Lippe died in 1888— as a result of wounds suffered during the Civil War.

1879: *AN ILLUSTRATED REPERTORY OF PAINS IN CHEST, SIDES AND BACK; their direction and character, confirmed by clinical cases*: Rollin R. Gregg, MD ✔
Duncan Brothers; 97 pages.
Surely one of the most unusual repertories published. This slim volume contains charts of the torso showing the location, direction, and character of the pain. Pains are described in the text and then illustrated. For example, in the plate on the following page, an arrow from the left side of the chest extending to the umbilicus and ending in a shape like pincers is labeled "Agar." and indicates that *Agaricus* has pinching pains in the place and direction shown.

The Heritage of Homœopathic Literature

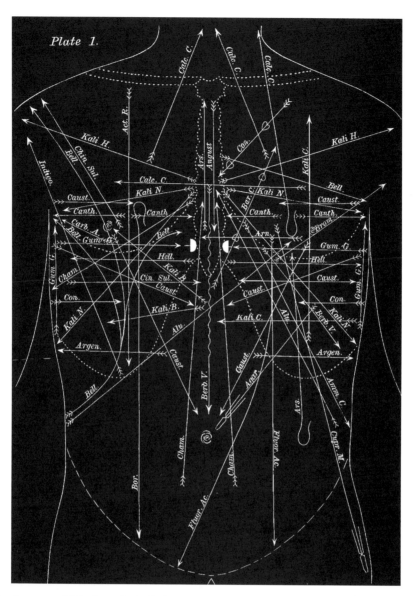

The book was republished as a limited edition in **1985** by Eclectic Medical Publishers in Portland, Oregon.

1879: *A REPERTORY OF MENSTRUATION*: William Jefferson Guernsey, MD ✔
Privately printed in Philadelphia; 17 pages.

1879: *UTERINE AND VAGINAL DISCHARGES*: William Eggert, MD
Boericke and Tafel; 543 pages.
"The present work is my private repertory. It was originally not intended for the press, had not my friends insisted upon its publication. I have revised, remodeled, added to, and expunged from it, in order to make it practical to the best of my ability… I have gathered from all obtainable sources, and introduced the verifications from my own experience during a period of twenty-five years and more…the whole homœopathic literature of this country and Europe has been diligently

searched in order to secure, if possible, the utmost perfection with regard to everything that is reliable and worthy of trust. For omissions and shortcomings, which in the face of the utmost care, may be detected here and there, I beg the indulgence of the profession."

1879: *A REPERTORY OF HEADACHES*: John C. King, MD
W. A. Chatterton; 297 pages.
King practiced in Circleville, Ohio. The work was done by the Allegheny County Materia Medica Club, which consulted "the standard works" of the day. The final edit was done by King. As for concomitant symptoms, he says: "A complete repertory of concomitant symptoms would be endless, an incomplete one worthless, thus none has been made."

1880: *THE SYMPTOM REGISTER*: Timothy F. Allen, MD ✔
Boericke and Tafel; 1331 pages.
This is the index and repertory to Allen's *Encyclopedia*. It is often seen in two parts, and offered as volume 11 and 12 of Allen's larger work.

When Kent assembled his Repertory, *he included some of the information from this work, but not all. Many times he put remedies from Allen's index that appear in very detailed sub-rubrics into more general rubrics, thus omitting useful information. Kent also omitted many smaller remedies for reasons of his own.*
When questioning the remedy selections of Erastus Case in his work Some Clinical Experiences, *I have found that many of the obscure symptoms he bases his remedy selection upon cannot be found in Kent's work, but are found in* The Symptom Register.

1880: *REPERTORY TO THE MODALITIES*: Samuel Worcester, MD ✔
Boericke and Tafel; 160 pages.
Derived primarily from Hering's *Condensed Materia Medica*. "This little book was originally compiled to meet a want felt in my daily practice. With its help, I have many times been able in a few moments to decide upon the indicated remedy, while, without it, a longer search would have been required than the busy physician is able, or the indolent physician, willing, to make.
"This book is arranged on a different plan… in nearly every instance the exact language of the text has been given, together with associated symptoms; thus enabling a more careful discrimination to be made."

1882: *A REPERTORY OF HAEMORRHOIDS*: William Jefferson Guernsey, MD ✔
(*Homœopathic Physician* reprint;) 25 pages.

1883: *A REPERTORY OF DESIRES AND AVERSIONS*: William Jefferson Guernsey, MD ✔
(*Homœopathic Physician* reprint); 16 pages.

1883: *REPERTORY TO THE SYMPTOMS OF INTERMITTENT FEVER*: William A. Allen, MD
Boericke; 107 pages.
"Dr. Allen was successful in curing Intermittent with the one remedy, and this is his working repertory."

1884: *COUGH AND EXPECTORATION*: Edmund Jennings Lee, MD, and George Henry Clark, MD ✱ ✔
A. L. Chatterton; 201 pages.
"Cough, with its attendant aches and pains, debility and emaciation, is one of the commonest complaints with which the physician has to deal. No excuse is necessary for the appearance of a volume whose sole aim is to assist the busy physician in treating a complaint so frequently met with, and often in such intractable forms. The numerous cough symptoms, before scattered through many volumes, are now for the first time brought together and properly arranged, so that the physician may readily find symptoms which before would have taken hours to discover."
28 authorities are consulted, including 28 volumes of the *North American Journal of Homœopathy*, and six volumes of Raue's *Annual Record*. Unmarked remedies come from Allen's *Encyclopedia*. All others are referenced as to the source. A 2nd edition was published by Clark in **1894** (238 pages), which included additions gleaned from journals and private correspondence.

1885: *A CARD REPERTORY FOR DIPHTHERIA*: William Jefferson Guernsey, MD
(*Homœopathic Physician* reprint); 25 pages.

1885: *REPERTORY OF ECZEMA*: Charles F. Millspaugh, MD
A. L. Chatterton; 43 pages.

A slim volume, of little use, since the same remedies appear in almost all the rubrics.

1886: *REPERTORY OF THE MOST CHARACTERISTIC SYMPTOMS*: George W. Winterburn, MD ✔
A. L. Chatterton; 182 pages.
A small Pocket *Repertory*. In the introduction to this pocket repertory Winterburn says:
"A very capable, conscientious, and experienced physician, a member of various homœopathic societies, said to me not long since, 'I don't take much stock in those things,' referring to repertories. I cannot understand such a remark, unless it is based on the mistaken idea as to the purpose the repertory is intended to serve. It is not a short-track method of practice and is of value to its possessor only in proportion to his intimate knowledge of materia medica. In the hands of an ill equipped physician it is little better that a Greek testament to a Choctaw; but as the profound student of the materia medica glances down the page, the apparently meaningless succession of abbreviations conjures up in his mind the pathognomonic pictures which these represent. As a memory refresher the repertory is of hourly service to the busy practitioner, and will enable him to select at the bedside, with certainty and confidence, the true drug-similar to the disease-condition before him."

The author claims to have saved several pages by shortening the abbreviations used. "Sulphur," seen in most books as "Sulph" has been shortened to "Sul," "Lycopodium" to "Ly," etc.

1887: *A COUGH TIME TABLE*: J. E. Winans, MD
(*Homœopathic Physician* reprint, Feb. 1887); 6 pages.

1887: *REPERTORY TO HAEMORRHAGES OF THE BOWELS*: J. V. Allen, MD
Supplement to the *Homœopathic Physician*, Volume 7; 2 pages.

1888: *REPERTORY OF THE URINARY SYMPTOMS*: Theodore J. Gramm, MD
Supplement to the *Medical Advance*; 52 pages.

1888: *PATHOGENIC AND CLINICAL REPERTORY OF THE MOST PROMINENT SYMPTOMS OF THE HEAD, WITH THEIR CONCOMITANTS AND CONDITIONS*: Charles Neidhard, MD
Boericke; 188 pages.
Neidhard has taken the most prominent symptoms from Allen's. Cured symptoms from his practice are in bold type and the remedies in italics. On occasion, the potency used to cure a specific symptom is indicated. "To them I have added my clinical experience of fifty years' extensive homœopathic practice. This very laborious work was undertaken principally with a view of assisting me in my own practice. On considering, however, that it might be of benefit to the profession generally, it is herewith presented to the public."

Neidhard was one of the first pupils of Hering at the Allentown Academy and was a founder of the American Institute of Homœopathy in 1844. Neidhard's personal notes are invaluable.

1888: *A REPERTORY OF GONORRHEA*: Samuel A. Kimball, MD ✔
Otis Clapp; 53 pages.
An extraction from Hahnemann, Hering, Lippe, and Allen.

I LOVE the idea that a repertory about gonorrhea is published by "Clapp."

1888: *REPERTORY OF HEART SYMPTOMS*: Edwin Snader, MD
Published by the *Medical Advance*; 112 pages.
The repertory was used as the 2nd part of Hale's *DISEASES OF THE HEART*, 3rd edition in **1889**.

1889: *GUERNSEY'S BÖNNINGHAUSEN*: assembled by William Jefferson Guernsey, MD
Globe Press, Philadelphia.
A limited edition. A slip repertory. A box 16.5" x 19.5" x 6. 50" compartments each containing 49 slips 13.5" long x 1.5" wide. Total of 2467 slips plus a 57 page book: *An Index to Guernsey's Bönninghausen.*
Says Erastus Case: "This needs to be used only in cases where it is very difficult finding the simillimum. Then it is the most expeditious mode of working out a case that I have ever known."

A forerunner of the computer repertory. Each slip of paper represented a single rubric, and had printed upon it, in a column, the grades of the remedies in alphabetical order. The first slip contained a columnar list of all the remedies. When the slips were all lined up next to the first slip, the gradings (1, 2, 3, 4) would line up with the remedy names. A visual scan would identify remedies appearing in the most rubrics in the case.

1889: *REPERTORY TO HERING'S CONDENSED MATERIA MEDICA*: J. C. Guernsey, MD, Charles Mohr, MD, E. R. Snader, MD
Globe Printing House, Philadelphia. 432 pages.

1889: *REPERTORY OF THE CHARACTERISTIC SYMPTOMS OF THE HOMŒOPATHIC MATERIA MEDICA*: Edmund Jennings Lee, MD
Published as a supplement to the *Homœopathic Physician*; 174 pages.
"The material used has been collected from all reliable sources. After the death of Dr. Constantine Lippe, all the manuscripts he had written for the second edition of his repertory was secured and included in this work. This repertory might, in fact, be considered as the second edition Dr. Lippe's book, with such additions and corrections as the present editor has made.
"The book includes over three hundred pages of notes from Dr. Edward Rushmore, and notes from Wesselhoeft's interleaved Repertory collected by Dr. Samuel Kimball. It also contains many additions from "Dr. Kent's Interleaved Repertory."
Shortly after the work was released, Lee became blind, and passed the project on to Kent.

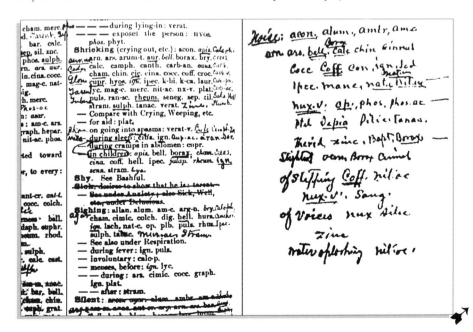

William Kirtsos has an edition of this book (illustration on the previous page) that belonged to Lee and was given to Kent. It contains many corrections and additions in Lee's fine hand, and then more corrections and additions in Kent's bolder hand. Many rubrics are crossed out, and others moved around. It was this Repertory that was used as the direct link between Lippe's work and the final work of Kent.

1889: *REPERTORY TO LABOR AND AFTER PAINS*: J. V. Allen, MD
Supplement to the *Homœopathic Physician*, Volume 9; 6 pages.

1889: *REPERTORY TO MASTITIS*: William Jefferson Guernsey, MD
Supplement to the *Homœopathic Physician*, Volume 9; 5 pages.

1890: *REPERTORY OF CONVULSIONS*: Ellis M. Santee, MD ✔
H. Hitchcock, New York; 85 pages.
Printed only on the right, leaving the left page for annotations.

c. 1890: *PSYCHISME ET HOMOEOPATHIE*: Jean-Pierre Gallavardin, MD
The book was republished in **1960** by Gallavardin's family.
Gallavardin believed that homœopathy could improve the character of people. The repertory deals with personality and psyche. Thus the headings are of the type: "quack; quack and liar; quack but sincere" etc.
Recent avarice toward donations: 1. Sulfur 2. Silicea 3. Puls. 4. Calc. c.
Insulted and blushing at other's behavior: Lycop. Anac.
The headings indicating *Ineptitude for…* were for disclosing a latent disposition. The headings indicating *Aptitude for…* were for developing or strengthening the natural disposition.
"Ineptitude for sculpture (the plastic arts): Nux v. Calc. c."
The second part of the work is a very small *REPERTORY OF PLASTIC MEDICINE*. Gallavardin used remedies to change the physical characteristics of people. He said that when you wanted to make a part bigger, the remedy should be given during the increasing moon. To diminish the plumpness of a part, the remedy should be given during the decreasing moon.
Buttocks very big: Nux
Cheeks very fat: Calc-c.Sulph, Puls.

Gallavardin's work was most interesting, and his REPERTORY OF PLASTIC MEDICINE is close to unbelievable. Although most of the newer repertories have included many of the additions from Gallavardin, many prescribers note his additions and discount them as "unreliable."

1890: *GENTRY'S CONCORDANCE REPERTORY OF THE MATERIA MEDICA*:
William D. Gentry, MD ✱ ✔
A. L. Chatterton; 6 volumes.
In the introduction, Gentry explains that in 1876 he was looking for a particular symptom— a dull frontal headache, worse in the temples, with aching in the umbilicus. After searching through repertories and materia medicæ for several days, he thought, "If we only had a repertory arranged on the plan of Cruden's *Concordance of the Bible* it would have to be necessary only to refer to the letter 'U' and under 'umbilicus' find at once the desired symptom." These massive volumes were the end product of that desire.

These volumes were not widely used. Julia M. Green characterized it as "absolutely worthless on account of bulk and repetition without useful method."
Of the work, Kent says, "…the most shameful work that ever appeared, and it is no wonder the author has gone over to Christian Science and abandoned medicine entirely. Not over 40 percent of the genuine materia medica is in this pretended complete work, while one half of Gentry's symptoms cannot be found in any materia medica. It is a mess of trash."
As an experiment, Dr. K-H. Gypser noted the symptoms that appear at the top right page of every 100 pages, and checked them for accuracy. He could trace them all back to provings and reliable sources. Who to believe? Was Kent simply trashing the competition?

1892: *A REPERTORY FOR DIPHTHERIA*: William Jefferson Guernsey, MD
Published in the *IHA Transactions,* 1892; 12 pages.

1892: *NOTES ON SCIATICA*: B. Simmons, MD
Supplement to the *Homœopathic Physician*, Volume 12. It has a 5 page repertory.

1893: *REPERTORY OF SYMPTOMS OF THE OVARIES*: Cyrus M. Boger, MD
Published in The *Homœopathic Physician,* Volume 13; 10 pages.

1893: *COMPLETE REPERTORY TO THE TISSUE REMEDIES OF SCHÜSSLER*: S. F. Shannon
Chain and Hardy, Denver, CO; 544 pages.
Reprinted by Boericke and Tafel in **1937**.

1894: *SENSATIONS AS IF*: A. W. Holcomb, MD
Medical Advance, Chicago; 130 pages.
The original work which was later expanded by H. A. Roberts.

1894: *BEE-LINE REPERTORY*: Stacy Jones, MD
Boericke and Tafel; 210 pages.
A fascinating little book that combines therapy within the repertory. Set out in an alphabetical order, there is a section on "Diet" in the "D" section, a discussion of "Dose" right after the rubric for "Dissecting knife cut," and instruction for getting foreign objects out of the ear under "Ear, in the." Many therapeutic dosages are contained within the rubrics.

1894: *REPERTORY OF FOOT SWEATS*: Olin M. Drake, MD
Published in The *Homœopathic Physician,* Volume 14; 7 pages.

1895: *REPERTORY OF SPASMS AND CONVULSIONS*: A. W. Holcomb, MD
Published in The *Homœopathic Physician,* Volume 15; 21 pages.

1895: *COUGH BY LYING*: Willard Ide Pierce, MD
Supplement to the Nov. 1895 *North American Journal of Homœopathy*; 12 pages.

1895: *REPERTORY OF SCARLET FEVER*: Edward Rushmore, MD.
Published in The *Homœopathic Physician,* Volume 15; 12 pages.

1895: *REPERTORY OF APPENDICITIS*: William A. Yingling, MD
Published in The *Homœopathic Physician,* Volume 15; 11 pages.

1896: *A REPERTORY OF THE GUIDING SYMPTOMS*: Calvin Knerr, MD ❋ ✔
F. A. Davis and Co.; 1232 pages.
Knerr, a pupil of Hering (and his son-in-law) compiled this repertory from Hering's 10 volumes. It is a bulky volume that has been characterized as not being useful in everyday study but valuable as a reference repertory for deeper comparative research.

Although it mixes pathogenic and clinical data, it contains several rubrics that cannot be found anywhere else. The biggest stumbling block to its use is the overly complex and graphically difficult layout. With the advent of having it on computer and being able to search for words and phrases, much of that difficulty has been overcome.

1896: *A REPERTORY OF TONGUE SYMPTOMS*: M. E. Douglas, MD
Boericke and Tafel; 190 pages.
No introduction included. Title page simply says "M. E. Douglas, M.D., Baltimore, MD"

1896: *HEART REPERTORY*: John Henry Clarke, MD
Gould; 30 pages.

1897: *REPERTORY OF WARTS AND CONDYLOMATA*: Olin M. Drake, MD
Published in the *Hahnemannian Advocate,* April 1897; 10 pages.

1897: *THE BED FEELS HARD*: H. C. Morrow, MD
Published in The *Homœopathic Physician,* Volume 17; 7 pages.

1897: *REPERTORY OF THERAPEUTICS OF THE EYE*: C. C. Boyle, MD
Published in the *Homœopathic Physician,* Volume 17; 2 pages.

1897-1899: *REPERTORY OF THE BACK*: E. H. Wilsey, MD
Published in *The Homœopathic Physician*; over 3 years (volumes 17-19); approx. 280 pages.
It was subsequently published by Boericke and Tafel as a single volume of 263 pages.

1897-1899: *A REPERTORY OF HOMŒOPATHIC MATERIA MEDICA*: James Tyler Kent, MD ✱ ✔
Examiner Printing House, Lancaster, PA; 1349 pages.
This has become the archetypal and definitive repertory. Kent attempted to pull together all the repertories that were in existence at that time. After several years of work he realized that there was no way to bring together works which approached the subject from so many different points of view. He abandoned that project and started again— this time with the original provings and information gathered till that time.
The work existed as an interleaved book in the office of his Post-graduate School. His students asked him to make it generally available. It was issued as one section at a time. Originally it was printed in 12 fascicles, sold individually as they were compiled and printed. It was not until 1900 that all 12 sections were bound together into a single book. The result was the repertory that is still in use today by homœopaths the world over.
The second edition (1380 pages) was printed in **1908**; the 3rd edition (1423 pages) was printed by Ehrhart and Karl in **1924**. Kent said, "The third edition completes my life work." It was proofed by his wife Clara Louise Kent, MD. All subsequent editions were printed by Ehrhart and Karl. The 4th edition was issued in **1935**; The 5th edition in **1945**; the 6th edition in **1957**. There were no changes made in the content after the 3rd edition.

Ehrhart and Karl printed one of the editions on "Bible Paper" allowing its thickness to be reduced from 2 1/2" to a bit less than 1 1/2". The book came in a slipcase. Henry N. Williams has the only copy of this edition I have ever seen.

In 1930, a young Elizabeth Wright, spoke to the IHA about "Revamping the Repertory" outlining some of the shortcomings of the work. The text of her talk was printed in the November 1930 issue of the Homœopathic Recorder. *These were the faults she saw with Kent's work:*
1. Many rubrics are out of place— pulse is under generals instead of being with the heart, lips are under the face instead of the mouth, etc.
2. There is no section for circulatory system, glandular system, lymphatic system, or nervous system.
3. Certain headings are misplaced: i.e., awkwardness under generals when it is a mental, desires and aversion under stomach when they should be in generals, etc.
4. Pathological, diagnostic, and objective symptoms are scattered throughout. They should be in a separate section.
5. Many common symptoms (such as vomiting, restlessness, etc.) are so large as to be useless.
6. Repetitions abound. They should be cross-referenced.
7. There are many more remedies that need to be included.
8. Confusion over the rubrics being "aggravated from" whereas "ameliorations" are clearly mentioned.
9. Many rubrics could be eliminated as being useless.
10. Lack of an index and good cross-referencing.

She proposed working on a new, abridged edition which would, she hoped, be printed on bible-paper and bound in two small volumes like the Boericke Book— The first volume being Generals and the second Particulars.
It is of note that George Royal commented when he asked Kent why he had not provided an Index, Kent replied, "A man with brains won't need it."
Many of Wright's ideas have finally been implemented in the Complete *and* Synthesis *Repertories— but the books have become larger instead of smaller as Wright intended.*

1898: *REPERTORY FACIAL AND SCIATIC NEURALGIAS:* F. H. Lutze, MD ✔
Boericke and Tafel; 296 pages.
The full title is THERAPEUTICS OF FACIAL & SCIATIC NEURALGIA WITH CLINICAL CASES AND REPERTORIES.

1898: REPERTORY OF RHEUMATISM, SCIATICA, AND ETC.: Alfred Pulford, MD ✔
Krammes, Tiffin, Ohio; 211 pages.
Aggravations of the parts, General aggravations, and Accompanying symptoms (vertigo, sleep, dreams, etc.)

1899: *REPERTORY OF THE URINARY ORGANS*: Alonzo Richard Morgan, MD
Published in *The Homœopathic Physician*, Volume 19; 2 pages.
This work was greatly expanded by the author and published by Boericke and Tafel in **1899** as *REPERTORY OF URINARY ORGANS AND PROSTATE GLAND*, (318 pages).

1900: *REPERTORY OF THE CYCLOPEDIA OF DRUG PATHOGENESY*: Richard Hughes, MD ✔
F. Gould; 476 pages.

1900: *A SYSTEMATIC, ALPHABETIC REPERTORY OF HOMŒOPATHIC REMEDIES*:
C. von Bönninghausen, edited by Cyrus M. Boger, MD
Boericke and Tafel; 269 pages.
The first English translation of Bönninghausen's seminal work.

1904: *CLINICAL REPERTORY OF MATERIA MEDICA*: John Henry Clarke, MD
Homœopathic Publishing Co.; 346 pages.
A clinical repertory containing *five* repertories: clinical, causation, temperaments, clinical relationships, and natural relationships. Based on the information in his three volume *DICTIONARY* and arranged by clinical symptom. Remedies in italics are found in *THE PRESCRIBER.*

1905: *CHARACTERISTICS AND REPERTORY OF BÖNNINGHAUSEN*: Cyrus Maxwell Boger, MD ✱ ✔
Boger, Parkersburg, WV; 857 pages.
A condensation of all Bönninghausen's work into a single volume. The Repertory section contains the *Pocket Book,* the *Asoric* and *Antipsoric* repertories, the repertory part of *Intermittent Fever,* and *The Sides of the Body.*
In reference to Dunham's annotated copy, Boger says: "An annotated copy presented by the author to the late Dr. Carroll Dunham later became the property of Dr. H. N. Guernsey and is now in the possession of his son, Dr. Joseph C. Guernsey, whose courtesy enables me to incorporate it in its entirety in the present work." All the additions by Dunham are marked with an asterisk (*).
The book was enlarged with Boger's notes, and reprinted by Roy in Calcutta in **1937**.

This is the book called "Bönninghausen" in the computer repertories. It is not *readily usable with the method outlined in the* Therapeutic Pocket Book.

1906: *HOMŒOPATHIC MATERIA MEDICA WITH REPERTORY*: Oscar Boericke, MD ✔
Boericke and Runyon; 1049 pages.
The Materia Medica, by William Boericke, MD, was issued in 1901. The repertory was added to the

3rd edition in 1906. The repertory is constructed differently than that of either Kent or Bönninghausen, and takes a bit of work to become familiar with. Nevertheless, its small size and fairly complete coverage— especially for acute disease states— makes it a most popular book to this day.

Because the book contains both a materia medica and repertory, and is pocket sized as well, I thought it would be an ideal book to use at the National Center Summer School introductory course. Realizing I was going to have to teach the use of this repertory to the students, and knowing that Henry N. Williams, MD often used the book when on house calls, I phoned him to ask if he had any pointers about the construction of the repertory or any helpful hints about its use. His laconic reply: "The structure becomes very clear after you use it for a few years."

1907: *COUGH BETTER AND WORSE*: Willard Ide Pierce, MD
Privately printed; 92 pages.
Derived from Allen's *Handbook*. "…everyone is confronted by the indefiniteness of many of our symptoms. This comprises the only difficulty in arranging a satisfactory repertory, for not only must a certain symptom be placed under several heading to insure of it being under the proper one, but frequently one would include a symptom that another would exclude."

1908: *CLINICAL REPERTORY*: P. W. Shedd, MD ✱ ✔
Boericke and Tafel; 233 pages.
It includes a *Repertory of Time Modalities* by Dr. Ide of Stettin, Germany, whose work was translated for the book. "To authors whose compilations in various languages have afforded data, due thanks are rendered. Originality in homœopathic materia medica is not the invention of new things, but a more helpful arrangement of durable pathogenic and clinical facts."

1910: *TIMES OF THE REMEDIES*: Cyrus M. Boger, MD ✔
Published by the International Hahnemannian Association, Derby, CT; 14 pages.

1912: *A CARD REPERTORY*: Margaret L. Tyler, MD
Unknown publisher and number of cards.
Kent did not think highly of the project and it was abandoned. Said Kent in a letter to Tyler, "Your cards will destroy the highest ideal of Hahnemann, and my teaching as it aims to fit and adjust remedies to the masses instead of to each one. The card system destroys growth and progress that must come from working out the case, every case, in the work of every beginner. Give a beginner a card system and that will be the end of him. He will not grow. He will not learn or master the materia medica. I once planned a similar scheme, but I soon saw that I must work out every case, making use of the fullest repertory accessible; curtailing nothing less I miss something important, and this meant a life charged against my conscience… Your card system will make mediocres out of good men as it will pervert advancement, growth, maturity in our pupils… You are doing as I used to do. You are hunting for labor saving machines. These machines are useful in everything but art. They are as ruinous to the art of prescribing as they are to music. I want to see my pupils in your country become more than mediocre in their old age."

A very rare card repertory. I have seen only one copy. The harsh words that Kent uses against the card-repertories, could also be used, today, against computer repertories. If the student does not spend the time in case taking and analysis before going to the repertory, the result will always be disappointing. The computer repertories are, of course, much more complete than a card repertory could ever be, yet if they are just used by those "hunting for labor saving machines" the results will be the same as Kent described.

1916: *DISEASES OF THE RESPIRATORY ORGANS*: F. H. Lutze, MD
Journal Publishing Club, NY, NY; 100 pages.
A short repertory compiled by a follower of Kent who worked in Brooklyn, NY.

1920: *CARD REPERTORY*: Enrique Jiminez-Nuñez
The card repertory was conceived in Costa Rica by Jiminez in 1910, and he began to make his own

cards. He based his work on Bönninghausen's *Therapeutic Pocket Book*. The final repertory had 2593 cards. He received a U. S. Patent in 1925.

Jimenez's son, Marco, took up the work and in **1948** produced a "Practical Homeopathic Repertory" consisting of 552 cards. See the 1948 entry.

1922: *SYMPTOM REGISTER*: Richard Field, MD (a card repertory) ✱
Private; 254 pages (book), 6460 cards comprising 383 remedies.
Although Field included many rubrics from Boger, he generally limited his remedies to grade 2 and 3 in Kent, so many possible remedies fell by the way, and according to some, the results were "not always satisfactory." The book contains the rubric and remedy codes (Part I) and a four-drawer wooden box filled with the cards (Part II).

1926: *THE GENERAL ANALYSIS*: Cyrus Maxwell Boger, MD (a card repertory)
Boger, Parkersburg, WV; 17 pages. 304 cards with 222 remedies.
A condensation of Boger's prior work.
"I have nearly all the card indices, but could not use them to advantage, so I slowly worked out one to suit myself. It was first printed in book form, for pocket reference and later transferred to punched cards to insure greater facility in use. The production of these cards was very troublesome until I found a firm that gets out statistical cards indices for the government. It agreed to print my rubrics of the forms and to punch them accurately as per sample. The continued use of these cards slowly evolved a system which depends upon a three-fold classification of symptoms: first, fundamental, constitutional, or life time effects; second, the present display which is a fresh or acute outburst of the deeper lying tendencies; and third, the modalities. As you see, its basis is essentially that of the philosophy of the *Organon*." — pg. 730 Oct. 1932 *Homœopathic Recorder*

A very useful work. Because of the "general" nature of the arrangement, this is not seen as an "end-all" substitute for a more detailed repertory, such as Kent's. It is too bad that the punch-card technology that produced it is no longer readily available. It would be a great addition to any practitioner's desk.
A number of years ago I showed the card repertory to Richard Pitcairn, a homœopathic veterinarian. He found it to be of great use because it is all "generals"— the information you can usually get in veterinary cases. He developed the repertory as a Macintosh Hypercard program, but few were interested.

1929: *CORRECTIONS TO KENT'S REPERTORY*: J. S. Pugh, MD
Published in the *Homœopathic Recorder*; 6 pages.
Pugh, Austin, and Gladwin had copies of Kent's hand corrected third edition. These were the corrections. A number of remedies were added— although it seems as if the remedies themselves *were* in the *Repertory*, but their names did not appear in the list of Remedy Abbreviations.

1932: *ADDITIONS TO KENT'S REPERTORY*: Cyrus M. Boger, MD ✔
Published by the *Homœopathic Recorder 1931-1932*; 132 pages.

1935: *THE PRINCIPLES AND PRACTICALITY OF BÖNNINGHAUSEN'S THERAPEUTIC POCKET BOOK*:
H. A. Roberts, MD and Annie C. Wilson ✔
Boericke and Tafel; 76 pages.
This exposition of the *Therapeutic Pocket Book* method was printed as a limited edition (200 copies), and then was bound into all *Therapeutic Pocket Book* editions (The 1891 T. F. Allen translation) sold by Boericke and Tafel after 1935.

1937: *SENSATIONS AS IF*: Herbert A. Roberts, MD ✔
Boericke and Tafel; 519 pages.
An enlarged edition of a work begun by Dr. A. W. Holcomb and published under the auspices of *The Medical Advance* in 1894. Roberts drew information from an interleaved copy of Holcomb's work that was compiled by Dr. W. A. Yingling, as well as from the works of Hering, Clarke, and Allen. The work is dedicated to Samuel Hahnemann, "the first to evaluate subjective symptoms." Roberts, aware of the shortcoming of this type of repertory, cautions to "Beware of the keynote that is not backed up by knowledge of, or reference to, the materia medica."

A very useful work. Although it has been absorbed into the larger repertories, it works best as a stand-alone volume. Hayes said of Case (who used the original volume by Holcomb) that he "chuckled about the things he found in it sometimes."

1939: *THE UNABRIDGED DICTIONARY OF SENSATIONS AS IF*: James W. Ward, MD ✔
Wobbers, Inc., San Francisco; 1637 pages.
A compilation of three books— Hahnemann's *Materia Medica*, Allen's *Encyclopedia*, and Clarke's *Dictionary*. Divided into two sections: Pathogenic symptoms— those seen through the provings, and Clinical symptoms— those verified through clinical experience.

The book has an index of the sources for each symptom, allowing the symptom to be referenced as to its exact source.

1939: *A REPERTORY OF LEUCORRHOEA*: Alfred Pulford, MD
Published in the *Homœopathic Recorder*, July 1939; 19 pages.

1948: *PRACTICAL HOMEOPATHIC REPERTORY IN COLORED AND PERFORATED CARDS*:
Marcos Jimenez, MD
Jimenez, Mexico City, Mexico. 126 pages.
The first 58 pages are in English. The remainder is the same in Spanish. This is the instruction book that accompanied the 552-piece card repertory. Describing Kent's *Repertory* as "complicated and difficult to master," the author says, "For the inexperienced, it is a maze where he is hopelessly lost, if a friendly hand does not aid him. To master it, many years of conscious patient study and experience are necessary; to repertorize a case, long, tedious, patient hours, and a careful selection of symptoms and drugs are necessary. To simplify, facilitate, and popularize the Homeopathic Repertorization, this *PRACTICAL HOMEOPATHIC REPERTORY IN COLORED AND PERFORATED CARDS* has been invented."
The repertory contains 552 cards, comprising 480 remedies. The grade of the remedy is indicated in color— red for 3, and blue for 2. Different sections have different colors; the mind section is on yellow cards, while the mouth, ear, nose, and throat are on blue cards. The cards contain the rubrics from Kent that the author believed were "most important and indispensable, that which cannot be omitted."

An attempt at a labor saving device which probably would have Kent rolling in his grave.

1950: *PUNCH CARD SPINDLE REPERTORY*: Robert H. Farley, MD
Published by the author, Philadelphia, PA.
190 cards of "general symptoms of the mind and body." 274 remedies.

1959: *CARD REPERTORY*: Dr. Jugal Kishore
Published by the author in India.
3497 cards.

1963: *THE CONCISE REPERTORY*: Dr. S. R. Phatak ✔
Sunanda Publishers, Bombay; 312 pages.
An alphabetized re-working of Boger and Bönninghausen. The author says, "No originality can be claimed except for presentation."

1965: *CARD REPERTORY*: Dr. Pichiah Sankaran
Published by the author in India.
389 cards.

1969: *CARD REPERTORY*: George Broussalian
Published by the author in France.
Kent's *Repertory* in 1861 cards.

1973: *THE SYNTHETIC REPERTORY*: ed. Horst Barthel, MD and Will Klunker, MD ✔
Published by Dr. med. Horst Barthel, Wiesbaden and Karl F. Haug Verlag, Heidelberg.
Three volumes compiled from the work of all the other repertory authors: Vol. I: Mental Symptoms (1102 pages) Vol. II: General Symptoms (774 pages) Vol. III: Sleeping and Sexual Symptoms (611 pages). Seemingly a very complete work, it has not resolved the problems that Kent found when trying to synthesize the repertories of his day. Although the sources of the rubrics are fully documented and the headings are in several languages, the work is more of a final reference rather than a day to day usable repertory.

The first attempt at synthesizing information that is found in the literature but not found in Kent's Repertory. It was the publication of this work that made people aware that other information was available that was not in Kent's repertory. Although it was difficult to use in daily practice, it formed the basis of a good portion of the computer repertories that were soon to come.

1974: *ADDITIONS TO KENT'S REPERTORY*: George Vithoulkas ✔
Privately published as a typewritten manuscript that was often duplicated. Based upon Boger's work with additions from Gallavardin and from Vithoulkas' practice. Published in **1989** by B. Jain; 89 pages.

1975: *CARD REPERTORY*: Hans Lees
Published by the author in Germany.
3,000 cards.

1978: *AUTOVISUAL REPERTORY*: Dr. Ramanlal Patel
Sai Homœopathic Publishing, Kerala; 144 pages.
The book is only the code for the contents of a large wooden box containing 5505 plastic strips (490mm x 6mm). Each strip represents a rubric, and has 435 grooves in it at right angles to its long axis, each groove representing a remedy. If a remedy is contained in the rubric, the groove is filled with color: grade 3 in Red, grade 2 in Yellow, and grade 1 in Black. The numbers on the strips are also color coded: Red being Generals, and Black being particulars.
The strips are put into a reading device which stacks them allowing the lines to be seen clearly. Having used the codes in the book to select the rubrics, one can now see that a number of lines are contiguous over (let's say) the line numbered 312. A search in the index will find the remedy of that number is *Nux vomica*.

The most complex way of using a repertory I have ever seen. The wooden box, filled with the 5505 plastic strips, is about 2 feet square and 7 inches deep. Made from a very dense native Indian wood, it weighs close to 90 pounds.

1980: *THE FINAL GENERAL REPERTORY*: Diwan Harish Chand, MD and Pierre Schmidt, MD ✔
National Homeopathic Pharmacy, New Delhi; 1423 pages.
This is Kent's *Repertory* edited and corrected by two Kentian experts. Kent made corrections into a few copies of his repertory. One was given to Alonzo Austin, and Austin passed it on to Pierre Schmidt. Schmidt also had Kent's copy of Hering's *Guiding Symptoms*.
In 1963 Dr. K. H. Mittal, from India, visited Schmidt and copied all the corrections into his repertory. When he left, he absconded with Kent's original.
In 1978, Dr. Ahmed Currim located Mittal, and Mittal told him that he had taken the original and cut it up and buried it.
In 1980, Currim was able to get the book from Mittal. It was in several thousand pieces. When I visited Currim in the late 1980s he showed the pieces to me. He was busy putting them together, like a jigsaw puzzle.
When Chand put together *The Final General Repertory*, he used a *copy* of Mittal's Repertory. This copy had been transcribed by a third party. It is not known how diligent this party was in the transcribing. Furthermore, Mittal had several annotations indicated as "KGS" which were copied from Kent's *Hering*. Some of these might have been added into the copy and, therefore, are not directly related to the repertory corrections.
This is one of the more bizarre episodes in homœopathic literature.

Although this book is still available it has been superseded, in large part, by the newer repertories like the Complete *and the* Synthesis. *If I had not seen the pieces in Currim's possession, I would have doubted the entire story. There were two other copies that were annotated by Kent. One went to Dr. Pugh in Texas, and one to F. E. Gladwin. The whereabouts of both of these books remains unknown.*

1980: *REPERTORY OF DESIRES AND AVERSIONS*: Dr. V. R. Agrawal ✔
Vijay Publications, Delhi; 46 pages.
A short repertory taken from the usual reliable sources— Hahnemann, Allen, Clarke, etc.

1981: *SEQUELAE*: Dr. G. S. R. Sastry
Curentur Homoeo Publishers, Hyderabad, India; 220 pages.
This interesting book is divided into three parts: After effects of diseases, After effects of conditions incidental to activities of life and diet, After effects of medicines— both allopathic and homœopathic. A large number of authors and works were consulted including Journals of the *American Institute of Homœopathy* from 1931 on, the *Homœopathic Recorder* from 1913 on, and the *British Homœopathic Journal* from 1948 on. A Second edition of 560 pages was issued in **1996**.

A useful repertory with information that is hard to find elsewhere.

1987: *REPERTORIUM GENERALE*: Jost Künzli, MD
Barthel and Barthel Publishing Corp; Berg am Starnberger See, Germany; 1172 pages.
An expanded Kent's *Repertory* compiled by a true homœopathic master. It contains many additions based on Künzli's experience and that of his teacher, Pierre Schmidt. Many rubrics have a "Black Dot" next to them— indicating that if this particular rubric is used in a case the curative remedy is certainly contained within that rubric.

Shortly after its publication, this book began to take the place of the basic Kent's Repertory *in the practices of many prescribers. One problem was that the pagination, because of the many additions, was different than the Kent book. This made it hard to use when teaching— when the pupils had an inexpensive Kent's* Repertory, *and the teacher was using the larger, newer work.*

1989: *REPERTORY OF PREGNANCY, PARTURITION, AND PUERPERIUM*: Alberto Soler-Medina, MD ✔
Haug Verlag; 76 pages.
"Pregnancy, parturition, and puerperium, which are such important moments in the life of a woman and for the newborn baby, are in my opinion, not developed, thoroughly and extensively

enough in Kent's *Repertory*. Therefore I think it is interesting to make up a compilation on these subjects, as treated by different authors, so as to give them the importance they deserve."

1990: *THE APPLIED REPERTORY*: Dr. Devika Aggarwal ✔
Homeopathic Publishing House, Bombay; 403 pages.
Pointing out that the plan of the repertory is "not coherent with case analysis and case synthesis," the author has synthesized several repertories into one encompassing the Mind section of *Kent*, the General modalities of *Bönninghausen*, the Pathological Generals of *Boger*, the Diseases of *Boericke*, and an updating of the whole from the *Synthetic Repertory* and Phatak's *Repertory*.
The book is laid out in 5 sections, each corresponding to a piece of the case:
General Modifying Factors; Miasms/ Pathological Tendencies; Mind; Physiological Generals/ Appetite/ Desires/ Aversions/ Sleep and dreams; Particulars: Organs, Systems, Fever

Not known in the USA, but used in India and Australia by many, those I have met who use this book can't say enough good things about it. For the best use, the case must be taken as outlined in the very detailed introduction, so the material gleaned will fall into the categories that comprise the above mentioned sections.

1992: *THE COMPLETE REPERTORY*: Roger van Zandvoort.
Based on Kent's *Repertory* in the MacRepertory computer program, this work includes many additions and corrections from numerous sources. The Mind Section was released on this date. The rest of the program was released in book form in **1995**.

1993: *THE HOMEOPATHIC MEDICAL REPERTORY*: Robin Murphy, ND ✔
Hahnemann Academy of North America, Colorado; 1590 pages.
A re-working of the *Complete Repertory* but placed into alphabetical order. Contains modern terminology and diagnostic rubrics. There are many additions, but they are of unknown value since no "source" key is included, making it impossible to differentiate which remedies came from Kent which were added in the *Complete*, and which are Murphy's additions.

Well bound and printed on "Bible paper," the book has been criticized for the lack of "sources" and because of the alphabetical arrangement. In the experience of some, the arrangement makes it so easy to find possible rubrics that the need to search for, perhaps, a more inclusive one is obviated by the ease of finding the first. The result is that in the hands of a beginner or inexperienced person, rubrics are found which are "close enough" but not necessarily the most precise rubric needed for a successful prescription. Although the arrangement of the Kent work might seem confusing, constant use of it inculcates a sense of exactness in rubric selection which is obviated by an alphabetical arrangement.

1993: *THE SYNTHESIS REPERTORY*: Frederik Schroyens, MD ✔
Homeopathic Book Publishers, London; 1720 pages, plus 111 page appendix.
Derived from the *RADAR* computer program, contains many additions to Kent's *Repertory* on which it is based.

1995: *THE COMPLETE REPERTORY*: Roger van Zandvoort ✔
IRHIS; 2800 pages.
Printed as a single volume or as three individual parts.

The COMPLETE *and the* SYNTHESIS *have become the standard as we enter the new millennium. Both are available for computer use. The structure of them are slightly different, and a careful reading of the introductions to each will give an outline of how each was constructed. They both follow the Kent structure, although a number of changes suggested by Elizabeth Wright in 1930 have finally been incorporated into the works.*

1999: *THE PHOENIX REPERTORY*: Dr. J. P. S. Bakshi ✔
Cosmic Healers, Pvt. Ltd, New Delhi; 2287 pages in two volumes.
A compilation derived from many sources. *ReferenceWorks* was used to source many symptoms, as was the *Complete* and the *Synthesis*.

2000: *BÖNNINGHAUSENS THERAPEUTISCHES TASCHENBUCH*: (German version)
edited by Klaus-Henning Gypser, MD ✔
Johannes Sonntag Verlagsbuchhandlung, Stuttgart; 502 pages.
Starting from a data-base of the *Pocket Book* that was compiled by George Dimitriadis in Sydney, this work was then further refined with the advice from a group of seven others in Germany.

THE BÖNNINGHAUSEN REPERTORY; THERAPEUTIC POCKET BOOK METHOD: (English version)
edited by George Dimitriadis ✔
Hahnemann Institute, Sydney; 287 pages.
A complete re-edit of Bönninghausen's *Pocket Book* undertaken by a team in Sydney, Australia over a period of five years, with contributions by K-H. Gypser and his team in Germany. To discuss the details is not possible in this short paragraph. The English work and the German work are a bit different in format and since the German work is in the original language there does not have to be the lengthy explanations (a 69 page appendix in the English book) as to how each rubric was translated.

Two incredibly thorough works. Once can only hope that a new generation (after a gap of almost 75 years) will begin to use the profound methodology of Bönninghausen. An excellent omen at the start of the new millennium!

Computer Repertories: A Commentary

Although the card repertories were the forerunners of the computer repertories, I have chosen to keep them within the repertory section— they were, after all, paper, manual, and not etheric.

Anyone who has ever looked at a repertory (which is simply, as Hahnemann conceived, an index to the materia medica) can understand it is a prime candidate for being accessed through a data sorting program. It was not until the mid–1980s and the development of personal computers, that several people, almost simultaneously, began developing computer based repertories. The first program, a very simple one called *Lamnia*, was developed in Australia. It used a very abbreviated repertory based on Kent's work.
As the conception of the computer-assisted repertory developed, several programs gained prominence: *MacRepertory* (USA), *RADAR* (Belgium), *CARA* (UK) and *Hompath* (India). Others, some not as "full-featured," are also on the market: *Homeopathy@Work, Homeopathic Assistant, PC Kent* (an outgrowth of the Broussalian card repertory), and *Polycrest*, among others.
An obvious outgrowth of entering all the information from a known repertory (such as Kent's) into a computer data base, is that additions can be made to the data base which can then serve as a source for a new printed repertory.
These new "book" repertories were released in the 1990s— *The Complete Repertory* by Van Zandvoort grew out of the *MacRepertory* program, while the *Synthesis Repertory* by Schroyens, grew out of the *RADAR* program.
When the team at the University of Namur began to develop the *RADAR* program, they realized the benefit of being able to search the materia medica itself for specific phrases. When the first *RADAR* was released by Archibel in 1987 in included the materia medicæ of Hahnemann, Clarke, T. F. Allen, and Hering in its searchable database.
By 1990, Kent Homeopathic Associates released *ReferenceWorks*, a searchable database of over 500 books, which grew to 900 titles by 2000.
By 1990 Archibel had issues a similar program called *ExLibris* with 47 volumes, and by late 2000 it had been replaced with *Encyclopedia Homeopathica*, a library of 440 titles (and growing), with a much better search engine.

The ability to search for phrases within what amounts to almost all major homœopathic literature (including some journals), is certainly an amazing power to have at one's fingertips. And the advances in technology which allows it all to be carried in a laptop computer no bigger than a thick writing pad, are truly miraculous.

But with the up side, there is a down side: a whole generation has stopped reading the primary texts. (See commentary at the end of the Appendix by Woodbury.)

Doing a search for a unique symptom in a database of homœopathic books, is akin to searching in a literature database for the phrases "while their hostess told them of increasing families upon Bear Creek," and "I know if I went riding with you I should not have an immature protector." If the database is large enough you will find that they were both from Owen Wister's *The Virginian*. What can that tell you? Does it tell you anything about the story? Does it tell you the plot? Does it outline the characters?

It is certainly useful that one can find a symptom spoken of in exact terms in the *Materia Medica* of E. A. Farrington, but the result is the finding of pieces and never being able to understand the wholeness of Farrington— how he developed his thoughts, how he structured the remedies, etc., and it is the wholeness of the man and his thinking which has lead prior generations to consider him as great. Now, he is just a name— known but not understood. And as long as we pick his work apart, out of context, we will never understand his greatness.

This is the failure of computer repertories/materia medicæ-- they can give us results without wholeness.

The Programs

1986: *MACREPERTORY*
Kent Homeopathic Associates, San Rafael, CA; 500MB
The Core program offers 6 repertories and 31 materia medicæ. The full complement is 17 repertories and 48 materia medicæ. *MacRepertory* requires between 300-500MB. PC and Mac.

1986: *THE HOMPATH*
Dr. Jawahar J. Shah, Mumbai, India; 1GB
Has seven modules including repertories and materia medica. PC only.

1987: *RADAR* (Rapid Aid in Direct Access to Repertorization)
Archibel, Assesse, Belgium; 1.5GB
The *Synthesis* repertory became the basic repertory in 1993. With version 8.0 (on computer) the end user can select exactly those authors and additions he would like to see in his repertory. He can create an infinite combination of views based on any combination of authors he would like. 1.5GB needed for whole package of RADAR and EH. PC only.

1988: *CARA* (Computer Assisted Repertorial Analysis)
Miccant, Nottingham, UK; 750MB
Upgraded in 1991. Contain an abbreviated materia medica— 65 books standard with an optional 15 more.

1990: *REFERENCEWORKS*
Kent Homeopathic Associates, San Rafael, CA; 1.2GB
There are, at present, 425 books available. It requires 500MB for the "core library" and 1.2GB for the full edition. PC and Mac.

Therapeutics

Therapeutics

The great majority of books written about homœopathy are therapeutic books— the clinical use of the remedies. Bradford lists 135 books that are about therapeutics, 47 of which are listed here. Books about therapeutics generally present a limited materia medica based upon an allopathic diagnosis, i.e., which remedies would help which disease.

For the purposes of this book, those works that are listed as "therapeutics" would usually have the word "therapeutics" in the title (e.g., *The Therapeutics of Intermittent Fever; The Therapeutics of Yellow Fever*) or the entire focus of the book is about treating a condition (e.g., Cholera; Diarrhea, etc.). The materia medica contained therein is limited to those symptoms and modalities that pertain to the stated condition.

By their very nature, a good number of therapeutic books include minimal repertories. Unlike materia medicæ where the book is read to glean information about the totality of a remedy, a therapeutics book usually has one aim— to shortcut the way to the remedy for the suffering individual.

While a number of these books encompass the entire range of clinical possibilities, there is a further division between those that combine diagnostics with therapeutics (Raue, Jahr) and those that simply state the name of the condition (Clarke's *Prescriber*, Lilienthal's *Therapeutics*, Tyler's *Pointers to the Common Remedies*) and present differentials through which the most appropriate remedy may be selected. The former category was usually used as texts at schools for the teaching of Pathology and Diagnostics and integrating it with homœopathic therapeutics, while the latter were simply references for daily prescribing.

Another category of books are those which were primarily physiology and pathology texts, and these I have listed in the "Anatomy, Pathology, and Diagnosis" section. In my differentiation of them I looked at how much therapeutic advice was given in the book. For example, while the books of Jahr and Raue discuss pathology and diagnosis, in the end they are concerned with therapeutics, while the books of Arndt and Goodno concentrate on the pathology and diagnosis, giving little mention to therapeutics.

Most of the "domestic manuals" that have appeared are also, basically, therapeutic books. Often, the only quality that separates them is the language; the "domestic manual" is sometimes more accessible to the layman and there is more instruction concerning what other general health measures might be used for a specific condition. The "domestic manuals" usually have a general introduction to the principles of homœopathy, and offer advice on hygiene and diet. If the work in question did not specify that it was intended solely as a domestic guide (e.g., Hering's *Domestic Physician*), I placed in the Therapeutic section.

Most works listed here need no further commentary as their titles are self explanatory. Many are concerned with epidemic diseases we no longer see— cholera, typhoid, malaria, and many types of fevers. Others have maintained their clarity and continue to be useful, yet even those are often lacking. Because of the nature of materia medica, a "condition" might have any number of remedies indicated. We find, in many of these works, the indications offered in the differentials are often for common symptoms, and using the work will still leave one with the necessity of going back to the materia medica to choose between those remedies that are the most similar to the case. Another problem, as many homœopaths have found, is the main complaint (the condition for which the book is being searched) might often be an acute exacerbation of an underlying chronic condition that needs a remedy outside of those listed in such a work in order to effect a total cure.

Therapeutics

1831: *SPECIAL THERAPY OF ACUTE AND CHRONIC DISEASES: EDITED ACCORDING TO HOMŒOPATHIC PRINCIPLES AND PUBLISHED BY FRANZ HARTMANN*: Franz Hartmann, MD (*Specielle Therapie acuter und chronischer Krankheiten: nach homoeopathischen Grundsaetzen bearbeitet und herausgegeben von Franz Hartmann*). Weigel, Leipzig eventually published the whole series: Volume I: Chapter I: About the fevers, **1847**, p. 1 - 271 Chapter II: About the acute eruptions of the skin and inflammations, **1847**, p. 273 - 572. Volume II: Chapter I: Chronic diseases I, **1848**, p. 1 - 310 Chapter II: Chronic diseases II, **1848**, p. 312 - 703.

The Heritage of Homœopathic Literature

These books were translated into English by Charles Hempel and published by William Radde. Volume I was published in **1847**, chapters I and II as separate volumes. In **1849** Radde published Volume II as two separate volumes. After this the *Acute and Chronic Diseases* were sold as Volume 1-4. The third volume of the series concerning mental diseases was published in Germany in **1853** and issued again, edited by G. H. G. Jahr in **1854**. It was translated into English by John Galloway, MD, and published by Henry Turner in **1857** (482 pages). It was never printed in the United States.

Upon the publication of this book, Hahnemann wrote to Hartmann: "Owing to the difficult nature of our homœopathic method of treatment, which requires so much thought and subtle differentiation for it to be successfully practiced, to try and popularize and render it empirical to the extent you intend, seems an impossible and unnecessary task, even harmful in the hands of the laity who have received no training." Hahnemann's warning went unheeded, and many books on "therapeutics" followed.

1833: *DIE DYNAMIK DER ZAHNHEILKUNDE BEARBEITET NACH DEN GRUNDSÄTZEN DEN HOMÖOPATHIE* (*The Dynamics of Dentistry According to the Principles of Homœopathy*): Salomo Gutmann Kollmann, Leipzig; 168 pages.
Gutmann located in Leipzig in 1816 and sought out Hahnemann, thinking that there might be a use for homœopathy in dentistry. He was a member of the prover's union.
This is the first work about homœopathy in dentistry. It is essentially a materia medica followed by a repertory. It has never been translated into English.

1838: *HOMŒOPATHIC PRACTICE OF MEDICINE:* Jacob Jeanes, MD
A. Waldie, Philadelphia; 391 pages.
"…to present to the American physician as complete a book on practical homœopathic medicine as can be done in the present state of the science… A very small edition of this work is published as the demand cannot be expected to be very extensive."
The first American book written about homœopathy. Jeanes, a native of Pennsylvania, learned German to read books on homœopathy. A short section of homœopathic theory is followed by a basic therapeutic text: conditions are named and remedy differential are presented along with cured cases.
This book was translated into German in **1842**.

Jeanes was a founder of the Homœopathic Medical College of Pennsylvania with Hering and Williamson.

1841: *DISEASES OF THE ALIMENTARY CANAL AND CONSTIPATION, TREATED HOMŒOPATHICALLY*:
W. Broackes
J. Dobson; 134 pages.

1847: *DISEASES OF THE EYE TREATED HOMŒOPATHICALLY*: Alexander C. Becker, MD
Radde; 77 pages.

1849: *THE HOMŒOPATHIC TREATMENT OF CHOLERA*: Benjamin Franklin Joslin. MD
William Radde; 144 pages.
Included a Repertory. Reprinted in **1885** as a supplement to The *Homœopathic Physician*, with notes from P. P. Wells.

1850: *JAHR'S CLINICAL GUIDE OR POCKET REPERTORY*: G. H. G. Jahr
Radde; 409 pages.
Translated from the German by Charles J. Hempel, MD.
"For the Treatment of Acute and Chronic Diseases." Says the translator: "This work is not to be confused with the original Manual of Jahr."
In **1869**, a second edition was published by Boericke and Tafel, and edited by Samuel Lilienthal, MD (624 pages). It was this book that became, in **1878**, Lilienthal's *HOMŒOPATHIC THERAPEUTICS*.

1852: *ELEMENTS OF HOMŒOPATHIC PRACTICE OF PHYSIC:* Joseph Laurie, MD
Matthew and Houard, Philadelphia, PA; 642 pages.
Also published with an Appendix on Intermittent fever by J. S. Douglas, by Radde; 939 pages.

1853: *DR. FRANZ HARTMANN'S DISEASES OF CHILDREN AND THEIR HOMŒOPATHIC TREATMENT*:
Franz Hartmann, MD
Radde; 516 pages.
Translated from the German by C. J. Hempel.

1853: *HOMŒOPATHIC TREATMENT OF INTERMITTENT FEVER*: James S. Douglas, MD
William Radde; 108 pages.
Included a repertory.

1855: *THE HOMŒOPATHIC GUIDE IN ALL DISEASES OF THE URINARY AND SEXUAL ORGANS, INCLUDING THE DERANGEMENTS CAUSED BY ONANISM AND SEXUAL EXCESSES*:
William Gollman, MD
Rademacher and Sheek; 309 pages.
Translated from the German by C. J. Hempel.

1856: *THE HOMŒOPATHIC TREATMENT OF DISEASES OF FEMALES, AND INFANTS AT THE BREAST*: G. H. G. Jahr ✔
Radde; 422 pages.
Translated from the German by C. J. Hempel.

1857: *SPECIAL THERAPEUTICS ACCORDING TO HOMŒOPATHIC PRINCIPLES: VOLUME 3: MENTAL DISEASES*: Franz Hartmann, MD
Henry Turner; 482 pages.
Translated by John Galloway. From the 1854 German edition edited by G. H. G. Jahr.
A translation was done by Hempel for Radde in 1856, but it was considered inferior to the Galloway translation. This work was reprinted in a facsimile version in the late **1980s** in Canada.

I had heard about the reprint and ordered a copy. It was an EXACT facsimile of the original— so exact, that it did not even have a page describing who republished it and when!

1860: *ON THE EFFICACY OF CROTALUS HORRIDUS IN YELLOW FEVER, ALSO IN MALIGNANT, BILIOUS, AND REMITTENT FEVERS*: Charles Neidhard, MD
Radde; 82 pages.

1864: *HOMŒOPATHY IN VENEREAL DISEASES*: Stephen Yeldham, MD
Henry Turner; 120 pages.
This was never published in the US.

1865: *CLINICAL LECTURES ON THE TREATMENT OF RHEUMATISM, EPILEPSY, ASTHMA, FEVER*:
Rutherford Russell
Leath and Ross; 399 pages.

1866: *A SYSTEMATIC TREATISE ON ABORTION*: Edwin M. Hale, MD
C. S. Halsey; 347 pages.
Says Bradford, "On account of some obscure wording on p. 319 of this work, Dr. Hale was accused, by some of the profession, of advising, under certain circumstances, the induction of abortion. To make his meaning clear, printed slips were issued, to be pasted over the obnoxious words."

1867: *THE APPLICATION OF THE PRINCIPLES AND PRACTICE OF HOMŒOPATHY TO OBSTETRICS, AND DISORDERS PECULIAR TO WOMEN AND YOUNG CHILDREN*: Henry N. Guernsey, MD ✱ ✔
Boericke; 752 pages.
2nd edition in **1873**, 3rd edition **1878**. Subsequent editions unchanged.
Usually called simply "Guernsey's Obstetrics", it is still in print. It covers all aspects of obstetrics including details of the female anatomy and physiology. It contains some excellent chapters on the care of the child for the first few months of life, and treatment of common childhood diseases. Said a review from the turn of the century, "A prominent obstetrician, who had every book on the subject published, told us that he refers to 'Guernsey' oftener than to any other in his big library. The reason for this is that Homœopathy changes not."

1868: *SPECIAL PATHOLOGY AND DIAGNOSTICS, WITH THERAPEUTIC HINTS*:
Charles G. Raue, MD ✱ ✔
Boericke; 644 pages.
"When I was called upon to lecture on special pathology and diagnostics about four years ago, I looked around for a work which would furnish the essential points of these branches of medical education, together with homœopathic therapeutics, in a concise manner and up to the latest researches; but I looked in vain. I was obliged to prepare my own material." This is the text that Raue used with his classes at Hahnemann Medical College in Philadelphia. It was reprinted in **1881** with 1072 pages, in **1885** with 1094 pages and again in **1898** with 1039 pages.

1869: *HOMŒOPATHIC THERAPEUTICS OF DIARRHEA*: James B. Bell, MD ✱ ✔
A. J. Tafel; 168 pages.
Subsequent editions were published by Boericke and Tafel in **1881** and **1888**. It contains an extensive repertory. The format of the book was subsequently used by many other authors. From a review in the *Hahnemannian Monthly*, "If there is a homœopathic physician who is not familiar with this work we simply say get this book and you will have at hand, in practical shape, all that is really valuable in Homœopathy in the treatment of this line of trouble."

One reviewer said that this book "saved thousands of lives."

1869: *THE SCIENCE OF THERAPEUTICS ACCORDING TO THE PRINCIPLES OF HOMŒOPATHY*:
Bernard Baehr, MD ✱ ✔
Boericke and Tafel; Volume 1, 635 pages. Volume 2, 752 pages.
A translation of *Die Therapie: nach den Grundsätzen der Homöopathie*, published by Weigel (Leipzig , **1862**). The introduction in the American edition calls it "a work of no ordinary merit" and suggests it will take the place of Hartmann's *Acute and Chronic Diseases*. The first 55 pages concern homœopathic philosophy. The rest is a listing of disease conditions followed by homœopathic therapeutical suggestions. Said Raue, "You can depend on what old Baehr says." And this from a review, "If a man wants to get to the scientific bottom of homœopathic therapeutics he would do well to carefully study this standard book. It is done with German thoroughness."

1869: *THERAPEUTIC GUIDE*: G. H. G. Jahr. ✱ ✔
Radde; 364 pages.
"The Most Important Results of More Than Forty Years of Practice; With Personal Observations regarding truly reliable and practically verified curative Indications in Actual Cases of Disease." Also known as "Jahr's Forty Years of Practice," this manual is written in a narrative style using an alphabetical order of the "condition. "I do not offer anything but what my own individual experience during a practice of forty years, has enabled me to verify *absolutely decisive* in choosing the proper remedy. The reader will easily comprehend that, in carrying out this plan, I had rigidly to exclude all cases which I had no experience *of my own* to offer." Reprinted **1873**, **1887**, **1935** by Boericke and Tafel.

Although the title is characteristically long, the book contains a mass of useful information. Said one reviewer, it was "…agreeable, chatty, and full of practical observation." Most I know who have bothered to read it are amazed at the useful information they can glean from its pages.

1869: *THE HOMŒOPATHIC TREATMENT OF SYPHILIS, GONORRHOEA, SPERMATORRHOEA AND URINARY DISEASES*: Dr. J. Ph. Berjeau ✔
A. J. Tafel; 256 pages.
Translated by J. H. P. Frost. This is a revision of the first English edition of **1856**.

1869: *A MANUAL OF THERAPEUTICS*: Richard Hughes, MD ✔
Henry Turner and William Radde; 540 pages.
Published simultaneously in the UK and the USA, this book was seen as Volume II of *A Manual of Homœopathic Practice*, the first being his book on *Pharmacodynamics*, published a year earlier. The author, in a narrative style, discusses the therapeutics of a variety of diseases. It is based on lectures he gave to his students.

1870: *HOMŒOPATHIC TREATMENT OF HOOPING COUGH*: C. von Bönninghausen
Henry M. Smith and Bro; 199 pages.
Translated by Carroll Dunham.
Contains a repertory. "In as much as we, homœopathists, treat concrete diseases and not abstract names, so it follows that a work on Hooping Cough may be equally available and useful as a guide in the treatment of any and every cough of a spasmodic nature, whether it receives the name of Hooping Cough or not."

1871: *ON INTERMITTENT FEVER AND OTHER MALARIOUS DISEASES*: Israel Shipman Pelton Lord, MD
Boericke and Tafel; 341 pages.
A record of over 200 cases cured with homœopathy and a discussion concerning the selection of the remedy.

One of the more unusual books about therapeutics. In the introduction, the author presents a number of cases and discusses in great detail which remedies come up for every symptom as found in the 1853 work of Douglas and the Repertory of Jahr, and why this "numerical counting" will not always yield the best remedy. The idea is interesting, but the writing is very dense and the points made are confusing. When the author discusses the actual cases, we find him giving two or more remedies in alternation, and usually without explanation.

A number of years ago I was contacted by a person who, it turned out, was a relation to Dr. Lord and found an unpublished manuscript written by him in an old trunk. It appeared to be more confusing than the first.

1871: *APPLIED HOMŒOPATHY OR SPECIFIC RESTORATIVE MEDICINE:* William Bayes, MD
Henry Turner; 171 pages.
Based on the therapeutic successes of the author in his 14 years of practice. 118 remedies are discussed in terms of their therapeutic use.

1871: *THERAPEUTIC KEY; OR PRACTICAL GUIDE FOR THE TREATMENT OF ACUTE DISEASES*:
Isaac D. Johnson, MD ✔
Boericke (USA); 179 pages.
By **1892** it was in its 16th edition and had been expanded to 400 pages. He wrote two other domestic books: *A GUIDE TO HOMEOPATHIC PRACTICE* (**1879**; 494 pages) and *COUNSEL TO PARENTS, AND HOW TO SAVE THE BABY* (**1889**; 224 pages).

1872: *LEUCORRHOEA, ITS CONCOMITANT SYMPTOMS AND ITS HOMŒOPATHIC TREATMENT*:
Alvin Matthew Cushing, MD ✔
T.P. Nichols, Lynn, MA: 70 pages.

1873: *THE TREATMENT OF TYPHOID FEVERS, WITH A FEW ADDITIONS:* Constantine Hering, MD
Boericke and Tafel; 24 pages.
Subsequently integrated into Hering's *Analytical Therapeutics*, it was republished, with many additions, in **1896** by the *Homœopathic Physician*.

1873: *THERAPEUTICS OF INTERMITTENT FEVERS:* C. von Bönninghausen
Boericke and Tafel; 243 pages.
Translated from the German by Augustus Korndoerffer, MD.

1873: *THE HOMEOPATHIC TREATMENT OF SURGICAL DISEASES*: J. Grant Gilchrest, MD
C. S. Halsey; 421 pages.
2nd edition in **1880** by Duncan Brothers; 464 pages.
"When the author first attempted a systematic arrangement of this great study, but few in our profession were willing to concede the efficacy of medicinal treatment in surgical affections, even those who were well grounded in the faith."
The book was translated into French, Spanish, Italian, and German.

1876: *HOMŒOPATHY IN ITS RELATION TO THE DISEASES OF WOMEN:* Thomas Skinner, MD ✔
Porter and Coates, Philadelphia; 74 pages

1876: *OPHTHALMIC THERAPEUTICS*: George S. Norton, MD and T. F. Allen, MD
Boericke and Tafel; 269 pages.
The New York Ophthalmic Hospital was founded in 1852, under allopathic management and achieved "indifferent success." In 1867 it came under homœopathic management with T. F. Allen at the helm. This book is an outgrowth of the success the hospital was able to claim. The book was enlarged to 342 pages and reprinted in **1882**. A further edition was offered in **1896**.

1878: *A TREATISE ON TYPHOID FEVER AND ITS HOMŒOPATHIC TREATMENT*: Cav. Francesco Panelli
Duncan Brothers; 297 pages.
This work was translated from the Italian by George Shipman. It contains a repertory.

1878: *HOMŒOPATHIC THERAPEUTICS*: Samuel Lilienthal, MD ✱ ✔
Boericke and Tafel; 710 pages.
Based on the earlier work found in Volume I of Jahr's *Manual*, this work has been updated by one of the grand old prescribers. It is a listing of "conditions" and a remedy differential. For example, the listing of APHONIA (loss of voice) is followed by a detailed description of 31 remedies from Aconite to Sulphur— all of which have that particular symptom. Said Charles Gatchell in a review, "…it is an extraordinarily useful book and those who add it to their library will never feel regret…" By **1915** it was in its 4th edition with 1,154 pages.

I first became acquainted with this book when I visited the Hahnemann Clinic in Berkeley in 1982. It was described as the book to which they referred when answers could not be found elsewhere. As we look back over all the therapeutics books ever written this one was probably the best. In a review, Samuel A. Jones says, "For the fresh graduate this book will be invaluable… to the older one who says he has no use for this book, we have nothing to say. He is a good one to avoid when well, and to dread when ill."

1878: *ON STERILITY*: Edwin M. Hale, MD
Boericke and Tafel; 298 pages.
The full title is "The Medical, Surgical, and Hygienic Treatment of Diseases of Women, especially those causing Sterility, the Disorders and Accidents of Pregnancy, and Painful and Difficult Labor."

1879: *ON THE TREATMENT, DIET, AND NURSING OF YELLOW FEVER*: William H. Holcombe, MD
Boericke and Tafel; 20 pages.
The author practiced in Mississippi, and was on the state Yellow Fever Commission.

1879: *HEADACHES AND THEIR CONCOMITANT SYMPTOMS, WITH A COMPLETE AND CONCISE REPERTORY-ANALYSIS*: John C. King, MD
W. A. Chatterton; 297 pages.
235 pages of materia medica and 62 pages of repertory.

1879: *THERAPEUTICS OF INTERMITTENT FEVER:* H. C. Allen, MD ✔
Drake's Homœopathic Pharmacy, Detroit; 232 pages.
The first part is a Materia Medica with differential comparisons and example cases. The last 81 pages of the book are a repertory. Says the author, "A somewhat extended personal acquaintance has convinced me that but comparatively few of our practitioners use a repertory in selecting the remedy; hence a bracketed comparison has been substituted in its place, as more likely to meet the wants of the majority." Reprinted by Boericke and Tafel in **1884**.

1880: *DIPHTHERIA; ITS CAUSES, NATURE, AND TREATMENT*; Rollin Robinson Gregg, MD
Matthews Bros and Bryant; Rochester, NY; 133 pages.

1880: *THE HOMŒOPATHIC TREATMENT OF DIPHTHERIA*: DeForest Hunt, MD
Lyons and Eaton, Grand Rapids, MI; 102 pages.
"An outline of Pure Homœopathic Treatment," by a lesser known homeopath.

Egbert Cleave, in his BIOGRAPHY OF HOMŒOPATHIC PHYSICIANS, says of Hunt, "…a thorough homœopathist according to the teachings of Hahnemann, has no sympathy with anything like mongrelism or compromise with those well-defined principles of the healing art."

1880: *SAFETY IN CHOLERA TIMES*: Boericke and Tafel
Boericke and Tafel; 63 pages.
No named author. A small "popular " text, aimed at both the practitioner and layman.

1880: *CURABILITY OF CATARACTS WITH MEDICINES*: James Compton Burnett, MD ✔
Homœopathic Publishing Co.; 133 pages.

The first of a series of 23 small books about therapeutics written by this fine English homœopath.

1880: *ON THE PREVENTION OF HARE-LIP, CLEFT PALATE, AND OTHER CONGENITAL DEFECTS*: James Compton Burnett, MD ✔
Homœopathic Publishing Co.; 26 pages.

1881: *THE MEDICINAL TREATMENT OF DISEASES OF THE VEINS*: James Compton Burnett, MD ✔
Homœopathic Publishing Co.; 189 pages.

1881: *A TREATISE ON DIPHTHERIA; ITS HISTORY, ETIOLOGY, VARIETIES, PATHOLOGY, SEQUELAE, DIAGNOSIS AND HOMŒOPATHIC THERAPEUTICS*: A. McNeil, MD
Duncan Brothers; 145 pages.

1882: *PHTHISIS PULMONALIS; OR, TUBERCULAR CONSUMPTION*: Gershom Nelson Brigham, MD
Boericke and Tafel; 244 pages.
The first specific book written about this pervasive disease.

1883: *THERAPEUTICS OF CHOLERA*: Dr. P. C. Majumdar
Boericke and Tafel; 102 pages.

1883: *UTERINE THERAPEUTICS:* Henry Minton, MD ✔
A. L. Chatterton; 710 pages.
Considered the definitive work on the subject. A very good repertory appears at the end of the book.

Kent considered this work, "most excellent."

1885: *LECTURES ON CLINICAL OTOLOGY:* Henry M. Houghton, MD
Otis Clapp and Son; 260 pages.
Lectures (illustrated by cases) delivered to the senior class at NY Homœopathic Medical College. Also included are therapeutic hints, and an excellent repertory.

1885: *THE PRESCRIBER; A DICTIONARY OF THE NEW THERAPEUTICS*: John Henry Clarke, MD ✔
Keene and Ashwell, London; 213 pages.
A pocket sized clinical repertory that contains dosage suggestions. "Without a doubt this is the best book published for beginners in homœopathic prescribing… the next time you feel too fagged out to make a thorough study of the remedy for some puzzling case, you will have something you have longed for."
The book was updated by Clarke in **1925**— 40 years after its release. Now, 75 years later, it is still in print and in daily use.

One of the best books concerning therapeutics. Its small size makes it an easier book to consult than Lilienthal's larger work. I have known many prescribers who were lead to the correct remedy by the differentials offered by Clarke.

1885: *VALVULAR DISEASE OF THE HEART FROM A NEW STANDPOINT*:
James Compton Burnett, MD ✔
Leath and Ross; 72 pages.

1886: *THERAPEUTIC METHODS; AN OUTLINE OF PRINCIPLES OBSERVED IN THE ART OF HEALING*:
Jabez Dake, MD
Otis Clapp and Sons; 195 pages.
Dake taught at Hahnemann Medical College in Philadelphia. A College Textbook edition was offered in **1889**.

1886: *DISEASES OF THE SKIN FROM THE ORGANISMIC STANDPOINT*:
James Compton Burnett, MD ✔
Homœopathic Publishing Co.; 140 pages.
This book was enlarged to 240 pages and published as a second edition in **1893** with the title, *DISEASES OF THE SKIN: THEIR CONSTITUTIONAL NATURE AND CURE.*

1887: *DISEASES OF THE SPLEEN*: James Compton Burnett, MD ✔
James Epps; 164 pages.

1887: *THE MEDICAL GENIUS: A GUIDE TO THE CURE*: Stacy Jones, MD
John C. Winston and Co., Philadelphia, PA; 320 pages.
Dedicated to those "who prefer curing diseases, to contending about dogma." Reprinted by Boericke and Tafel through the 1920s.
An alphabetical listing of remedies (often by their common name; *Gelsemium* is listed under "Yellow Jessamine") and cures containing homœopathic, allopathic, and eclectic information. Said a reviewer: "A gentleman once told the writer of a case in which three liberal homœopathic physicians were in consultation and pronounced it hopeless— it was an acute case— but the *Medical Genius* yielded a remedy known to none of them that saved the patient's life. A book of what might be termed unconventional lore."

1888: *THE HOMŒOPATHIC TREATMENT OF RHEUMATISM*: Daniel C. Perkins, MD
Boericke; 180 pages.
Therapeutics and Repertory.

1888: *FEVERS AND BLOOD POISONING, AND THEIR TREATMENT WITH SPECIAL REFERENCE TO THE USE OF PYROGENIUM:* James Compton Burnett, MD ✔
James Epps; 56 pages.

1888: *TUMOURS OF THE BREAST AND THEIR CURE*: James Compton Burnett, MD ✔
James Epps; 213 pages.

1889: *CATARACT ITS NATURE AND CURE:* James Compton Burnett, MD ✔
Homœopathic Publishing Co.; 208 pages.

1889: *ON FISTULA AND ITS RADICAL CURE BY MEDICINES*: James Compton Burnett, MD ✔
James Epps; 141 pages.

1889: *ON NEURALGIA: ITS CAUSES AND REMEDIES:* James Compton Burnett, MD ✔
Homœopathic Publishing Co.; 168 pages.

1890: *CONSUMPTION AND ITS CURE BY ITS OWN VIRUS:* James Compton Burnett, MD ✱ ✔
Homœopathic Publishing Co.; 181 pages. This book was expanded to 295 pages and published four years later in **1894** as *EIGHT YEARS EXPERIENCE IN THE NEW CURE OF CONSUMPTION*.

1890: *THE HOMŒOPATHIC TREATMENT OF ALCOHOLISM*: Jean Pierre Gallavardin, MD ✔
Boericke and Tafel; 136 pages.
Translated from the French by Iraneaus D. Foulon. Written by a prominent French homœopath, this book has been considered the major work on the subject. It was reprinted by East-West Publication, Katonah, NY, in **1976**.

1891: *THE GREATER DISEASES OF THE LIVER*: James Compton Burnett, MD ✔
Homœopathic Publishing Co.; 186 pages.

1892: *RINGWORM: ITS CONSTITUTIONAL NATURE AND CURE:* James Compton Burnett, MD ✔
Homœopathic Publishing Co.; 126 pages.

1892: *OPHTHALMIC DISEASES AND THERAPEUTICS:* Arthur B. Norton, MD ✔
Boericke and Tafel; 555 pages.
A new, improved edition of the older work (1882). George Norton, the author of the original work, was the older brother of the present author. A 2nd edition was issued in **1898**, a 3rd edition in **1902**. It is *the* book on the subject "at the hands of an author whose name is a guarantee for first-class work."

1892: *THE HOMŒOPATHIC THERAPEUTICS OF HAEMORRHOIDS*: William Jefferson Guernsey, MD ✔
Boericke and Tafel; 142 pages.

1893: *CURABILITY OF TUMOURS*: James Compton Burnett, MD ✔
Homœopathic Publishing Co.; 345 pages.

1895: *DELICATE, BACKWARD, PUNY AND STUNTED CHILDREN*: James Compton Burnett, MD ✔
Homœopathic Publishing Co.; 164 pages.

One of my favorite homeopathic titles. No "political correctness" here. The title "Children with Developmental Challenges" just doesn't have the same ring!

1895: *GOUT AND ITS CURE*: James Compton Burnett, MD ✔
James Epps; 180 pages

1895: *A HANDBOOK ON THE DISEASES OF CHILDREN AND THEIR HOMŒOPATHIC TREATMENT*:
Charles E. Fischer, MD ✔
Medical Century; 905 pages.
H. C. Allen and J. W. Hawkes "confirmed" the therapeutics. In the preface, the author says, "In treatment, a stricter loyalty to Hahnemann's law and established practice of the early fathers than is now generally practiced, is observed."

A very valuable work.

1895: *ACCOUCHEUR'S EMERGENCY MANUAL*: William A. Yingling , MD ✔
Boericke and Tafel; 323 pages.
Therapeutics of labor, with a short repertory appended. "Dr. Yingling has compiled a book that will be useful as long as babies are born into the world."

Still as useful as when it was written over 100 years ago. The introduction is well worth reading, especially the section about the time until reaction happens when prescribing in emergency situations.

1896: *ORGAN DISEASES OF WOMEN*: James Compton Burnett, MD ✔
Homœopathic Publishing Co.; 156 pages.

1896: *THE PRACTICE OF MEDICINE; A CONDENSED MANUAL FOR THE BUSY PRACTITIONER*:
Marvin A. Custis, MD
Boericke and Tafel; 367 pages.
Bound in flexible leather, this is a pocket manual similar to Gatchell's work, with the remedy listings containing pointers quoted from Baehr, Farrington, Lilienthal, Jahr, and others.

1897: *VACCINOSIS AND ITS CURE BY THUJA*: James Compton Burnett, MD ✔
Homœopathic Publishing Co.; 145 pages.

1898: *CHANGE OF LIFE IN WOMEN*: James Compton Burnett, MD ✔
Homœopathic Publishing Co.; 185 pages.

1898: *ESSENTIALS OF HOMŒOPATHIC THERAPEUTICS*: Willis A. Dewey, MD ✔
Boericke and Tafel; 285 pages.
"Being A Quiz Compend Of The Applications Of Homœopathic Remedies To Diseased States." The companion edition to his *THE ESSENTIALS OF MATERIA MEDICA*.

These two "Essential" books are a summary of what Dr. Dewey expected his students to know when they finished their four year education at the University of Michigan Homœopathic Medical Department at Ann Arbor, Michigan. Not only are they excellent study guides but are still appropriate for their intended use as quiz compends.

1898: *NERVOUS DISEASES WITH HOMŒOPATHIC TREATMENT*: Joseph O'Connor, MD
Boericke and Runyon; 416 pages.

1898: *THERAPEUTICS OF FACIAL AND SCIATIC NEURALGIA WITH CLINICAL CASES AND REPERTORIES:* F. H. Lutze, MD ✔
Boericke and Tafel; 296 pages.
Says homœopathic literature expert Chris Ellithorp, "It is set up like *Bell on Diarrhoea*. A great book by an overlooked great. It should be in print, if it is not. I have the only copy I have ever seen, a signed presentation copy from the author."

1898: *A HANDBOOK OF THE DISEASES OF THE HEART AND THEIR HOMŒOPATHIC TREATMENT*: Thomas Cation Duncan, MD
Halsey Brothers; 114 pages.
Concise clinical outlines of "diseases" followed by therapeutics— classification of heart remedies and characteristics of heart remedies.

1898: *THE HOMŒOPATHIC THERAPEUTICS OF DIPHTHERIA*: Cyrus M. Boger, MD ✔
Cochran, Lancaster, PA; 82 pages.
Set up like Bell's *Diarrhea*, with leading remedies and indications, followed by a repertory.

1899: *CATARRH, COLDS, AND GRIPPE, INCLUDING PREVENTION AND CURE, WITH CHAPTERS ON NASAL POLYPUS, HAY FEVER, AND INFLUENZA:* John Henry Clarke, MD ✔
Boericke and Tafel; 122 pages.
1st American. Original publication date in the UK unknown.

1899: *POCKET BOOK OF MEDICAL PRACTICE*: Charles Gatchell, MD
By the author, Chicago; 384 pages.
A 5th edition in **1903** was published by Era Publishing in Chicago. An 8th edition was printed by Boericke and Tafel in **1911**, an 11th edition in **1934**.
"This work is designed to be a pocket companion for the general practitioner. The presumption is that those who make use of it have a thorough and comprehensive knowledge of medicine, and refer to it only for the purposes of refreshing the memory."
The disease name is presented, followed by a brief view of the etiology, the symptoms, possible complication, sequelae, and prognosis, followed by therapeutics (both allopathic and homœopathic) and general measures of diet, sanitation, etc.

An amazing amount of information tucked into a 4" x 7" pocket book. Akin to the present day allopathic Merck Manual, *it presents a useful differential of homœopathic therapeutics. Its usefulness can be appreciated by the large number of editions printed. It is one of those homœopathic volumes often found at used book sales.*

1900: *LEADERS IN TYPHOID*: E. B. Nash, MD ✔
Boericke and Tafel; 135 pages.
A small materia medica of the remedies useful in typhoid, with clinical suggestions from the author's extensive experience.

1901: *ENLARGED TONSILS CURED BY MEDICINE:* James Compton Burnett, MD ✔
Homœopathic Publishing Co.; 100 pages.

1901: *MENTAL DISEASES AND THEIR MODERN TREATMENT*: Selden H. Talcott, MD ✔
Boericke and Runyon; 352 pages.

Although the title might hold hope, there is little useful in the contents of this small volume, other than giving the reader a view into early 20th century thought on mental diseases. Talcott was the teacher of "mental diseases" at New York Homœopathic Medical College and was the superintendent for the Homœopathic Hospital for the Insane at Middletown, New York. The book discusses the special needs of a mental hospital. A brief materia medica is appended. Having seen some of the records of Middletown, I would say that Talcott's successes were based more upon good general care than upon the homœopathic treatment.

1901: *PRACTICAL HOMŒOTHERAPEUTICS*: Willis A. Dewey, MD ✱ ✔
Boericke and Tafel; 379 pages.
"The indications for the remedies given are those born of the experience of the foremost prescribers." Said one reviewer, "The book strikes me as being the most satisfactory work of the kind I ever

saw." Another said, "You want it handy. Right on the nearest corner of the middle shelf of your bookcase."
A 2nd edition was published in **1914**, enlarged to 426 pages.

1902: *DISEASES AND THERAPEUTICS OF THE SKIN*: James Henry Allen, MD ✔
Boericke and Tafel; 353 pages.
Allen was the teacher of Skin Diseases at the Hering Medical College in Chicago.

1902: *THERAPEUTICS OF FEVERS:* Henry C. Allen, MD ✔
Boericke and Tafel; 542 pages.
A materia medica of remedies useful in the treatment of fevers. Characteristics and differentials are offered, as is a repertory.

1903: *HAY FEVER: ITS PREVENTION AND CURE*: Perry Dickie, MD
Boericke and Tafel; 168 pages.
The review in the *Medical Advance* said, "It is the weakest apology for a monograph on a disease, where help is so sadly needed by every homœopathic physician, that has appeared from the press of B&T in many years."

A loser. While cleaning out the attic of B&T in 1992 I found about 50 of these books, uncut and unbound.

1903: *A CLASSIFIED INDEX OF THE HOMŒOPATHIC MATERIA MEDICA FOR UROGENITAL DISEASES*: Bukk G. Carleton, MD and Howard Coles, MD
Boericke and Runyon, NY; 158 pages.
"Compiled from Hahnemann, Allen, Hale, Jahr, Hering, Farrington, Cowperthwaite, and many others… symptoms pertinent to these diseases arranged… upon a somewhat new repertory plan."

1906: *BEFORE AND AFTER SURGICAL OPERATIONS*: Dean T. Smith, MD ✔
Boericke and Tafel; 260 pages.
"A guide for the care of surgical cases in private homes."
"The room in which the operation is to be done should be well lighted and capable of being made clean. The kitchen or the dining room is most suitable."

A view into times past. We forget that the "operating room" of the hospital is a rather recent arrival. The author has some good suggestions about the therapeutics of post-operative pain. He advises the use of morphine only if the health of the patient would be worse without it.

1906: *WHAT TO DO FOR THE HEAD*: George E. Dienst, MD ✔
Boericke and Tafel; 184 pages.
Symptoms of the head with leading remedies.

1907: *WHAT TO DO FOR THE STOMACH*: George E. Dienst, MD ✔
Boericke and Tafel; 202 pages.
"A careful arrangement of the most important symptoms of diseased conditions of the stomach and the remedy indicated for the cure of these symptoms."

Dienst was a pupil of Kent, taught at the Hering Medical College in Chicago, and served as the first Dean of the American Foundation Post-graduate course in 1922.

1908: *THE CURE OF TUMOURS BY MEDICINES WITH SPECIAL REFERENCE TO THE CANCER NOSODES*: John Henry Clarke, MD ✔
James Epps; 196 pages.

1909: *LEADERS IN RESPIRATORY ORGANS*: E. B. Nash, MD ✔
Boericke and Tafel; 188 pages.

Another wonderful yet brief work from this grand homœopath.

1911: *THE TESTIMONY OF THE CLINIC*: E. B. Nash, MD ✔
Boericke and Tafel; 209 pages.
A collection of 100 cases, many from Nash's practice, showing the effectiveness of homœopathy in clinical use.

A fascinating reference of interesting cases from some of the great prescribers of the time. Much can be learned by going through the cases with a repertory and materia medica in hand.

1911: *MENTAL DISEASES AND THEIR HOMŒOPATHIC TREATMENT*: William Morris Butler, MD
Boericke and Runyon; 504 pages.
"For the Student and Practitioner of Medicine." Mental diseases, as classified by Kraepllin, are discussed, and remedies are suggested. The book is illustrated with photos of patients at the New York State Asylum for the Insane at Middletown, NY.
"The homœopathist needs no assistance from any other school of medicine to combat this most dreaded foe of humanity… Any physician who carefully studies his cases and applies his materia medica according to the laws laid down by Hahnemann need seek no assistance from opiates, hypnotics, and anodynes."

1913: *HOMŒOPATHY IN MEDICINE AND SURGERY*: Edmund Carleton, MD ✽ ✔
Boericke and Tafel; 311 pages.
"The author's aim was to avowedly always exemplify the practical— the clinical side of medicine. Leaving the theoretical and didactic side to others, he felt that his work, name, and fame were gained at the sick bedside… we can learn the theory, materia medica, and pathology from books and colleges. The clinic gives us diagnosis, surgery, and familiarity with the disease and its course. It should also give us the practical knowledge of therapy. Does it? Candor would compel most of us to reply, No. To fill this gap is the purpose of this book."

Edmund Carleton was one of the second generation of homœopaths in the USA. He knew Wells, Biegler, Bayard and Swan. He was one of the staunch Hahnemannians of the IHA. This book is a narrative of his clinical experiences and contains gems on almost every page. Where else would you find that Lac caninum *was made from the milk of Mrs. Bayard's spaniel whose "affection for the human race was unusually strong"? This book is, in the words of Chris Ellithorp, "another neglected gem."*

1916: *SOME CLINICAL EXPERIENCES*: Erastus E. Case, MD ✔
Emerson, Hartford, CT; 226 pages.
Erastus Case was a perennial presenter at the IHA meetings, and this book is a collection of material, much of it direct from his printed cases. He was acclaimed as one of the great clinicians, and his selection of curative remedies often baffled those of his day. The book was reprinted by Van Hoy Publishers in **1991**, with many additions by the editor, Jay Yasgur.

The original of this little red volume has remained a highly treasured prize in homœopathic collections. Jay Yasgur has not only added some wonderful other articles by and about Dr. Case, but he has restored the "discussions" which often followed the presentations, and which Case did not include in his original book. Much can be learned from this book, especially if one is curious enough to do the digging that Case did to find the reasons for giving the remedy.

1916: *THERAPEUTICS OF THE RESPIRATORY SYSTEM*: M. W. VanDenburg, MD
Boericke and Tafel; 782 pages.
The last section contains an extensive repertory.

1917: *MATERIA MEDICA FOR NURSES:* Benjamin Woodbury, MD ✔
Woodside Press, 200 pages. 2nd Edition by Ehrhart and Karl, **1922**. Reprinted by Van Hoy Publishers in **1992**.
The first 45 pages are homœopathic theory; pages 46-168 are materia medica; pages 169 -195 are therapeutic hints.

In the recent reprint, the editor, Jay Yasgur, added 100 pages of material— 12 additional papers published by Woodbury.

1919: *THERAPEUTICS OF THE RESPIRATORY ORGANS:* Francois Cartier, MD ✔
Boericke and Tafel; 297 pages.
Translated by Carl L. Williams.

1927: *THE CANCER PROBLEM: SOME DEDUCTIONS BASED ON CLINICAL EXPERIENCE:*
R. M. Lehunte Cooper
John Bale and Sons, London; 29 pages.
A discussion of the causes and therapeutics of cancer, by the son of the noted British physician, Dr. Robert Cooper, the founder of arborvital therapeutics.

1928: *LEADERS IN PNEUMONIA:* Alfred Pulford, MD and Dayton Pulford, MD ✱ ✔
Published by the authors, Dayton, OH; 100 pages.
A materia medica of the remedies most useful in pneumonia along with a short repertory. Originally printed on "bible paper" and designed to be carried in the pocket.

1928: *HOMŒOPATHIC THERAPY OF THE DISEASES OF THE BRAIN AND NERVES:*
George Royal, MD ✔
Boericke and Tafel; 360 pages.
Divided into four sections: "The algias," "The itisis," "Functional changes," "Structural changes." There are many examples of cases and the attendant homœopathic therapeutics.

1928: *TEN REMEDIES INDICATED IN THE TREATMENT OF SCARLET FEVER AND ITS COMPLICATIONS:* Elizabeth Wright, MD
Reprint from *Hahnemannian Monthly*, May, 1928; 18 pages.

1930: *A HANDY BOOK OF REFERENCE:* George Royal, MD ✔
Boericke and Tafel; 323 pages.
The first five chapters are about homœopathic philosophy and the last seven are of clinical therapeutics, as seen through examples from the author's practice. Some of the chapters are re-worked articles Royal published, based on his presentations at conferences.

A delightful look into the thought process of a teacher of homœopathy at one of the last homœopathic colleges at the State University of Iowa. Royal had a unique way of thinking about it all— attempting to integrate "modern" knowledge into his understanding of homœopathy. It is not a well known book, and deserves to be read by a wider audience.

1939: *THE RHEUMATIC REMEDIES:* Herbert A. Roberts, MD✔
Homœopathic Publishing Company; 234 pages.
A specific materia medica of only those remedies which have rheumatic symptoms.

1939: *CHILDREN'S TYPES:* Dr. Douglas Borland, MD ✔
British Homœopathic Association; 54 pages.

1939: *INFLUENZAS:* Dr. Douglas Borland, MD ✔
British Homœopathic Association; 20 pages.

1939: *PNEUMONIAS*: Dr. Douglas Borland, MD ✔
British Homœopathic Association; 76 pages.
All Borland's pamphlets are derived from a series of lectures given to the Faculty of Homœopathy.

c. 1939: *POINTERS TO THE COMMON REMEDIES*: Margaret L. Tyler, MD ✔
British Homœopathic Association.
Nine short pamphlets comprising a series of differentials. Originally published in the magazine *Homœopathy*.

Six of these "pointers" are found in the second part of Shadman's Who is Your Doctor and Why? *The full collection is available as a unit from Indian publishers. These are well ordered differentials which are valuable for practitioners at all levels of expertise.*

1950: *HOMŒOPATHY FOR MOTHER AND INFANT*: Douglas Borland, MD ✔
British Homœopathic Association; 20 pages.

1955: *MARASMUS AND RICKETS WITH COMMON DISEASES OF ADULTS AND CHILDREN*:
Dr. P. S. Kamthan ✔
B. Jain; 207 pages.
Republished in **1971** under the title *THERAPEUTIC GUIDE TO COMMON DISEASES OF INFANTS, CHILDREN, AND ADULTS*.
"…a companion volume to the Materia Medica (without which we are sure to go adrift)…" Although many authorities are directly quoted, the book reflects over 20 years of prescribing experience.

1965: *DRAINAGE IN HOMŒOPATHY (DETOXIFICATION)*: E. A. Maury, MD ✔
Health Science Press; 60 pages.
Translated from the French by Mark Clement. An exposition of the therapeutic concept of "organ drainage" with a list of remedies that are associated with each tissue, organ, or organ system. Differentials are also included.

Although some homœopaths have adopted the idea of "organ drainage" this is not *considered "homœopathy" by most Hahnemannian prescribers.*

1967: *HOMŒOPATHY IN EPIDEMIC DISEASES*: Dorothy Shepherd, MD ✔
Health Science Press; 100 pages.
A collection of her writings on the subject, published posthumously.

One of the few works that discusses epidemic diseases, their treatment, and the concept of homœopathic prophylaxis.

1970: *QUICK BEDSIDE PRESCRIBER:* Dr. J. N. Shinghal ✔
Harjeet, New Delhi; 572 pages.
Originally published in **1959** in a much condensed version. It has been republished several times since. In 1938 the author spent time with Dr. S. C. Sircar, the grand Indian homœopath. This book is based on the author's personal experiences and is compiled very similarly to Clarke's *Prescriber*. It also includes chapters on homœopathy in pediatrics and homœopathy in surgery. Says the author, "I lay no claim to originality."

This was one of the first books I obtained, after seeing it on the shelves of several homœopaths who spoke of its value. Yes. It is like Clarke's work. But there is enough of another viewpoint in it to be valuable in its own right.

1977: *TREATISE ON DYNAMIZED IMMUNOLOGY:* Dr. O. A. Julian ✔
Traité de Micro-immunothérapie dynamisée. Matière médicale
Biothérapiques-nosodes: Librairie Le François, édit. Paris 1977.

Published in English by Jain in **1988**; 716 pages.
The first part of the book discusses the history and concepts of treating disease with nosodes. Pages 167-559 are a materia medica of 66 nosodes.

1977: *EMERGENCY HOMEOPATHY AND FIRST AID*: Paul Chavanon, MD and René Levannier, MD
Thorsons; 177 pages.
First published in France **1973** as *Mémento Homoeopathique d'urgence* by Editions Dangles.
The first page is a diagram of how the remedy, when placed under the tongue, arrives via the bloodstream to the heart. A presentation of a very physiological understanding of homœopathy. Despite its title, this is a therapeutics book and not a domestic manual.

1980: *THE ESSENTIALS OF THERAPEUTICS*: Jacques Jouanny, MD
Editions Boiron, Lyons; 418 pages.
This, like its companion volume *THE ESSENTIALS OF HOMEOPATHIC MATERIA MEDICA* holds fast to the "Hahnemannian" concepts discarding the more "spiritual" works of Kent and Vithoulkas. In this light it could be considered a descendant Richard Hughes' work— the leading proponent of pathologic prescribing in the 19th century. The remedies are discussed in terms of specific actions, and dosages are suggested based on physiological and pathological involvement. The potencies suggested are all 30c or below, and dosages are quite standardized, as is the practice in France. The book is filled with photographs of the visual pathology of various ailments.

A very "French" view of homœopathy. The doses are given by prescription, e.g., for this *condition, give* this *remedy, in* this *potency, for* this *number of days. Often the doses are given weekly with an intercurrent nosode once a month— certainly Pluralist and not Unicist prescribing. The photographs of the skin conditions may be somewhat useful although, in the view of some prescribers, the remedies suggested have not been curative of similar looking conditions.*

1980: *HOMEOPATHIC PRESCRIBING*: Noel Pratt ✔
Beaconsfield; 68 pages.
"Intended for the student of homœopathy who requires short lists of remedies for most of the common ailments… Primarily for qualified physicians." It has one line indications in a list of differentials. It was republished in **1985** with 15 more pages, the addition comprising a discussion on "constitutional types."

This is a typical "useless book" of which we have seen many during the last 20 years as homœopathy continues its resurgence. The information presented is almost too brief to be of consistent value, and moves the practitioner back to prescribing on a "single keynote" instead of understanding the fullness of a case. The "constitutional" pages added to this new edition can be very misleading to the prescriber who possesses a limited understanding of homœopathy.

1981: *HOMEOPATHY IN PRACTICE:* Dr. Douglas Borland, edited by Dr. Kathleen Priestman ✔
Beaconsfield; 173 pages.
Published posthumously, the first 100 pages are a narrative about remedies and their therapeutic use, and the last 70 pages are a materia medica.

1983: *THE DENTAL PRESCRIBER*: Dr. Colin Lessell ✔
British Homœopathic Association; 22 pages.
"…intended for the general dental practitioner, the dental specialist, and the homœopathically oriented patient."

Although articles had appeared as early as the 1890s about the danger of dental amalgams, and numerous articles have appeared about dentistry, this is the first modern work, albeit small in scope, solely discussing homœopathy in dental practice.

1986: *HOMEOPATHIC PRACTICE IN CHILDHOOD DISORDERS*: Denis Demarque, MD, et. al.
Centre d'etudes et de documentation homeopathiques, Lyons; 151 pages.
First published in France, **1980**. Translated by Dany Clausen.
Demarque is joined by Drs. Michel Aubin, Pierre Joly, Yves Saint-Jean, and Jacques Jouanny, each writing a chapter or two on specific disorders and their treatment. The approach, of course, is French— the use of unit-dose tubes, or remedies repeated for set time frames.

1986: *MANAGEMENT OF OTITIS MEDIA WITH EFFUSION IN HOMEOPATHIC PRACTICE*: Randall Neustaedter, OMD ✔
American Institute for Homeopathy: 28 pages.
Reprinted from the *JAIH*, Vol. 79, no. 3 and 4.
A brief review of the pathophysiology of otitis, and a review of the main remedies used.

1988: *KENT'S COMPARATIVE REPERTORY OF THE HOMŒOPATHIC MATERIA MEDICA*:
Rene Dockx, MD and Guy Kokelenberg, MD ✔
Homeoden Bookservice, Ghent, Belgium.
A large, loose-leaf book which was designed to be added to. Each rubric is described as to its meaning, and extensively cross referenced. Often there is a differential between the remedies in the rubric explaining exactly how that remedy manifests that symptom. Most of this work has been incorporated into the newer books.

Although titled "repertory," this is a therapeutics book, in that it presents differentials of the remedies found in the rubrics of Kent's Repertory.

1988: *HOMEOPATHY IN PEDIATRIC PRACTICE*: Hedwig Imhäuser, MD ✔
Haug Verlag; 236 pages.
First published in Germany in **1969**.
Translated by Sigrid Penrod, ND. Based on "experiences from my practice." A formulaic guide with a lot of "give this for that."

The book contains an interesting chapter on Autohemic therapy— the use of the patient's blood, potentized. Since homœopathy is about using remedies based upon the symptoms elicited in provings, the use of autogenic substances cannot be considered homœopathy, although some "homœopaths" do use such methods.

1992: *HOMEOPATHIC EMERGENCY GUIDE*: Thomas Kruzel, ND ✔
North Atlantic Books; 366 pages.
This book "fills a need for those who have not quite mastered the art of repertorization and case analysis." A condition is named and remedy differential provided. An earlier 220 page version, *ACUTE HOMEOPATHIC PRESCRIBER*, was published by Medicina Biologica (Portland, OR) in **1988**.

A very easy volume to access, with clearly presented information. Each section describes the "condition" followed by the various possible remedies (with their modalities) and a list of rubrics to consult in Kent's Repertory. The book also contains nine flow charts prepared by Stephen Messer, ND, and a magnificent introduction by Andre Saine, ND.

1992: *HOMEOPATHIC MEDICINES FOR PREGNANCY AND CHILDBIRTH*: Richard Moskowitz, MD ✔
North Atlantic Books; 288 pages.
The author describes the book as "…a kit of basic remedies and enough of a methodology to help people get started using them…the book is a 'primer'… intended to be used by the beginner in homœopathy, both lay and professional, as a basis for further study." The work is presented in three sections: a basic introduction to the principles of homœopathy, a condensed materia medica of 25 remedies, and a discussion of common problems illustrated by cases from the author's extensive experience.

The author has told me that he wrote the book after struggling with Yingling's ACCOUCHEUR'S EMERGENCY MANUAL, and realizing that there might be a better way to present the information to a contemporary audience.

1995: *A TEXTBOOK OF DENTAL HOMOEOPATHY*: Dr. Colin Lessell ✔
C. W. Daniel; 224 pages.
A complete modern work on the application of homœopathy to oral medicine, general dentistry, and oral surgery.

1997: *HOMEOPATHY FOR THE MODERN PREGNANT WOMAN AND HER INFANT*:
Sandra Perko, PhD ✔
Benchmark Publications, San Antonio, TX; 415 pages.
"A Therapeutic Practice Guidebook for Midwives, Physicians, and Practitioners."

A well written and useful guide.

1997: *HOMEOPATHY IN PRIMARY CARE*: Bob Leckridge, BSc, MB, MFHom.✔
Churchill Livingstone, New York; 281 pages.
Intended for "any health care professional working within a primary care setting…" A guide to the uninitiated, well written and explained. It contains clinical indications for using homœopathy in a primary health care setting, including four categories of treatment differentials: Where there is no effective allopathic treatment for the condition; When it is an unsafe situation to use allopathic treatment; Where the patient would have an unacceptable side-effects profile; Where it would be beneficial for the patient to reduce their allopathic medication. These differentials are followed by a simple materia medica with basic indications.

An excellent introduction to homœopathy for the busy General Practitioner.

1997: *HOMEOPATHIC HANDBOOK FOR POISON IVY AND POISON OAK:* Joel Kreisberg, DC ✔
Private, Chatham, NY; 52 pages.
A well organized domestic guide. There is an excellent discussion about the importance of understanding the disease picture and matching it to the remedy picture. The descriptive definitions of the condition are exceptionally clear.

1998: *THE HOMEOPATHIC TREATMENT OF ECZEMA:* Robin Logan, FSHom. ✔
Beaconsfield; 152 pages.
Recognizing that writing about a "condition" is not compatible with the general standards of "classical" homœopathy, the author discusses techniques of casetaking and analysis he has used to treat cases of this "disease" and discusses the specifics of treatment, the materia medica of several "useful" remedies, and ties it all together with illustrations from 22 cases.

A useful book and a "must have" for the practitioner who is struggling with difficult skin cases.

1998: *THE DESKTOP COMPANION TO PHYSICAL PATHOLOGY:* Roger Morrison, MD ✔
Hahnemann Clinic Publishing; 605 pages.
"A concise yet thorough differential for each of the main pathologies encountered in homœopathic prescribing." The book was written with three criteria in mind:
1. To cue the practitioner toward likely remedies for the condition
2. As a study guide to bring main points of the remedy into focus
3. To give advice about treatment, based on the author's experience.
Each "disease" is described, followed by sections on management, therapeutic tips, repertory rubrics, and remedy differentials.

An excellent addition to Morrison's previous well received Desktop Guide to Keynote and Confirmatory Symptoms.

1998: *THEMATIC REPERTORY AND MATERIA MEDICA OF THE MIND SYMPTOMS*:
José Antonio Mirilli, MD ✔
IRHIS: 1138 pages.
In the introduction, the author raises four points: 1. Symptoms, by being severed and classified in alphabetical order, lose their dynamic expression. 2. Symptoms come from several sources of different languages and organizations, and are, thus, not related. 3. Symptoms taken from the Pure Materia Medica are not totally represented in rubrics. 4. There is a great difference in vocabulary between the repertory and the materia medica.
In compiling the work, the author attempted to satisfy these points by referencing the symptoms in the repertory back to the original source in the provings.

Although called a "Repertory" and "Materia Medica," this book is similar to the work of Dockx and Kokelenberg, in that the prime aim is to show the exact differentiation of remedies that appear in the same rubric. Each symptom, as seen through the repertory rubric, is annotated as to its source. Each major "theme" (i.e., "Anger," "Conscience," etc.) is followed by a listing of the remedies, giving the source of the proving, and the exact symptom as reported. A very useful work to establish the fine distinctions between rubrics, as well as a work from which one can study pure materia medica.

1999: *THE HOMEOPATHIC TREATMENT OF INFLUENZA*: Sandra Perko, PhD. ✔
Benchmark Publications, San Antonio, TX; 383 pages.
The first part of the book is a good history of influenza including the pandemic of 1918. The second part discusses possible therapeutic interventions.

Domestic Manuals

Domestic Manuals

Since the remedy selected for homœopathic treatment is dependent upon the symptoms presented, homœopathy becomes an ideal system for self help in domestic emergencies. One must remember that there was little medical help available in the 1850s— be it for pioneers crossing the USA, for farmers in the UK, or for those emigrating to less inhabited parts of the world. The self help books often came with an accompanying kit of remedies and provided a good level of health care for much of the population. A sense of how many of these books were used can be had from looking at the following listing and seeing how many of these manuals were reprinted over the years. All totaled, many millions were sold.

The majority of the self help books took the approach of "for this symptom, give this remedy." The intent of these books is best summed up by Joseph Laurie, MD, who states in his introduction to HOMŒOPATHIC DOMESTIC MEDICINE: "I nowhere enjoin the layman who has the means and immediate access to efficient homœopathic profession, to undertake the treatment of dangerous disease without it; I only endeavor, in a measure, to provide for those who do not possess such advantages."

Many of the books were titled "For the Physician and Families," thus blurring the possible intent of the book. For our purposes in the present work, if it said "Family" it has been placed under the "Domestic" heading.

Most of these references, from the oldest to the newest, share a commonality of layout. They begin with an explanation about what homœopathy is, and what the remedies are. They address health in general, and often give common sense advice as to diet, sleep, hygiene, etc. They discuss the concept of disease and the differences of perceiving it through the homœopathic and the allopathic models. The bulk of the work concerns "conditions" (Abscess, Colds, Gastro-Intestinal problems, etc.) and presents a differential of remedies useful in treatment. This is usually followed by a brief Materia Medica of the remedies discussed, and then a short Repertory and/or Clinical Index may be offered.

For the purposes of this work, I have separated those books that, although aimed at the domestic market, are primarily therapeutic books. These works move straight into "conditions" and offer no beginning advice. Examples of such books would be THE PRESCRIBER by J. H. Clarke, or HOMEOPATHIC EMERGENCY GUIDE by Thomas Kruezel. These books will be found in the "Therapeutics" section.

A brief look at dates of publication shows that most self-help manuals were written during the 1850s and 1860s. Most enjoyed a long life through reprints or further editions. Bradford lists 64 books that were domestic guides, 32 of which are included here.

It was only in the late 1970s that new domestic manuals began to appear. Many of these ventured far from the intent of "domestic medicine." For example, in EVERYDAY HOMŒOPATHY, David Gemmell writes, under the heading "Colitis": "First Aid treatment has no part to play here. The patient must be in the care of a physician." This is then, surprisingly, followed by a listing of possible remedies to use for the condition and their differentials. Similarly, the best selling book by Dr. Andrew Lockie, contains suggestions for remedies for such conditions as Bulimia, Manic Depression, Pneumothorax, Parkinson's Disease, etc. — certainly not conditions that should be treated on a "domestic" basis.

Recently, with the technology of color printing getting less expensive, a new kind of book has surfaced— something between a "domestic" and a "popular" work. These have wonderful color photos of the remedy sources, old paraphernalia, portraits of old homœopaths, and pictures of people suffering or being treated for sprains, fractures, sore throats, and all the rest. Some books suggest prescribing on the "visual" constitutional type, with beautiful photographs of the "types." These books, in my opinion, do a disservice to homœopathy by trivializing it and bringing it into the realm of entertainment similar to books of "armchair astrology." They look good on the surface yet have little depth.

Happily some "domestics" discuss only those conditions which are self-limiting and self-treatable. They attempt to educate the public in the proper and reasonable use of remedies under rational constraints.

A final note: While many of the therapeutics texts are written by practitioners who author them out of their own experience, many of the domestic manuals— especially as we approach contemporary times— are mere pastiches of previous work, regurgitated through another's pen.

Domestic Manuals

1826: *HOMÖOPATHISCHER HAUS-UND REISEARZT* (*Homœopathic Domestic and Traveling Physician*):
Carl Caspari, MD
Baumgaertner, Leipzig; 122 pages.
2nd edition in **1829**; 122 pages, edited by Franz Hartmann; 4th edition in **1833**; 198 pages, edited by Franz Hartmann; 11th edition in **1873**; 312 pages, edited by Heinrich Goullon.

1835: *THE HOMŒOPATHIST OR DOMESTIC PHYSICIAN:* Constantine Hering, MD ✔
J. G. Wesselhoeft, Philadelphia; 177 pages.
The second part, containing 290 pages, was published in **1838**.
The first "self help" book published in the USA. The early editions gave no names of remedies. This book was sold with a box of 42 remedies that were numbered to match the prescriptions in the book. In one remedy-case, prepared by Rademacher, the bottles were only "an inch in length and filled with infinitesimal pills."
The book went through a number of revisions during Hering's lifetime and was republished by a number of people— C. L. Rademacher, Koehler, and Boericke and Tafel. The 4th edition in **1848** contained a chapter on "diseases of females" by Walter Williamson, MD. The book was concurrently printed in Germany in **1835**. Subsequently it was translated into Spanish and French. The book is still in print. Although often quoted as the first self-help manual, it was antedated by Caspari's *Homöopathischer Haus-und Reisearzt* that was translated into English in **1852**.

The book had its start in a manual written by Hering for the use of those he was leaving behind in Surinam when he moved to the USA. Hering, the "father" of American homœopathy, was considered a master homœopath and he was certainly more of a practitioner than a writer. Most of his writings were about rather "dry" information— materia medica in the form of his Analytical Therapeutics, Condensed Materia Medica, *and his massive* Guiding Symptoms. *This book is the only one of his works that talks directly about basic therapeutics, and gives insight into how he thought, what he saw as important in a case, and how he differentiated remedies. Although the writing is rather stilted by current standards, the information contained is quite valuable, especially if it is studied with a repertory and a materia medica in hand.*

1839: *DOMESTIC HOMEOPATHY:* John Epps, MD
John Epps, London; 200 pages.
Subtitled, "Rules for the Domestic Treatment of the Maladies of Infants, Children, and Adults, and for the Conduct and Treatment during Pregnancy, Confinement, and Suckling." The first American edition, an exact reprint of the London edition was issued by Otis Clapp & Sons in **1843**. The 5th American, edited and enlarged by John A. Tarbell, MD, contained 382 pages and was published in **1853**.

1839: *DOMESTIC HOMŒOPATHY*: Paul F. Curie, MD
Jasper Harding, Philadelphia; 250 pages.
"When olfaction is advisable, one or two globules of the selected remedy should be placed in a small vial and its aperture be applied to the nose of the patient for a few seconds, or for a minute or two as the case may require." — page 22

A very early and very scarce book.

1841: *AN EPITOME OF HOMŒOPATHIC DOMESTIC MEDICINE:* Joseph Laurie, MD ✔
Leath and Ross, London; uknown pages.
"A complete guide to medical practice." The potencies suggested are usually 3, 6, 12 (all centesimal) although 30 and 200 are mentioned at times. It is interesting that the number of globules taken for a specific condition was stressed, and dosages were written as a fraction with the number of globules indicated by zeros in the numerator and the potency as the denominator. Thus, two granules of

the 3rd potency was written as 00/3 and four granules of the 6th potency was written as 0000/6. There were several editions of this volume produced. The first American edition in **1843** (230 pages) was offered by Radde and edited by A. G. Hull ("Hull's Laurie"). Hull noted that Hering's *Domestic Physician*, by then, was out of print. Thirty years later, in **1871**, Robert McClatchey edited yet another edition of "Hull's Laurie" that had 1044 pages. Says Bradford, "So rapid was the sale that the 4th edition was issued in **1872**. The 12th was issued in **1892**."

The nomenclature for the number of globules and potency of the remedy was common at the time. We see it in reports in Stapf's Archiv *and it is also seen in both Hahnemann's and Bönninghausen's casebooks.*
The major books that appeared to be used for "domestic medicine" were Hering's, Laurie's, Pulte's, and Ruddock's. This statement is based upon how many of these volumes are seen as used books versus others of a similar nature.

1846: *THE HOMEOPATHIC DOMESTIC PHYSICIAN*: Charles Hempel, MD
Radde; 184 pages.
In 1853, Hempel produced a German language edition.

1849: *THE POCKET HOMEOPATHIST AND FAMILY GUIDE*: John A. Tarbell, MD
Otis Clapp; 67 pages.
Four edition published between 1849 and 1874.

1850: *THE HOMŒOPATHIC DOMESTIC PHYSICIAN:* Joseph Hypolyte Pulte, MD ✔
H. W. Derby & Co.; 556 pages.
"Containing Treatments of Diseases; with popular explanations of Anatomy, Physiology, Hygiene and Hydrotherapy." It was reported that the first edition— a printing of 1000 books— was sold out in three days. 71 remedies are listed as well as 4 tinctures (*Arnica, Symphytum, Ruta, Urtica*). The mineral and animal remedies were in the 6th potency and the vegetable remedies were in the 3rd. *Coffea, Belladonna,* and *Cina* were in both the 3rd and 200th.
By **1886** the 13th edition was issued. Bradford says, "This book had an extensive sale. The London reprint has reached in England and the Colonies fifty thousand copies, and the Spanish translation as many."
An interesting addition was published by G. W. Smith in **1888**: the 370 page *DOMESTIC COOKBOOK; A COMPANION TO PULTE'S DOMESTIC PHYSICIAN* written by Mrs. Pulte.

1851: *A POCKET MANUAL*: Joel Bryant, MD ✔
William Radde; 352 pages.
See the entry in the "Repertory" section. Although sold as a domestic manual, it was set out as a repertory but included descriptions of diseases as well as a section on poisons and antidotes.

1852: *HOMEOPATHIC DOMESTIC PHYSICIAN*: Carl Caspari, MD
Rademacher and Sheek, Philadelphia; 475 pages.
Translated from the 8th German edition. "Directions to enable patients living at a distance from a Homeopathic Physician to describe their symptoms."

1852: *FAMILY GUIDE TO THE ADMINISTRATION OF HOMŒOPATHIC REMEDIES:* H. V. Malan, MD
Radde; 112 pages.
Published by Radde in **1853** in Spanish.
A pocket guide (3" x 5") covering 27 remedies.

1853: *WOMAN'S MEDICAL GUIDE:* Joseph Hypolyte Pulte, MD
Moore, Anderson, Wilstach, and Keys, Cincinnati, OH; 336 pages.
"Containing Essays on the Physical, Moral, and Educational Development of Females, and the Homœopathic Treatment of their Diseases in all Periods of Life, together with the Directions for the Remedial Use of Water and Gymnastics."

1853: *THE HOMŒOPATHIC PRACTICE OF MEDICINE*: Martin Freligh, MD
Lamport, Blakeman, and Law, New York, NY; 576 pages.
"Designed as a text-book for the student, a concise book of reference for the profession, and Simplified and Arranged for Domestic Use. " Charles T. Hulbert became the publisher after the 7th edition. Six editions were issued in Spanish. An abridged version was issued in **1856**.

1853: *HOMEOPATHIC DOMESTIC PRACTICE*: Egbert Guernsey, MD
Radde; 581 pages.
"Containing chapters on Anatomy, Physiology, Hygiene and an Abridged Materia Medica." It went though 11 editions and was translated into four languages.

The North American Journal of Homœopathy said, in 1857, that this was one of the best for its "superior literary finish."

1854: *MANUAL OF HOMEOPATHIC PRACTICE FOR THE USE OF FAMILIES AND PRIVATE INDIVIDUALS:* Alvan Edward Small, MD
Rademacher and Sheek; 831 pages.
15 editions were issued. This book was abridged to 126 pages and published in **1855** as *THE POCKET MANUAL OF HOMEOPATHIC PRACTICE*. Dr. Small assisted in the preparation of *WARREN'S HOUSEHOLD PHYSICIAN*, 984 pages, a highly used domestic manual of allopathic care that included a homœopathic section written by Dr. Small.

1855: *GENTLEMAN'S HANDBOOK OF HOMEOPATHY*: Egbert Guernsey, MD
Otis Clapp; 255 pages.
"Especially for Travellers and for Domestic Practice." A 2nd edition was published by Radde in **1857**.

1856: *HOMŒOPATHY SIMPLIFIED*: John A. Tarbell, MD
Otis Clapp; 360 pages.
"Domestic Practice Made Easy; containing Explicit Directions for the Treatment of Disease, the Management of Accidents, and the Preservation of Health."

1856: *HUMPHREYS' MANUAL OF SPECIFIC HOMEOPATHY*: Frederick Humphreys, MD
Published by the author in Auburn, NY; 148 pages.
By 1892 there were, reports Bradford, ten revised editions. The early editions sold between 10,000 and 20,000 copies annually. By the time the 10th edition was published, 2,500,000 were being sold annually. Bradford estimates that 15 million copies were made in English, French, German, and Portuguese, of which about 12 million were in the USA.
Humphreys formulated a line of "specifics" (combination remedies) and for doing so was expelled from the AIH in 1855. The book consists of a listing of the "specifics" (No. 1. Inflammations, Congestions, Fevers; No. 4. Diarrhea, Summer Complaints; etc.) followed by a therapeutic guide i.e., for this, take that. The formulation of the "specific" is not revealed in the books.

1856: *THE HOMŒOPATHIC POCKET COMPANION*: Martin Freligh, MD
Charles T. Hulbert; 291 pages.
"A Simplified Abridgment of the Homœopathic Practice of Medicine, designed especially for the use of Families and Travellers." The 11th edition was printed in **1890**. The author says he took out all that is "historical and theoretical and therefore of interest solely to the professional reader" from his previous book, leading to this best selling abridgment.

1856: *HOMÖOPATHISCHEN HAUS UND SCHIFFSARZT (The Home and Ship doctor/Physician)*:
Ludwig Reichenbach
Spamer, Leipzig; 261 pages.
Contains an appendix about the homœopathic treatment of domestic animals.

Just the work needed for the long sea voyages to and from the Continent!

1857: *PROFESSOR REMSEN'S HOMŒOPATHIC FAMILY GUIDE FOR TRAVELLERS, ETC.*: J. B. F. Remsen
Remsen, New York; 50 pages.
One of the first "covers" of the successful line of "New Era" kits being marketed by Humphreys. The book came with a box of combination remedies.

1859: *ACUTE DISEASES AND THEIR HOMEOPATHIC TREATMENT*: Jabez P. Dake, MD
J. G. Backofen and Son, Pittsburgh, PA; 77 pages.
A 5th edition was published by William Gamble and Co. in Nashville in **1871**.

1859: *THE HOMŒOPATHIC SURGICAL ADVISOR AND TRAVELLER'S COMPANION*: A. Z., MD
Boericke; 85 pages.
The author, identified only as "A. Z, MD," says that the work is intended to give clear and easily understood instructions for the treatment of accidents, when no medical attendance can be procured, or when the accidents are of such a nature that professional aid is not deemed necessary."

1860: *PRACTICAL HOMEOPATHY*: James S. Douglas, MD
Milwaukee, private by the author; 86 pages.
"Adapted to the Comprehension of the Non-professional and for Reference by the Young Practitioner. Including a number of most valuable New Remedies and Improvements, in the Treatment of numerous Diseases, not in general use." A 6th edition, enlarged to 129 pages was published by C. S. Halsey in **1862**. the 14th edition was published by Lewis Sherman in **1882**. In commenting on the need for this volume, the author treats us to the following paragraph, aimed at Frederick Humphreys, and his line of "specifics":
"The reputation of homœopathic remedies has become so general, and the demand for them so great, that the country is becoming flooded with Homœopathic quackery, under the name of "Specific Homœopathic Remedies," no one knowing what they are but him who prepares them. When a bottle or box is exhausted, the owner has no resource but to send to the getter-up of these nostrums, or some of his agents to get it replenished. The unfortunate example of this mode of quackery has been set by a medical man in the East, who has thereby forfeited his standing in the profession, and been, very properly, expelled from the American Institute. His example is being followed by others, who have a higher regard for their own pockets than for their professional reputations or the interests of the public."

1862: *MANUAL OF HOMŒOPATHIC THEORY AND PRACTICE DESIGNED FOR THE USE OF PHYSICIANS AND FAMILIES*: Arthur Lutze
Radde; 742 pages.
Translated by Charles Hempel.
Reprinted in **1870**. The original German edition was printed in **1860**, and had sold 60,000 copies at the time of the English translation. The original book contained a section describing the use of two remedies simultaneously, and quoted an exchange between Hahnemann and Aegidi as the source of the information. This section had been pulled from the translation and printed separately at the front of the book with a commentary by William Radde.

The business of the Hahnemann/Aegidi affair and the use of double remedies has persisted to this day, and is usually quoted by those who use combinations. There are letters from Aegidi describing his abandonment of this practice, but these were unknown to Lutze when the book was written.

1863: *A GUIDE FOR EMERGENCIES*: Henry B. Millard, MD
C. T. Hulbert; 136 pages.
"Containing the Homœopathic Treatment of Such Diseases as Require Immediate Attention, and of Such as may be Treated Without the Assistance of a Physician; and also containing the Treatment of Cases of Poisoning and of every common Variety of Accidents. For the use of Families."
The 3rd edition was published in **1871**. The author says that many under his care have asked

about having such a book in their homes, and stresses it is an *emergency* manual, not a manual for diseases in general of which there is "no lack of works on domestic practice."

c. 1864: *STEPPING STONES TO HOMEOPATHY AND HEALTH*: E. Harris Ruddock, MD ✔
W. Butcher, London; unknown pages.
By the 7th edition in **1872**, 60,000 had been sold. The first American edition was by C. S. Halsey in **1870** (241 pages), and was based on the 6th London edition. A second edition was issued in **1872** because the plates of the first were lost in the Great Chicago Fire. A "New American Edition" was offered in **1890** by Boericke and Tafel with a chapter on "Diseases of Women" by William Boericke, MD.
Ruddock wrote a number of domestic manuals. His most well known was THE HOMŒOPATHIC VADE MECUM OF MODERN MEDICINE AND SURGERY (the 6th edition in London was printed in **1876**). By 1893, the *VADE MECUM* had sold 95,000 copies. It was reprinted in **1884** as *RUDDOCK'S FAMILY DOCTOR* and published by Gross and Delbridge (734 pages). It included "notes and additional chapters by James E. Gross."
Unfortunately, the original publisher of Ruddock's work in the UK, the Homœopathic Publishing Company, never put dates on any of the books, and Ruddock never dated his introductions. One can assume that the books were written between 1860 and 1870; certainly no later than 1875, the date of Ruddock's death.
His other works include THE LADY'S MANUAL (**c. 1865**) published in the USA by C. S. Halsey (231 pages) in **1870**, and *THE DISEASES OF INFANTS AND CHILDREN AND THEIR HOMŒOPATHIC AND GENERAL TREATMENT* published at an unknown date in the UK with an edition by Boericke and Tafel in **1901**.

1868: *HOMŒOPATHIC HOME AND SELF TREATMENT OF DISEASE. FOR THE USE OF FAMILY AND TRAVELLERS:* Charles Woodhouse, MD
Published by the author in Rutland VT; 180 pages.
"We think we have made some important improvements…" The book contains information about 41 remedies. Says the author, "Many persons must or will doctor themselves, more or less, for various considerations and there seems to be no good reason why they should not, if they would take the pains to get instruction in this important matter."

1870: *MATERNITY: A POPULAR TREATISE FOR YOUNG WIVES AND MOTHERS*: Tullio S. Verdi, MD
J. B. Ford and Co., New York; 451 pages.
Enlarged and re-published in **1893**.

1872: *HUMPHREYS' HOMEOPATHIC MENTOR:* Frederick Humphreys, MD
Humphreys Specific Homœopathic Medicine Co.; 352 pages.
An expanded version of his *SPECIFICS*, with the first part of the manual dealing with general health matters, hygiene and diet, and the second part concerning therapeutics using "Specifics."

1879: *TRAVELLER'S MEDICAL REPERTORY AND FAMILY ADVISOR FOR HOMŒOPATHIC TREATMENT OF ACUTE DISEASES*: William Jefferson Guernsey, MD
Boericke and Tafel; 36 pages.
A materia medica of 24 remedies followed by a 19 page repertory.

1879: *A GUIDE TO HOMEOPATHIC PRACTICE*: Isaac D. Johnson, MD ✔
Boericke and Tafel; 494 pages.
"Designed for the Use of Families and Private Individuals." This book was offered by Boericke and Tafel with a box of remedies.

It was Johnson's Guide *that young Arthur Grimmer memorized by the time he was seven years old, and he was able to use it for prescribing in emergencies when his parents were away. Grimmer went on to become a physician and took over Kent's practice in Chicago in 1916.*

1885: *DOMESTIC GUIDE TO HOMŒOPATHIC TREATMENT, ALSO THE HYGIENIC MEASURES REQUIRED IN THE MANAGEMENT OF EPIDEMIC CHOLERA*: Joseph A. Biegler, MD
Schlicht and Field, Rochester, NY; 57 pages.

1886: *SEXUAL ILLS AND DISEASES; A POPULAR MANUAL:* Anonymous
Boericke and Tafel; 160 pages.
Information culled from several sources; the compiler is not identified. The preface, in reference to many other books on the subject, says "the moral advice may be excellent, but people do not buy medical books for it." Descriptions of "Sexual Ills" are offered (Masturbation, Nymphomania, Satyriasis) and general advice is given. The second part of the book is a short materia medica.

1887: *THE ELEMENTS OF MODERN DOMESTIC MEDICINE*: Henry G. Hanchett, MD ✔
Charles T. Hulburt; 337 pages.
"A plain and Practical Handbook Describing Simple Diseases, their Safe Home Treatment, the Signs that a Physician is needed, and the Procedure until the Doctor arrives."
"The world is chiefly filled up with sick folk. The drug stores are startlingly abundant, and crowded with a bewildering array of mysterious concoctions, most of them dangerous, intended for the relief of the sick. The people are trying to cure themselves, and are listening to the advice of friends and neighbors, of quack advertisements and newspaper puffs, and are putting into their stomachs gallons of stuff of whose composition and qualities they know nothing, and from which they often-times suffer more than from their original diseases."
The author, allowing that physicians are readily at hand in most cities, says that a "physician's first duty is to give advice and instruction…" and that "…most diseases tend toward recovery, that there is an inborn tendency in the human family to help itself out of any difficulty…" presents the book as one offering lots of basic domestic advice, but not much in the way of homœopathic therapeutics.

The copy in my library is signed, "To my friend, Dr. Stuart Close, with compliments of the author."

1887: *PRACTICAL GUIDE TO HOMEOPATHY*: A. Worthington, MD
Otis Clapp and Son; 175 pages.
"The necessity for a work of this kind will be more apparent, when we bear in mind that a large portion of the population of the United States are not within reach of homeopathic physicians..." A small (3 1/2" x 5 1/2") pocket manual describing the use of 28 homœopathic remedies.

1891: *THE TEXT BOOK FOR DOMESTIC PRACTICE:* Samuel Morgan, MD
Hahnemann Publishing House; 191 pages.
"Being plain and concise directions for the administration of homœopathic medicines in simple ailments." A small (4" x 5 1/2") pocket manual. Explaining his reasons for writing the book, the author mentions the conventional use of cathartics, liniment, and other remedies used at home. He says, "… to calculate the medicines employed in domestic practice to relieve complaints which are too trivial to call in medical assistance and who does not know many instances where the haphazard administration of such remedies does infinitely more harm than good."

1893: *SPECIAL DIAGNOSIS AND HOMŒOPATHIC TREATMENT OF DISEASE FOR POPULAR USE*:
Tullio S. Verdi, MD
Boericke and Tafel; 579 pages.
"Including such functional disturbances as are peculiar to girls and to maternity." An enlarged version of *MATERNITY*, published in **1853**. "Knowledge should be the right of many rather than the privilege of a few; hence, the author is more willing to instruct than command. If in the development of this work he has succeeded in putting this principle into practice, he will need no praise, for in its success he will have found his reward."

1890: *DICTIONARY OF DOMESTIC MEDICINE*: John Henry Clarke, MD ✔
Homeopathic Publishing Co.; 363 pages. Published by B & T in **1901**.
"Many non-medical readers of *THE PRESCRIBER* having requested me to bring out a more popular and elementary work on the same lines of arrangement…" Very similar to his previous work but gives description of the conditions being studied.

A wonderful little book containing clear definitions of the conditions and occasional helpful hints.

1908: *A NURSERY MANUAL*: Ruel Benson, MD ✔
Boericke and Tafel; 175 pages.
"The Care and Feeding of Children in Health and Disease." Benson was a lecturer on Diseases of Children at NY Homeopathic. "This book was originally written for the use of my own patients and nurses, among whom I have found a constant demand for such information as the book contains."

1940: *THE LITTLE HOMEOPATHIC PHYSICIAN*: William Gutman, MD ✔
Boericke and Tafel; 41 pages.
A materia medica followed by a therapeutic section, followed by sickroom advice. It was reprinted by Boericke and Tafel in **1961** and was one of the few self-help books available during the period from 1940 to 1960.

1945: *HOMEOPATHY FOR THE FIRST AIDER*: Dorothy Shepherd, MD ✔
Homœopathic Publishing Co.; 72 pages.
A brief exploration in the chatty, narrative style that is typical of the author. It contains useful information laced with case experiences.

c. 1950: *CHILDREN'S TYPES*: Dr. Douglas Borland ✔
British Homeopathic Association; 54 pages.
The original printing was of a series of lectures on the subject at the London Homœopathic Hospital. This book is an extraction of that information. Although having the same title, they are two very different works.

1950: *HOMEOPATHY FOR MOTHER AND INFANT*: Dr. Douglas Borland ✔
British Homeopathic Association; 20 pages.
The first part is a lecture given in 1929 at the London Homœopathic Hospital. The second part is simply an extraction of the information into an easier to use form. This work *might* have been published earlier, but no earlier copies are known.

1950: *ESSENTIALS OF HOMEOPATHIC TREATMENT*: H. Fergie Woods, MD
Homœopathic Publishing Company; 78 pages.
A brief materia medica of 81 remedies with a "rapid repertory" which is, essentially, a clinical index. It *could* be looked at as a therapeutic text, but the intention was for the domestic market.

1950: *HOMEOPATHY*: Garth Boericke, MD
AIH; 23 pages.
"The object of this pamphlet is to bring to the attention of the intelligent layman homeopathic methods which he can use himself without harmful effects for many of the common complaints and minor illnesses of everyday life." A quick guide to a few remedies for cold, croup, and indigestion.

1960: *THE HOME PRESCRIBER*: A. Dwight Smith, MD ✔
Ehrhart and Karl; 43 pages.
One of the few works written during the 1950s and 1960s.

A. Dwight Smith was a grand old homœopath, a member of the IHA. He practiced in Glendale, CA.

c. 1960: *HOMEOPATHIC TREATMENT IN THE NURSERY*: H. Fergie Woods, MD ✔
British Homœopathic Association, London; 12 pages.

1976: *A DOCTORS' GUIDE TO HELPING YOURSELF WITH HOMEOPATHIC REMEDIES*:
James Stephenson, MD ✔
Parker Publishing, West Nyack, NY; 197 pages.
Re-published by Thorsens in **1984**. "This book attempts to present a difficult medical specialty in a simple form for home use… do not let its simplicity make you over-confident. You are not qualified to treat difficult constitutional cases of illness in yourself or in others."

One of the first "self-care" books written as homœopathy was rising from the doldrums, this book never received any acclaim from the community. One reason, perhaps, is that it is written in a narrative style, with therapeutics, case examples, health advice, all mixed together; the essential information being difficult to extract. The author, a respected homœopath from New York and a pupil of Elizabeth Wright Hubbard, expressed disappointment that the work was not better received.

1976: *BEFORE THE DOCTOR COMES:* Donovan Cox and T. W. Hyne Jones
Thorsens; 48 pages.
"Written exclusively for home use." A thin book written by "Two London businessmen" who have "derived benefit" from the application of homœopathy.

1977: *THE AMAZING HEALER ARNICA, AND A DOZEN OTHER HOMEOPATHIC REMEDIES*:
Dr. A. C. Gordon Ross
Thorsons; 96 pages.

c. 1970: *FIRST AID HOMEOPATHY IN ACCIDENTS AND AILMENTS:* Dr. Douglas M. Gibson ✔
British Homœopathic Association; 84 pages.
The 6th edition bears an imprint of **1977**. A very clear first aid guide.

This was one of the first books I bought when I started studying homœopathy and have always found to be serviceable. I've learned a lot since I first bought it, but I find it is the book I go to in first-aid situations when I'm unsure.

1978: *HOMEOPATHIC REMEDIES FOR PHYSICIANS, LAYMEN, AND THERAPISTS*: David Anderson, MD, Dale Buegel, MD, Dennis Chernin, MD
Himalayan Press, Honesdale, PA; 140 pages.
One of the first self-help books published in the "homœopathic revival." It was republished in an amended and enlarged form (250 pages) in **1991** as *HOMEOPATHIC REMEDIES FOR HEALTH PROFESSIONALS AND LAY PEOPLE*: David Anderson was not a part of this effort. The third author on the new edition was Blair Lewis, PA.

1979: *HOMŒOPATHIC PRESCRIBING; REMEDIES FOR THE HOME AND SURGERY*:
Dr. Adolph Voegeli
Thorsens; 94 pages. Translated from the German by Geoffrey A. Dudley.
Originally published in Germany in 1964 as *die korrekte homöopathische Behandlung in der täglichen praxis*.

1980: *HOMEOPATHIC MEDICINE AT HOME*: Maesimund B. Panos, MD and Jane Heimlich ✔
Jeremy Tarcher; 287 pages.
A basic domestic manual, written in a chatty style that makes use of the 28 remedies that were sold in a domestic kit by the National Center for Homeopathy. It was, in essence, the manual for the kit. It has some very clear charts with therapeutic differentials.

Written by an experienced family physician in collaboration with a professional writer, it was the first homœopathy book that had major distribution at the time the homeopathic resurgence was beginning in the USA. It

The Heritage of Homœopathic Literature

has been published in other countries and translated into a number of other languages. Jane Heimlich is the wife of physician Henry Heimlich, MD, inventor of the Heimlich Maneuver, an important 1st aid measure to help people who are choking on food.

1982: *HOMŒOPATHIC MEDICINE: A DOCTOR'S GUIDE TO REMEDIES FOR COMMON AILMENTS:*
Trevor Smith, MD ✔
Thorsons; 256 pages.
"A practical guide book to basic homeopathy written for the family by a practicing physician."

The first of a series of "self-help" books by the author.

1983: *HOMEOPATHIC REMEDIES FOR CHILDREN:* Phyllis Speight ✔
Health Science Press; 96 pages.
Pages 11-64 is materia medica; pages 65-94 is a repertory

Phyllis Speight and her husband Leslie were lay-people in the UK who carried on a practice, ran a publishing business, and taught many courses. They were two of the many responsible for keeping homœopathy alive in the UK during the 1940s and 1950s.

1984: *EVERYBODY'S GUIDE TO HOMEOPATHIC MEDICINES:*
Dana Ullman, MPH and Stephen Cummings, MD ✔
Jeremy Tarcher; 312 pages.
Along with the Panos book, one of the first "domestics" at the beginning of the homœopathic resurgence. It is clearly formatted and each therapeutic division contains a section titled, "Beyond Home Care." It was republished in **1997** as a revised edition with 63 more pages.

Not quite as "chatty" as the Panos book, this book followed well on the heels of the Panos/Heimlich book and had enough added information to be valuable in itself or as an addition to the Panos work. The "Beyond Home Care" section is extremely valuable and clearly states what the limits of self-care are.

1984: *A WOMAN'S GUIDE TO HOMŒOPATHIC MEDICINE: SELF HELP IN THE TREATMENT OF GYNÆCOLOGICAL AND RELATED FEMALE AILMENTS:* Trevor Smith, MD ✔
Thorsens; 176 pages.

1984: *THE HOMŒOPATHIC TREATMENT OF EMOTIONAL ILLNESS:* Trevor Smith, MD ✔
Thorsens; 208 pages.

One of the first books that began to suggest "self-treatment" for conditions that are not really amenable to self-care. Included are suggestions for remedies to be used for schizophrenia, obsessional states, depression, withdrawal, and a host of other mental and emotional conditions. It would be one thing if the book was written as a text that discussed the problems and how homœopathy has been shown to help, but the book is clearly labeled as "A Self-Help Guide to Remedies Which Can Restore Calm and Happiness" and, as such, oversteps its bounds.

1985: *HOMŒOPATHY FOR WOMEN'S AILMENTS:* Phyllis Speight ✔
Health Science Press; 150 pages.
38 remedies. Pages 15-103 is materia medica; pages 105-144 is a repertory

1986: *THE FAMILY GUIDE TO HOMEOPATHY:* Alain Horvilleur, MD ✔
Health and Homeopathy Publishing, Arlington, VA; 249 pages.
Translated from the French by D. Clausen.
A unique alphabetical arrangement. Remedies, biographies, medical definitions, therapeutic categories, and history are set out in alphabetical order; e.g., "Flea bites, Flu-like symptoms, *Fluoricum acidum,*

Formica rufa, Fractures..."— all in order. It contains many illustrations.

Many of the illustrations are meaningless and seem like "filler." Why use a whole page for a picture of a woman smiling, while the caption talks about the need for good tooth care? This book was an attempt by Boiron Pharmacy to get people in the USA interested in homœopathy, and was introduced shortly after Boiron came into the American marketplace after they purchased the homœopathic pharmacy of J. Borneman and Sons. Because of cultural differences (French/American) it lost something in the translation and did not have much appeal in the USA market. In an attempt to add information about homœopathy in the USA, I was asked to help with the writing and editing, but the final result left much to be desired.

1986: *HOMEOPATHIC GUIDE FOR THE FAMILY:* Allan Neiswander, MD
American Foundation for Homeopathy, Alhambra, CA; 123 pages.
A basic therapeutic guide with a brief materia medica.

1987: *CURING COLIC AND LACTOSE INTOLERANCE:* Jana Shiloh ✔
Rocky Mountain Homeopathics, Boulder, CO; 43 pages.
Excellent charts with useful differentials of 25 remedies.

1987: *EVERYDAY HOMOEOPATHY: A SAFE GUIDE FOR SELF-TREATMENT:* Dr. David Gemmell ✔
Beaconsfield; 184 pages.
Reprinted, with some additions, in **1997**.

There is a real double standard here. For example, in the "Colitis" section, there is this statement: "First Aid treatment has no part to play here. The patient must be in the care of a physician." Then follows a listing of possible remedies for use in the condition.

1989: *THE FAMILY GUIDE TO HOMEOPATHY: THE SAFE FORM OF MEDICINE FOR THE FUTURE*:
Dr. Andrew Lockie ✔
Hamish Hamilton, London; 400 pages.
"Loosely based on Ruddock's *Domestic Physician,*" this book follows the general outline of other domestic manuals. When discussing "Ailments and Diseases" several codes are used to suggest conditions where emergency help is needed *now*, where one should consult a physician if no improvement is seen in two hours, etc.

Another book with a wide double standard. Many of the categories (such as Bulimia, Manic Depression, Pneumothorax, Parkinson's) have suggestions for remedial self-help, although it is mentioned that a medical practitioner might be consulted.

1990: *THE COMPLETE HOMEOPATHY HANDBOOK:* Miranda Castro, FSHom. ✔
St. Martin's Press; 253 pages.
"Safe and effective ways to treat... a wide range of everyday complaints." Says the author, "I am concerned that people who are using homeopathic medicine should know their potential and use them with respect, especially since they are now sold over-the-counter in most chemists and health food shops, with very few guidelines." The book contains an explanation of homœopathy, a materia medica and repertory, and a therapeutics section titled, "Diseases you can treat using this book."

Probably one of the best of the new "self help" books; well written, easy to understand and very clear guidelines about the limits of what is "self-treatable."

1991: *HOW TO USE HOMOEOPATHY:* Dr. Christopher Hammond
Element, Dorset, UK; 148 pages.
Presents therapeutics as a series of tables for each condition: The remedies listed in the columns,

and the symptoms and modalities listed in the rows. A much expanded re-do of a work published by Caritas Healthcare in **1988**.

One more "new book" that matches symptoms to conditions, in an overly simplistic way.

1991: *SPORTS AND EXERCISE INJURIES:* Stephen Subotnick, DPM ✔
North Atlantic Books; 391 pages.
The first book to discuss this specific subject from the homœopathic viewpoint.

1992: *HOMEOPATHIC MEDICINE FOR CHILDREN AND INFANTS:* Dana Ullman, MPH ✔
Jeremy Tarcher; 256 pages.
A specific focus which includes theory, therapeutics, and materia medica.

1993: *HOMEOPATHY FOR PREGNANCY, BIRTH, AND YOUR BABY'S FIRST YEAR*:
Miranda Castro, FSHom ✔
St. Martin's Press; 318 pages.
Similar to her previous book, but more specific in its focus.

1993: *HOMEOPATHY FOR COMMON AILMENTS:* Robin Hayfield, RSHom ✔
Frog Ltd., Berkeley, CA; 95 pages.
37 common ailments with remedy differentials and a materia medica of "constitutional" types. Beautiful full color photographs of the remedy sources.

1995: *CONSUMER'S GUIDE TO HOMEOPATHY*: Dana Ullman, MPH ✔
Jeremy Tarcher; 410 pages.
"The definitive resource to understanding homœopathic medicine and making it work for you." This work explains the philosophy of homœopathy, gives a brief history of the movement, explains the pharmacy process, and gives some hints for possible remedies to be used for a variety of conditions.

1996: *HEALING WITH HOMEOPATHY: THE NATURAL WAY TO PROMOTE RECOVERY AND RESTORE HEALTH*: Wayne Jonas, MD and Jennifer Jacobs, MD ✔
Warner Books; 349 pages.
A book by a major publisher containing a bit more about what homœopathy is and a bit less of how to do it. There a summary chart of conditions with modalities, and an appendix listing all the major research papers done up to that time. There is no separate materia medica, although there is differential materia medica under each "condition."

At the time the book was written, Dr. Jonas was the director of the Office of Alternative Medicine at the National Institutes of Health (NIH) and Dr. Jacobs was the author of the first homœopathic double-blind trial to be published in a conventional medical journal.

1996: *HOMEOPATHY CHILDBIRTH MANUAL*: Betty Idarius, LM, CHom. ✔
Private by the author, Ukiah, CA; 160 pages.
"A practical guide for labor, birth, and the immediate post-partum period."

1997: *HOMEOPATHIC SELF CARE: THE QUICK AND EASY GUIDE FOR THE WHOLE FAMILY*:
Judyth Reichenberg-Ullman, ND and Robert Ullman, ND ✔
Prima Publishing, Rocklin, CA; 433 pages.
Saying that "some books are written by authors who have no clinical experience," this is a "book that a bleary-eyed, half-awake parent could pick up in the middle of the night." Having exceptional visual clarity, each condition contains a description of the symptoms, possible medical complications, hints on what to look for, listen for, and ask— with remedy differentials where appropriate and a

listing of the remedies most used, general pointers, and finally a chart showing the remedy differentials. This book was followed, in **2000**, by *WHOLE WOMAN HOMEOPATHY (The comprehensive Guide to treating PMS, Menopause, Cystitis, and Other Problems— Naturally and Effectively)*. 345 pages, authored by Judyth Reichenberg-Ullman, ND.

1998: *MENOPAUSE AND HOMEOPATHY: A GUIDE FOR WOMEN IN MID-LIFE*: Ifeoma Ikenze, MD ✔
North Atlantic Books; 144 pages.

1998: *HELP! AND HOMEOPATHY: WHAT TO DO IN AN EMERGENCY BEFORE 911 ARRIVES:* Eileen Nauman, DIHom, EMT and Gail Derin-Kellog, OMD, EMT ✔
Blue Turtle Publishing (Cottonwood, AZ); 310 pages.
An outline of conditions including a definition, an emergency medical response, and possible remedies to use. The book has an excellent index.

Most books say, "This condition is an emergency. Get the person to the hospital." This book simply adds, "and give them this remedy on the way." Written by two people who are both familiar with homœopathy and have worked as Emergency Medical Technicians, the information is well presented and very valuable.

2000: *PRACTICAL HOMEOPATHY*: Vinton McCabe ✔
St. Martin's Press, NY; 592 pages.
"My hope in putting this together was to provide the beginner with one book that would be of help for the period of time before they go out to get their first full length materia medica and repertory." The first part of this work is called "The Role of the Physician" and takes a look at what homœopathy is and how it is practiced. It takes many aphorisms from the *Organon* and elaborates upon these— discussing the meaning of the word "physician" and how it differs from the word "doctor," and how anyone who makes use of any sort of medicinal substance—allopathic or homeopathic—to treat another is taking on the role of the physician, and, therefore, needs to understand the process and the guiding philosophy, case taking and case management.
The second section can be seen as a brief repertory for acute care and discusses those symptoms that are visible and tangible (Sensations, Discharges, Discolorations, Distortions) and therefore of the most help in treating the acute case. This is followed by a "traditional" domestic section of conditions and the remedies that they suggest. Finally, there is a brief materia medica that lists the 60 remedies that are most commonly used in the home.
The endnotes include information on dosage and potency, diet during treatment (based on Johnson's guide from the 1870s), a glossary of terms and a suggested case taking form.

The author is a homœopathic educator who has been involved in study groups for about 20 years.

Veterinary Manuals

Veterinary Manuals

In 1820, Johann Joseph Wilhelm Lux (1743-1849), a veterinary surgeon in Leipzig, began to experiment with the use of homœopathy in his veterinary practice.

By the late 1830s there were a number of books available, mostly in German. By 1847, most of the German works had been translated and used in a number of English veterinary manuals. Most books dealt with animals of the farm. In 1863 John Moore wrote the first book exclusively about dogs.

It should be noted that most of the early veterinary manuals borrowed heavily from the works of Rückert, Günther and Schaeffer, and provided information that had been passed down from others, rather than stating anything new. It took a number of years before books were published that contained "new" first-hand practical experience.

The "specifics" of Humphreys were widely used, and through the 1920s, a number of zoos in the USA and the Ringling Brothers Circus used them for most of the animal care, as did the US Department of Interior and the US Cavalry.

Veterinary homœopathy almost disappeared through the 1930s (although it always maintained a tradition in Germany), and it was not until the works of George MacLeod were published in the mid 1970s that veterinary homœopathy began to experience its resurgence.

Veterinary Manuals

1836: *ZOOIASIS, OR HOMŒOPATHY IN ITS APPLICATION TO THE DISEASES OF ANIMALS*:
Wilhelm Lux
Kollmann, Leipzig ; unknown pages. *Zooiasis: oder Heilungen der Thiere nach dem Gesetz der Natur; ein Buch für Gutsbesitzer, unstudierte Viehärzte und Solche, welche allerley Zeitungen, worin homöopathische Kuren vorkommen, nicht lesen können.*
Lux, a veterinary surgeon in Leipzig, was the first to use homœopathy with animals, having begun that practice in 1820. This work took the form of a periodical, of which two volumes were published. Lux's work has not been translated into English.

1837: *HOMŒOPATHIC MATERIA MEDICA FOR VETERINARIANS*: Johann Carl Ludwig Genzke
Schumann, Leipzig; 440 pages. *Homöopathische Arzneimittellehre für Thierärzte: nebst Anweisung zur Bereitung der homöopathischen Arzneien und Hinweisung auf deren Anwendung in verschiedenen Krankheitsformen.*
The first book about using homœopathy with animals. It was never published in English.

1839: *PERCEPTION AND CURE OF THE MOST IMPORTANT DISEASES OF THE HORSE*:
Ernst Ferdinand Rückert
Klinkicht, Meissen; 279 pages. *Die Erkenntniß und Heilung der wichtigsten Krankheiten des Pferdes: nach homöopathischen Grundsätzen bearbeitet für Oeconomen und Pferdeliebhaber.* (Edited according to homœopathic principles for oeconoms [agrarians] and lovers of horses.)
The information from this work was used in a number of other veterinary works, but the book itself was never translated into English.

1846: *THE HOMŒOPATHIC FARRIER*: Christian Bush
Carlisle, PA; 136 pages.
"An Indispensable Assistant to those who Desire to Cure the Diseases of Horses with Ease, Success, Simplicity, and not much Expense."

1847: *NEW MANUAL OF HOMŒOPATHIC VETERINARY MEDICINE*: F. A. Günther
Otis Clapp; 408 pages.
"The Homœopathic Treatment of the horse, the ox, the sheep, the dog, and other domestic animals."

The Heritage of Homœopathic Literature

Translated from the 3rd German edition. "The want of a more extended guide in the English Language… has induced the translation of the present work." The translator is not identified.

1854: *THE HANDBOOK OF VETERINARY HOMŒOPATHY:* John Rush ✔
Rademacher and Sheek; 144 pages.
Originally published in London by Jarrold and Sons; (no date known). "The Homœopathic Treatment of the Horse, the Ox, the Sheep, the Dog and the Swine." The work was quoted in Ruddock's *Veterinary Guide*. It was re-printed five times by Boericke and Tafel between **1858** and **1911**. It is still in print.

1856: *NEW MANUAL OF HOMŒOPATHIC VETERINARY MEDICINE*: J. C. Schaeffer
Rademacher and Sheek; 331 pages.
Translated from the German by C. J. Hempel.
"An easy and comprehensive arrangement of diseases, adapted to the use of every owner of domestic animals, and especially designed for the farmer, living out of the reach of medical advice, and showing him the way of treating his sick horses, cattle, sheep, swine, and dogs in the most expeditious, safe, and cheap manner." Reprinted by Boericke and Tafel; in **1871** and **1880**.

1857: *THE HOMŒOPATHIC CATTLE DOCTOR*: Carl Ludwig Boehm
Heckenast, Pest; 147 pages.
Boehm also wrote THE HOMŒOPATHIC HORSE DOCTOR, in **1855** and THE HOMŒOPATHIC SHEEP DOCTOR in **1860**, all in German. The content was used in many other books, but the full texts were never translated to English.

1857: *OUTLINES IN VETERINARY HOMŒOPATHY*: James Moore
Henry Turner; 201 pages.
"Comprising Horse, Cow, Dog, Sheep, and Hog Diseases and their Homœopathic Treatment."

1860: *MANUAL OF VETERINARY SPECIFIC HOMŒOPATHY*: Frederick Humphreys
Humphreys; 250 pages.
"Comprising Diseases of Horses, Cattle, Sheep, Hogs, Dogs, and Poultry, and their Specific Homœopathic Treatment." Bradford (1892) reports that there have been four revised editions with about 250,000 copies printed. Humphreys' work concerned the use of "specifics" sold for "conditions" and available only from Humphreys Pharmacy in New York, as well as being sold in regular drug stores.

1861: *REPERTORY OF THE VETERINARY HEALING ART ACCORDING TO PRINCIPLES*:
Carl Ludwig Boehm
Meinhold, Dresden; 110 pages. German.

1863: *THE DISEASES OF DOGS AND THEIR HOMŒOPATHIC TREATMENT*: James Moore
Simkin, Marshall, and Co. London; 320 pages.
Saying that "no work exists in any language specially treating of the subject," the book is written with "the fruits of many years experience."

1867: *DIE HOMÖOPATHISCHEN THIER ARZNEIMITTEL*: Carl Ludwig Boehm
Braumüller, Vienna; 220 pages.
The physiological actions and clinical application of homœopathic remedies in veterinary practice.

1867: *RINDPEST*: A. B. Conger
Weed and Parsons, Albany, NY; 141 pages.
"First and Second Reports of Special Committee Appointed by the Executive Board of the New York State Agricultural Society on the Statistics, Pathology, and Treatment of the Epizoötic Disease Known as Rindpest."

Veterinary Manuals

Pages 101-115 discusses the successes in England and Belgium with homœopathic treatment. Though other methods are discussed, the sanction of homœopathic medicines is given by the Society. The New York State Homœopathic Medical Society lauded this as "official recognition" of homœopathy. Samuel Lilienthal is acknowledged as having translated a monograph by Jessen from the German on innoculation treatment of the rindpest done in Russia. The rest of the homœopathy quoted was mostly from Pope in England.

1870: *VETERINARY HOMŒOPATHY*: James S. Beach
C. S. Halsey; unknown pages
All printing plates and all books were destroyed in the Chicago Fire in 1871. The book was not re-printed.

1874: *A MANUAL OF HOMŒOPATHIC VETERINARY PRACTICE DESIGNED FOR HORSES, ALL KINDS OF DOMESTIC ANIMALS, AND FOWLS*: no author given
Boericke; 684 pages.
A condensation of a number of other works including all of *VETERINARY HOMŒOPATHY* by Leath and Ross, and the works of Moore, Günther, Träger, Boehm, Gooday, and others.

It is a beautiful large volume with gold embossed pictures of a horse and a cow on the leather spine (on the cover, second book from the right, top shelf). The paper, unfortunately, was not of good quality and all the volumes I have seen are very brittle and fragile. Unfortunately, it has never been re-printed. It might have been compiled by J. H. P. Frost, since his obituary says that he did a large veterinary book at about this time.

1878: *POCKET MANUAL OF HOMŒOPATHIC VETERINARY MEDICINE*: E. Harris Ruddock   ✔
Homœopathic Publishing Co.; 134 pages.
"Containing the symptoms, causes and treatment of the diseases of horses, cattle, sheep, swine, and dogs." This book might have been published earlier, but no records can be found. This edition was edited by George Lade, three years after Ruddock's death.

1878: *POULTRY PHYSICIAN*: Fr. Schröter
Boericke and Tafel; 92 pages.
"Plain Directions for the Treatment of the most Common Ailments of Fowls, Ducks, Geese, Turkeys, and Pigeons, based on the Author's large Experience and Compiled from the most reliable Sources. Translated from the German." "…as yet there existed no work on the treatment of numerous ailments peculiar to poultry by homœopathic remedies…"

1879: *HOMŒOPATHIC VETERINARY HANDBOOK*: J. W. Johnson, VS
Ohio Farmer Co., Cleveland, Ohio; 128 pages.
Written by the editor of the Veterinary Department of the *Ohio Farmer* (Cleveland) and the *Practical Farmer* (Philadelphia), two widely circulated farming magazines. "…the irrational brute has become the partaker of this Greatest Gift [homœopathy] of God to his creatures."

1884: *THE CAT AND ITS DISEASES:* Edwin M. Hale, MD
private; Chicago; 16 pages.
"'Silent Be; it was the Cat'— Dick Deadeye." Bradford identifies this work as a "reprint from the Compendium of Health; forming part 7 of that book."The *COMPENDIUM OF HEALTH* was authored by Hale and Charles A. Williams. It was sub-titled, *Pertaining to the Physical Life of Man and the Animals which Serve Him*. A book of 945 pages, it was published by the American Book Company in 1884.

1885: *HUMPHREYS' VETERINARY GUIDE*: Frederick Humphreys
Humphreys' Specifics; 70 pages.
A much condensed version of Humphreys' 1860 work. Bradford reports that, in 1892, they were selling about 350,000 copies a year. The book was still in print in **1923**.

1886: *DOGS IN HEALTH AND DISEASE AS TYPIFIED BY THE GREYHOUND*: John Sutcliffe Hurndall
E. Gould, London; 88 pages.

1890: *THE HOMŒOPATHIC VETERINARY DOCTOR*: George Hammerton
Gross & Delbridge; 435 pages.
"Giving the History, Means of Prevention and Symptoms of all Diseases of the Horse, Ox, Sheep, Hog, Dog, Cat, Poultry and Birds, and the most Approved Methods of Treatment." Illustrated.

1890: *THE HOMŒOPATHC CURE OF DOMESTIC ANIMALS*: M. A. A. Wolff
People's Health Journal; 12 pages.

1891: *THE POULTRY DOCTOR INCLUDING THE HOMŒOPATHIC TREATMENT AND CARE OF CHICKENS, TURKEYS, GEESE, DUCKS, AND SINGING BIRDS*: P. H. Jacobs ✔
Boericke and Tafel; 85 pages.
Reprinted in **1908**. P. H. Jacobs, of Hammondton, NJ, was the editor of the *Poultry Keeper*.

1892: *"INCURABLE" DISEASES OF BEAST AND FOWL*: James Moore
Boericke and Tafel: 30 pages.
Based on an earlier work of James Moore (date unknown) concerning the treatment of pneumonia in cattle, this small pamphlet was enlarged to include the treatment of several other "incurable" diseases—rindpest, glanders, roup, and hog cholera.

1895: *HOMŒOPATHY IN VETERINARY PRACTICE*: John Sutcliffe Hurndall, MRCVS
unknown publisher; 33 pages.
A narrative about the use of homœopathy in animals, more of a popular guide as to "why, " rather than an expositions as to "how."

1896: *VETERINARY HOMŒOPATHY IN ITS APPLICATION TO THE HORSE*:
John Sutcliffe Hurndall, MRCVS
Boericke and Tafel; 340 pages.
Published the same year in England. "I am informed that over large districts in the United States of America, the services of a qualified Veterinary Surgeon are not available simply because there is not one resident within a reasonable distance; I hope that in such district, especially, this book will prove of considerable service."

1902: *CATS. HOW TO CARE FOR THEM*: Edith K. Neel, MD
Boericke and Tafel; 48 pages. 2nd edition in **1907**.
The author was associated with Keuka Lake, NY Cat Kennels. *The Cat Journal* said in a review: "This little book should be in the hands of every cat lover and breeder…"

1903: *DOGS. HOW TO CARE FOR THEM IN HEALTH AND TREAT THEM WHEN ILL*:
Edward Pollock Anshutz
Boericke and Tafel; 100 pages.
"Doctor Kent of Chicago, has kindly reviewed this work, and added much original matter to it."

1909: *POCKET BOOK OF VETERINARY MEDICAL PRACTICE*: A. Von Rosenberg
Boericke and Tafel; 125 pages.
The author, a member of the Michigan State Veterinary Association, suggests that because horse and cattle are vegetarian and not addicted to liquor, spicy foods, etc., they are in a more natural condition to respond to small doses of medicine. "The author, having put this to a test in general practice, decided to record the results of his work and publish them for the benefit of all practitioners."

1911: *POULTRY SENSE: A TREATISE ON THE MANAGEMENT AND CARE OF CHICKENS*:
James P. Pursell
Published by the author, Sellerville, PA; 123 pages.

1929: *TREATMENT OF CANINE DISTEMPER WITH THE POTENTIZED VIRUS*: Dr. Horace B. Jervis
Ehrhart and Karl; 40 pages.
"… it is written in the hope that a good many Veterinarians may, perhaps, find it of interest sufficient to at least give it a trial."

1935: *SPEEDY DOG CURES*: F. J. Bennett
Homœopathic Publishing Co.; 40 pages.

1960: *TREATMENT OF CATS BY HOMEOPATHY*: K. Sheppard
Health Science Press; 62 pages.

1963: *TREATMENT OF DOGS BY HOMEOPATHY*: K. Sheppard
Health Science Press; 97 pages.

These two books by Sheppard (not to be confused with Dorothy Shepherd) were the first books offered for general sale as the resurgence of homœopathy began. In 1965, they were the books you bought if you wanted information about veterinary homœopathy.

1975: *HOMEOPATHY IN VETERINARY PRACTICE*: K. J. Biddis, MRCVS
Nelsons; 21 pages.
A very abbreviated materia medica and repertory.

1976: *HOMEOPATHIC TREATMENT FOR BIRDS*: Beryl Chapman ✔
C. W. Daniel; 64 pages.

1977: *TREATMENT OF HORSES BY HOMEOPATHY*: George MacLeod, MRCVS ✔
Health Science Press; 182 pages.
The second edition, published in that same year, was expanded to 264 pages.

The first of a series by this great homœopathic veterinarian. The books (unlike those by Day, Pitcairn, and later by Hamilton) say little about the theory and philosophy of homœopathy. These are therapeutics books, pure and simple; for this condition, look at these remedies. His subsequent books are listed below.

1981: *TREATMENT OF CATTLE BY HOMEOPATHY*: George MacLeod, MRCVS ✔
Health Science Press; 160 pages.

1981: *HOMEOPATHY FOR PETS*: George MacLeod, MRCVS
Homeopathic Development Foundation, London; 28 pages.

1982: *DR. PITCAIRN'S COMPLETE GUIDE TO NATURAL HEALTH FOR DOGS AND CATS*:
Richard H. Pitcairn, DVM, PhD and Susan Hubble Pitcairn ✔
Rodale Press, Emmaus, PA; 287 pages. Second edition printed in **1995**, 383 pages.
There have been three foreign translations: *Cani & Gatti in Buona Salute* (Italian), *Den Hund— Gesund auf natürliche Weise* (German), *Guia Del Dr. Pitcairn de Salud Natural para Perros y Gatos* (Spanish).

Dealing primarily with domestic household pets, it was published by Rodale Press, the publisher of Prevention *Magazine. Because of this, it was the first general veterinary book that was broadly marketed. It discussed many alternative therapies as well as diet, and homœopathy figured prominently.*

The Heritage of Homœopathic Literature

1983: *VETERINARY MATERIA MEDICA WITH REPERTORY*: George MacLeod, MRCVS ✔
Health Science Press; 206 pages.

1983: *HOMEOPATHIC TREATMENT OF DOGS*: George MacLeod, MRCVS ✔
Homeopathic Development Foundation, London; 138 pages.
Revised and updated by Health Science Press, **1989**, 232 pages, from the prior *DOGS: HOMEOPATHIC REMEDIES*.

1984: *HOMEOPATHIC TREATMENT OF SMALL ANIMALS*: Christopher Day, MRCVS ✔
Wigmore Publications, London; 153 pages.
The first modern text that went beyond the "therapeutic" approach of the other books and discussed the larger issues of health and disease in the homœopathic context. Day provides some interesting models of the workings of homœopathy and for the selection of the potency.

The models that Day has hypothesized are contained in the first 37 pages of the book and should be read by all interested in homœopathy, not just those interested in the veterinary application of the art.

1984: *HOMEOPATHIC FIRST AID TREATMENT FOR PETS:* Francis Hunter, MRCVS
Thorsens; 144 pages.

1985: *ANIMAL EMERGENCY HANDBOOK*: Gloria Dodd, DVM
Published by the Author, San Ramon, CA; 26 pages.

A guide to emergency care, using a 24 vial kit that was supplied with the book.

1990: *CATS: HOMEOPATHIC REMEDIES*: George MacLeod, MRCVS ✔
Health Science Press; 184 pages.

1991: *TREATMENT OF GOATS BY HOMEOPATHY*: George MacLeod, MRCVS ✔
C. W. Daniel; 192 pages.

1991: *YOUR HEALTHY CAT: HOMEOPATHIC MEDICINES FOR COMMON FELINE AILMENTS*:
Hans Gunther Wolff, DVM ✔
North Atlantic Books; 131 pages.
A translation of the original German work published in **1980** by Sonntag.

1994: *PIGS: A HOMEOPATHIC APPROACH TO THE TREATMENT AND PREVENTION OF DISEASES*:
George MacLeod, MRCVS ✔
C. W. Daniel; 168 pages.

1995: *HOMEOPATHIC TREATMENT OF BEEF AND DAIRY CATTLE*: Christopher Day, MRCVS ✔
Beaconsfield; 141 pages.
Like his earlier work, the first 39 pages contain a grand exposition about homœopathy, and some interesting models of potency selection, and levels of treatment. It is well written and could usefully be read by all.

1996: *HOMEOPATHIC FIRST AID FOR ANIMALS*: Kaetheryn Walker ✔
Healing Arts Press, Rochester, VT; 176 pages.
"Tales and techniques from a country practitioner."

1997: *CRIES OF THE WILD; A WILDLIFE REHABILITATOR'S JOURNAL*: Jeff Lederman ✔
Heritage House Publishing, Surry, BC, CANADA; 144 pages
The author is a wildlife rehabilitator who used homeopathy in his practice. The book consists of 20 essays, 16 of them about particular cases, including that of an eagle, a crow, a fox, a deer, and several seals.

Veterinary Manuals

1997: *HOMŒOPATHIC HANDBOOK FOR DAIRY FARMING*: Tineke Verkade, RCHom ✔
published by the author, Ohaupo, New Zealand; 68 pages.
The author is a practicing homœopath who began to help farmers with their herds after they had experienced successful homœopathic treatment themselves.

A delightful and informative basic-level book. Knowing that the book will probably be referred to under all sorts of inclement conditions, the pages are all laminated in plastic and the whole is ring bound.

1998: *COMPLEMENTARY AND ALTERNATIVE VETERINARY MEDICINE: PRINCIPLES AND PRACTICE*: Allen M. Schoen, DVM, and Susan G. Wynn, DVM, PhD, editors. ✔
Mosby, St. Louis, MO; 820 pages.
An academic book written for practicing veterinarians that contains four chapters on homœopathy written by Dana Ullman, Christopher Day, C Edgar Sheaffer, and Peggy Fleming. The book has valuable information on research and practical applications in veterinary care.

1999: *HOMEOPATHIC CARE FOR CATS AND DOGS: A COMPREHENSIVE GUIDE*:
Donald Hamilton, DVM ✔
North Atlantic Books; 482 pages.
The most up to date guide for the care of household pets. Like the books of Day, this work is steeped in the theory of homœopathy and the issues of health and disease before moving on to the question of therapeutics. The book takes a similar approach to that of Jahr over 150 years ago— starting with chapters on the systems (skin and ears, mouth, gums, teeth) before continuing with chapters on specific therapeutics conditions (abscesses, allergic reactions, etc.). Hamilton has protocols in each clinical chapter that inform the reader when their cat or dog may need professional attention. He also has a chapter on animal vaccination that is highly critical of common vaccination practice.

Anatomy, Pathology, Diagnosis

Anatomy, Pathology, Diagnosis

As homœopathy grew, so did the schools which taught it. Between 1848 and the turn of the century, 22 homœopathic colleges were opened in the United States. They were all medical colleges, granting their graduates the degree Doctor of Medicine. The graduates of these schools made their way into the community to become physicians alongside others, be they eclectic, homœopathic or allopathic.

Although many teaching clinical subjects at the homœopathic schools were often recruited from the general medical community, other clinical instructors came from within the homœopathic ranks. Some wrote texts that became the standard within the schools. Very similar to the conventional medical texts of the time, there are often subtle difference between those "practices" written by a conventional physician and those written by homœopathic physicians.

Most of these books were published by "homœopathic" publishing firms. Bradford lists 60 books published until 1892 that would be considered in this category. Eleven of them are listed here.

Many of the books contain therapeutic hints, but these are usually relegated to a paragraph at the end of the section which often simply lists some remedies useful in treating the particular "disease." The focus of these works is to provide detailed explanations of the disease in terms of etiology, pathology, and presentation.

These books offer a partial window into the state of medicine at that time. This often proves to be a source of fascinating reading.

Many of these books werere succinctly described by A. McNeil, MD, who spoke about "The Homœopathic Library" at the 1896 IHA Meeting. McNeil says:

"It would take too much time to go over the fields of surgery, obstetrics, diagnosis and pathology, and I will therefore leave this to others better acquainted with these subjects.

"I will only say that you should own at least one standard work on each of these subjects, which is fully up to date. As to these books a question arises on which there may be a difference of opinion. But I boldly assert that if you cannot get a book written by a real homœopath, that you can get works containing better descriptions of disease and of the necessary operative processes required written by allopaths than by polypaths. I refer to such works as Arndt's, Wood's, Goodno's, Hale's, etc. As far as the treatment taught in the latter I would not risk the lives and health of those confided to my care to such as these writers advise. Just think of confining your selection of remedies in pneumonia to four, and they not the most frequently useful."

Anatomy, Pathology, Diagnosis

1855: *SURGERY, AND ITS ADAPTATION TO HOMŒOPATHIC PRACTICE*: William Tod Helmuth, MD
Moss and Brother, Philadelphia; 651 pages.
The author put together this work to "satisfy the need for a work which would be adapted to the requirements of our school." Over 20 years later the author wrote of the work's shortcomings, saying, "being a recent graduate, the book was imperfect…" Those imperfections were corrected in his later, **1879** work.

1855: *THE HOMŒOPATHIC PRACTICE OF SURGERY AND OPERATIVE SURGERY*: B. L. Hill, MD
J. B. Cobb and Co., Cleveland, OH; 654 pages.
The first part of this work concerns the use of remedies in conditions which were considered only amenable to surgical treatment. The second part, "Operative Surgery," concerns itself with only surgery—mostly the setting of fractures and dislocations and removal of foreign bodies.

1867: *THE SCIENCE AND ART OF SURGERY*: Edward C. Franklin, MD
Missouri Democrat Book and Job Print, St. Louis; Vol. 1, 844 pages, Vol. 2, (**1873**) 865 pages.
"Embracing Minor and Operative Surgery; Compiled from Standard Allopathic Authorities, and adapted to Homœopathic Therapeutics, with a General History of Surgery from the Earliest

Periods to the Present Time, for the use of Practitioners and Students of the Homœopathic Practice of Medicine."
A 2nd edition (minus the sections on bandaging and minor surgery) was published in **1882**.

The author was one of the few (along with Verdi and Von Tagen) who was allowed to employ homœopathy during his service in the Civil War. In an extensive section in Volume 1 on "Gunshot Wounds," he relates how he was given charge of a ward at the Mound City Hospital in Illinois. He and his two assistants were given the wounded who were declared "hopeless" by the allopathic field surgeons. More than 30% of them recovered during homœopathic treatment.
Franklin's mortality rate was 7.9% as compared with the 11.5%-25% in the allopathic hospitals in St. Louis. He handled the severely wounded from a number of major battles. He presents several cured cases of bullet wounds treated solely with homœopathic remedies.

1875: *A RECORD OF THE SURGICAL CLINICS OF WILLIAM TOD HELMUTH, MD, HELD AT THE NEW YORK HOMŒOPATHIC MEDICAL COLLEGE DURING THE SESSION OF 1874-75*: Philetus J. Stephens
Published by the Author, New York; 207 pages.
The lectures delivered by Helmuth as he examined the cases in the surgical clinic.
"Among the lower classes, there are those who so frequently engaged in fighting that they become brutal, and snap like the lower animals, and their bite seems to be very poisonous. I have amputated more than one finger for such a wound."

1879: *A SYSTEM OF SURGERY*: William Tod Helmuth, MD
Boericke; 1000 pages.
The second book from Helmuth, now written with 24 more years of experience. Said one review, "Whether he likes it or not, every doctor will at some time be called upon to do a little surgery, in view of which no homœopathic physician can afford to be without Dr. Helmuth's great work, which is admirably adapted to the needs of the General Practitioner…Ever since it was issued the necessity for student or practitioner to invest in allopathic works on the subject ceased to exist."

1881: *BILIARY CALCULI*: C. H. Von Tagen, MD
Boericke and Tafel; 154 pages.

1882: *SUPRAPUBIC LITHOTOMY*: William Tod Helmuth, MD
Boericke and Tafel; 90 pages.
A historical study of the extraction of stones from the bladder by using an incision above the pubic bone, and practical advice about performing the operation. There are many colored illustrations and patient charts.

This volume was not a big seller. When I was helping Boericke and Tafel move from their Arch St. location in Philadelphia, I found about ten of these books, in mint condition— as good as the day they were printed.

1883: *KEY NOTES OF MEDICAL PRACTICE*: Charles Gatchell, MD
Gross and Delbridge; 217 pages.

1883: *VENEREAL AND URINARY DISEASES:* Temple S. Hoyne, MD
Halsey Brothers; 125 pages.
Lectures given on the subject between 1881 and 1883 to his classes in Chicago. "At the request of my publishers, who claim that a slight résumé of the remedies suitable for urinary disorders is greatly needed, I have added the last few pages."

1883: *DISEASES AND INJURIES OF THE EYE*: J. E. Buffam, MD
Gross and Delbridge; 428 pages.

1885: *A SYSTEM OF MEDICINE BASED UPON THE LAW OF HOMŒOPATHY*: Hugo R. Arndt, MD ✻
Boericke; In three volumes. Volume I, 960 pages, Volume II, 900 pages, Volume. III, 990 pages.
Of the book T. F. Allen said, "We shall advise it to our students in preference to any other system of practice." It contains complete etiology, pathology, and description of diseases, followed by a very short section on homœopathic therapeutics. It is primarily a clinical text.

1893: *DISEASES OF THE NOSE AND THROAT*: Horace F. Ivins, MD
F. A. Davis, Philadelphia, PA; 507 pages.
Divided into three sections: The Nose and its Diseases; The Pharynx and its Diseases; The Larynx and its Diseases. It has 129 illustrations, many showing instruments and how to conduct a proper exam. The therapeutics are generally homœopathic with substantial information about the disease and differentials.

1894: *THE PRACTICE OF MEDICINE*: William C. Goodno, MD
Hahnemann Press, Philadelphia; Volume I, 948 pages, Volume II, 981 pages.
Each disease condition is discussed in the following sequence: etiology; pathology and morbid anatomy; symptomatology; course, duration, etc.; diagnosis; prognosis; treatment.

1894 : *A TEXTBOOK OF GYNÆCOLOGY*: James Craven Wood, MD
Boericke and Tafel; 858 pages.
Revised and enlarged 2nd edition, **1898**, 964 pages. Said one review, "Professor James C. Wood has produced the best textbook on gynæcology that has ever been offered to the medical profession."

1895 : *A MANUAL OF GENITO-URINARY AND VENEREAL DISEASES*: Bukk Carleton, MD
Boericke and Runyon; 315 pages.

1895: *A HOMŒOPATHIC TEXTBOOK OF SURGERY*: Charles E. Fischer and T. L. MacDonald, editors.
Boericke and Tafel; 1661 pages.

1896: *MANUAL OF THE ESSENTIAL DISEASES OF THE EYE AND EAR*: Joseph H. Buffam, MD ✔
Gross and Delbridge; 315 pages.
"This Manual, written at the request of the author's classes, presents the essential diagnostic and therapeutic points of the various diseases of the Eye and Ear in such concise form as to enable the student and the general practitioner to readily obtain the more important details of the treatment of such diseases."

1897: *LECTURES ON NERVOUS AND MENTAL DISEASES*: Charles S. Elliott, MD
A. L. Chatterton; 912 pages.
The author, a teacher at the College of Homœopathic Medicine at Kansas City University, states he wrote the book to fully cover the field— "anatomy, physiology, pathology, and homœopathic therapeutics."

1897: *A PRACTICAL WORKING HANDBOOK IN THE DIAGNOSIS AND TREATMENT OF THE DISEASES OF THE GENITO-URINARY SYSTEM AND SYPHILIS*: George Parker Holden, MD
Boericke and Tafel; 441 pages.
An editing of the essays that first appeared as class notes by Francis E. Doughty, MD, during his lectures at New York Homœopathic Medical College. Dr. Doughty reviewed the manuscript before publication. A clinical work with only a suggestion of therapeutics.

1898: *RENAL THERAPEUTICS: INCLUDING ALSO A STUDY OF THE ETIOLOGY, PATHOLOGY, DIAGNOSIS, AND MEDICAL TREATMENT OF DISEASES OF THE URINARY TRACT*: Clifford Mitchell, MD
Boericke and Tafel; 365 pages.
A Clinical text. The majority of the therapeutics discussed are allopathic using orthodox (at the time) medicines. Dr. Mitchell wrote a number of texts concerning the urinary organs, *MANUAL OF URINARY ANALYSIS*, **1902**, 363 pages; *DISEASES OF THE URINARY ORGANS*, **1903**, 716 pages; *MODERN UROLOGY*, **1912**, 627 pages.

1898: *A PRACTICAL TREATISE ON THE SEXUAL DISORDERS OF MEN*: Bukk Carleton, MD
Boericke and Runyon; 169 pages.

1898: *MEDICAL AND SURGICAL DISEASES OF THE KIDNEYS AND URETERS*: Bukk Carleton, MD
Boericke and Runyon; 300 pages.
"Many professional friends have requested me to prepare and publish a practical working companion to my *Manual of Genito-Urinary and Venereal Diseases*…"
A second edition, with the new title *URIPOIETIC DISEASES* (384 pages) was published in **1900**. It included a section on disorders of the bladder.

1901: *PRACTICAL MEDICINE*: Frederic Mortimer Lawrence, MD
Boericke and Tafel; 521 pages.
"Intended for students, not advanced workers," the author concentrates on pathological processes rather than detail of morbid anatomy, "with the object of correlating the symptoms of the disease to the underlying changes." The book is, essentially, a condensed version of Goodno's two volumes.

1901: *PRACTICE OF MEDICINE CONTAINING THE HOMŒOPATHIC TREATMENT OF DISEASES*:
Dr. Pierre Jousset
A. L. Chatterton; 1115 pages.
Translated by J. Arschangouni. A clinical work. Based on the translation of the 2nd edition (**1877**) of the French work.

1902: *DISEASES OF THE LUNGS*: A. L. Blackwood, MD ✔
Halsey Brothers; 338 pages.

Blackwood wrote a number of similar books about the main organs, "Diseases of the Heart," etc.

1903: *DISEASES OF THE SKIN*: Henry M. Dearborn, MD ✔
Boericke and Runyon; 654 pages.
Detailed pathology of skin disorders. Homœopathic advice is limited to a single line or two, "study…" followed by a list of remedies. A good amount of the therapeutics involves topical applications or recommendations for exposure to "Roentgen Rays" (x-ray).

1903: *STEPPING STONES TO NEUROLOGY; A MANUAL FOR THE STUDENT AND GENERAL PRACTITIONER*: E. R. McIntyer, MD
Boericke and Tafel; 205 pages.
"The earnest requests, oft repeated and almost unanimous, coming from my students… that I put my lectures in book form is my apology for offering this little work to the profession." McIntyer taught Neurology at Dunham College in Chicago. "Homœopathic treatment is emphasized in all respects." The pathological explanations are followed by fairly well differentiated suggestions for remedy selection.

1905: *A TREATISE ON UROLOGICAL AND VENEREAL DISEASES*: Bukk G. Carleton, MD
Boericke and Tafel; 795 pages.
This work contains very detailed discussion of anatomy and pathophysiology of the urinary tract. The suggestions for therapeutics are, for the most part, allopathic, e.g., applications of iodine directly to the affected surface, with little homœopathy mentioned.

1909: *DISEASES OF THE PERSONALITY*: Th. Ribot
Boericke and Tafel; 142 pages.
Translated by P. W. Shedd. Originally published in France in **1884**, and published in England through several editions. Ribot was not a medical doctor nor homœopath; he was a psychologist and philosopher. This translation was made by Shedd because he believed that the material Ribot

offered was of great use to the homœopath. The minimal amount of therapeutics offered in the work are annotations by the translator, and *not* by the author. The ideas, in light of our current knowledge, make very interesting reading.

1910: *DISEASES OF THE DIGESTIVE SYSTEM*: E. O. Adams
Cleveland Homœopathic Publishing Co.; 349 pages.

1915: *PRACTICE OF MEDICINE*: Walter Sands Mills, MD ✔
Boericke and Tafel; 705 pages.
"Under 'treatment' I have referred to the generally accepted old school methods first. Finally I have added briefly the most frequently indicated homœopathic remedies…" In many cases, Mills simply says, "The homœopath will use the indicated remedy" with no further explanation.

While cleaning up at Boericke and Tafel in 1992, I found a number of books, wrapped in newspaper, still in the attic. They were unbound, not trimmed, and the boards (covers) had not been attached. A book bindery in the next block told me that whenever they had a sale of one of these books, they would have it finished at that time. There were about 70 copies of Mills' book in the attic. With this in mind, one might think that the publisher's sense of the market, and the actual market was quite different. It was not a big seller.

1916: *DISEASES OF THE NERVOUS SYSTEM*: John Eastman Wilson, MD
Boericke and Tafel; 682 pages.
Anatomy and pathology with a paragraph about possible therapeutics.

1917: *CLINICAL GYNÆCOLOGY*: James Craven Wood, MD ✔
Boericke and Tafel; 236 pages.

1923: *A TREATISE ON THE PRACTICE OF MEDICINE*: Clarence Bartlett, MD
Hahnemann Publishing, Philadelphia, PA; In three volumes. Volume 1, 743 pages; Vol. 2, 826 pages; Vol. 3, 676 pages.
A very detailed description of all conditions encountered in medical practice. Both conventional and homœopathic therapeutics are mentioned.

1929: *THE PRACTITIONER OTOLOGY*: Gilbert Palen, MD and Joseph Clay, MD
Boericke and Tafel; 240 pages.
A pathology text from the two main teachers of the subject at Hahnemann Medical College. Homœopathic therapeutics receives just a line or two.

Palen and Clay were professors of Otology at Hahnemann Medical College in Philadelphia.

1932: *DISEASES OF THE NOSE AND THROAT*: Joseph Clay, MD
Boericke and Tafel; 202 pages.

1991: *HOMEOPATHIC PEDIATRICS ASSESSMENT AND CASE MANAGEMENT*:
Randall Neustaedter, OMD ✔
North Atlantic Books; 337 pages.
A very complete work that contains excellent information on behavioral assessment, and emotional and physiological behavioral scales.

Pharmacy

Pharmacy

The grounding of homœopathic practice rests with the pharmaceutical substances used. Hahnemann, in his *Organon*, described the methodology for making the remedies and in his subsequent work, further discussed the process and the physical nature of the substance itself.

It is, obviously, important to document the processes through which the medicinal substances are derived. Within a short time of the birth of homœopathy, the first pharmacopœias were written. These outlined the pharmacy process and established standards which were to be followed in the production of homœopathic remedies.

While remedies made from minerals, salts, and elements can have their sources documented in conventional chemistry, those derived from plants (and animals) need to have detailed descriptions, of a visual and written nature. Some of the best "herbal botanicals" were spawned from homœopathy.

In 1805, Hahnemann published the results of his fifteen years of observation in his *Fragmenta de viribus medicamentorum positivis sive in sano corpore humano observatatis.* Text (269 pages), and index (470 pages), published in Leipzig. Between 1811 and 1832 his *Materia Medica Pura* and *Chronic Diseases* were published. In 1832 the first number of Stapf's journal *Archiv* was published. In all of these publications, general and special instruction was given for the preparation of remedies.

The first Dispensatory or Pharmacopœia was published by Dr. C. Caspari in 1825. Dr. Henry M. Smith, of New York, assembled a listing of the major homœopathic pharmacopœia published, and it was printed in the first few editions of the *Homeopathic Pharmacopoeia of the United States*. I have included most of the titles mentioned there.

A perusal of the listing will show that, for a while, there were *two* Pharmacopœia in the USA published simultaneously— *The American Homœopathic Pharmacopœia* and *The Homœopathic Pharmacopœia of the United States*.

There was a single factor that led to the two different references. This factor concerned the ability to create a uniform drug product.

For example, *The British Homœopathic Pharmacopœia* of 1882 developed a standard to measure the drug strength:

> "In every instance, the dry crude substance is to be taken as the starting point from whence to calculate its strength and, with very few exceptions, the mother tincture contains all the soluble matter of one gram of the dry plant in ten cubic centimeters of the tincture."

To develop the tinctures in this way, a sample of the plant must be weighed, then dried, and the amount of water the plant contains is figured as a proportion of the alcohol to the plant weight. All tinctures, made this way, have a drug strength of 1/10 or the equivalent of a 1X potency.

This methodology is quite different from that suggested by Hahnemann in the *Materia Medica Pura*, where he divided the plant remedies into "classes" depending on their moisture content. Class I is for "juicy plants" where the expressed juice is mixed with an equal part of alcohol, Class II has two parts of alcohol to three parts plant, Class III has two parts of alcohol to one part plant, and Class IV has five parts of alcohol to one part plant.

The American Homœopathic Pharmacopœia held to this Hahnemannian standard. When the American Institute of Homœopathy Committee on Pharmacopœia began to establish guidelines for its own book, it decided to adopt the British standard. The first *Homœopathic Pharmacopœia of the United States* was issued in 1897. Shortly after, the American *Homœopathic Pharmacopœia* printed the following:

> "[The British Pharmacopoeia] adopts the innovation of prescribing that the tinctures should contain in ten parts the soluble matter of one part of the dry plant. This rule if adopted, would necessitate a careful drying of all fresh plants in order to calculate their percentage of water. This, in our estimation, would needlessly complicate the process, it looks well enough in theory but is tedious and difficult of practical execution. In other respects this is a work

The Heritage of Homœopathic Literature

of great merit and bears evidence of very careful preparation and of high scholarship. In Dr. Schwabe's "Polyglotta" on the other hand, the rules laid down by Hahnemann for the preparation of the remedies are closely followed, and the remedies introduced after his time are brought under the same rules as far as practicable; however no descriptions of the plants are given, or of the chemical process. The *American Homœopathic Pharmacopœia* has been planned to include all medicinal substances used in homœopathy, either fully or partially proved, as well as others in actual use or occasional demand, to identify them accurately and concisely after the highest authorities, to give reliable working formulas for the preparation of the chemicals, and finally, to convert them into remedial agents in accordance with the rules laid down by Hahnemann."

Both books continued to be printed, but the 10th and final *American Homœopathic Pharmacopœia* was published in 1928. With the passage of the Food, Drug, and Cosmetic Act of 1938, *The Homœopathic Pharmacopœia of the United States* (HPUS) became the officially recognized manufacturing standard for homœopathic remedies.

With two Pharmacopoeia there was certainly a question as to which would become "official." It appears that there was an underlying power struggle between the physicians of the American Institute of Homeopathy and the manufacturing pharmacies. There was certainly a *sub rosa* political story behind it all. Jay Borneman remembers his pharmacist grandfather talking about the problems surrounding the adoption of the new standard.

Another casualty of homœopathy becoming "official" with the adaptation of the *HPUS*, was the dropping of all the older manufactured potencies from the pharmacy catalogs during the period of 1937-38. Until this time, a number of the pharmacies offered back stocks of potencies made by Jenichen, Swan, Fincke, Dunham, Lehrman, and others. After this date, no mention of older stocks were made, and the stocks themselves were lost, most likely discarded by the pharmacies.

Pharmacy

1825: *HOMÖOPATHISCHES DISPENSATORIUM FÜR AERZTE UND APOTHEKER*: Dr. C. Caspari
Baumgärtner, Leipzig; 67 pages.
"*Homœopathic dispensatory for medical doctors and pharmacists*." The first guide to making and dispensing the remedies. It was published as an expanded 2nd edition in **1828**.

1829: *HOMÖOPATHISCHE PHARMAKOPÖE FÜR AERZTE UND APOTHEKER Auch unter dem Titel Caspari's Homöopathisches Dispensatorium für Aerzte und Apotheker, worin nicht nur die bis jetzt bekannten, sondern auch die in Hofrath Hahnemann's neuestem Werke und die in Hartlaub und Trinks' Arzneimittellehre enthaltenen Arzneien aufgenommen worden sind. Herausgegeben von Dr. Franz Hartmann*: Franz Hartmann.
Baumgärtner, Leipzig; 144 pages.
"*Homœopathic pharmacopœia for medical doctors and pharmacists: Also under the title Caspari's homœopathic dispensatory for medical doctors and pharmacists, where not only the remedies known till now have been included but also the ones from Hofrath Hahnemann's newest work and the ones contained in Hartlaub and Trinks' Materia medica. Published by Dr. Franz Hartmann.*"
This was a 3rd edition of Caspari's work, and edited by Hartmann. The 4th edition was published by Baumgärtner in **1834** (164 pages); the 5th is unknown; the 6th edition in **1844** (241 pages); The 7th edition in **1852** (227 pages). A Latin edition was published the same year, and the 8th edition appeared in **1864** (108 pages).

1829: *DISPENSATORIUM HOMŒOPATHICUM*: Dr. C. Caspari
Baumgärtner, Leipzig; 58 pages.
Published in Latin.

1829: *ELEMENTI DI FARMACOPEA OMIOPATICA ESTRATTI DALLA MATERIA MEDICA DI S. HAHNEMANN*: Dr. Vincenzo la Raja
L'Esercizio della Clinica Omiopatica, Naples; 210 pages.
"Elements of the pharmacopœia extracted from the materia medica of Hahnemann." A second edition was published in **1838**.

1830: *MEDICAMENTORUM HOMŒOPATHICIS*: Dr. G. Widenmann.
Preparatio, Munich.

1834: *PHARMACOPŒIA HOMŒOPATHICA*: Frederick Foster Hervey Quin, MD
S, Higley, London; 165 pages.
Published in Latin.

1835: *PHARMACOPÉE HOMŒOPATHIQUE*: L. Noirot and Ph. Mouzin.
Djon and Paris; 460 pages.
This is incorporated in the second part of Jahr's *Manuel d'Homœopathique*.

1836: *AUSFÜHRLICHE BESCHREIBUNG SÄMMTLICHER ARZNEIGEWÄCHSE, WELCHE HOMÖOPATHISCH GEPRÜFT WORDEN SIND UND ANGEWENDET WERDEN. FÜR HOMÖOPATHIKER ZUR BENUTZUNG BEIM EINSAMMELN DER ARZNEIKÖRPER AUS DEM PFLANZENREICHE*: Eduard Winkler
Magazin fur Industrie und Literatur, Leipzig; 312 pages.
"Detailed description of all remedial plants which were homœopathically proved and are used. For homœopathicians to use when collecting the remedial bodies from the plant kingdom."

1836: *ABBILDUNGEN DER ARZNEIGEWÄCHSE WELCHE HOMÖOPATISCH GEPRÜFT WORDEN SIND UND ANGEWENDET WERDEN*: Eduard Winkler
Magazin fur Industrie und Literatur, Leipzig; 156 pages. 156 copper plates.
"Pictures of the remedial plants, which were homœopathically proved and are used."

1836: *HOMÖOPATHISCHE PHARMACOPÖE nach neuesten Erfahrungen der verschiedensten Thierärzte und Apotheker, enthaltend alle bis jetzt geprüfte und angewandte homöopatische, auch die von Dr. Lux potenzirten isopathischen Arzneistoffe*: Von Dr. A. Rollink
Adolph Reimann, Leipzig; 298 pages.
"Homœopathic pharmacopœia according to the most recent experiences of different veterinaries and pharmacists, containing all up to now proved and used homœopathic remedial substances, including the potentized isopathic remedial substances by Dr. Lux." Second edition in **1838**.

1838: *PHARMACOPOEA UNIVERSALIS, oder übersichtliche Zusammenstellung der Pharmacopöen. Mit einer Pharmacopöe der homöopathischen Lehre.*
Weimar.
"Pharmacopoeia universalis or lucid synopsis of the pharmacopœia. Together with a pharmacopœia of the homœopathic doctrine." In two volumes. This was the third edition. No record can be found of the first or second editions, nor of the author.

1840: *HOMÖOPATHISCHE ARZNEIBEREITUNGSLEHRE*: Joseph Benedict Buchner.
Verlag von George Franz, München; 419 pages.
"Homœopathic doctrine of the preparation of remedies." A second edition of 468 pages was published in **1852**.

1840: *NOUVELLE PHARMACOPÉE ET POSOLOGIE HOMOEOPATHIQUE OU DE LA PRÉPARATION DES MÉDICAMENTS HOMOEOPATHIQUES*: G. H. G. Jahr
J. B. Ballière, Paris; 328 pages.
A greatly revised edition was published in **1853**.

1842: *NEW HOMŒOPATHIC PHARMACOPOEIA AND POSOLOGY, OR THE MODE OF PREPARING HOMŒOPATHIC MEDICINES, AND THE ADMINISTRATION OF DOSES:* G. H. G. Jahr
J. Dobson; 306 pages.
Translated by James Kitchen, MD. The first pharmacopœia published in the United States.

1845: *HOMÖOPATHISCHE PHARMACOPOE in Auftrag des Central Vereins Homöopathischer Aerzte bearbeitet und zum Gebrauch der Pharmaceuten herausgegeben, mit einem Vorwort von Medicinalrath Dr. C. F. Trinks, Dresden und Leipzig:* Carl Ernst Gruner
Arnold, Leipzig.
"Homœopathic pharmacopœia, edited by order of the central union of homœopathic doctors and published for the use of pharmacists, by Carl Ernest Gruner, pharmacist in Dresden, with a preface of Medicinalrath Dr. C. F. Trinks, Dresden and Leipzig." A second edition "diligently revised and much extended" (259 pages) was printed in **1854**, and a third edition was published in **1864**.

1845: *HOMÖOPATHISCHE PHARMACOPOE:* De Horatiis.

1846: *HOMÖOPATHISCHE ARZNEIBEREITUNG UND GABENGRÖSSE:* Dr. Georg Schmid.
Braumüller u. Siedel, Vienna; 309 pages.
"Homœopathic preparation of remedies and size of doses."

1847: *NEUVA FARMACOPEA Y POSOLOGIA HOMEOPATICA, O MODO DE PREPARAR LOS MEDICAMENTOS HOMEOPATICOS Y DE ADMINISTRAR LAS DOSIS:* G. H. G. Jahr
Boix, Madrid; 340 pages.
The first pharmacopœia in Spanish.

1850: *NEW HOMŒOPATHIC PHARMACOPOEIA AND POSOLOGY; OR, THE MODE OF PREPARING HOMŒOPATHIC MEDICINES AND THE ADMINISTRATION OF DOSES:* G. H. G. Jahr and
C. E. Gruner
Radde; 359 pages.
"Compiled and translated from the German works of Buchner and Gruner and the French work of Jahr, with original contributions by Chas. J. Hempel, MD. "

1852: *FLORA HOMŒOPATHICA:* Edward Hamilton, MD ✔
H. Ballière, London; 523 pages.
Illustrations and descriptions of 66 medicinal plants used as homœopathic remedies. This is both a botany book, and a materia medica with information about the symptomatology of poisonings, and records of cases where the remedy was successfully employed, as well as a description of the homœopathic uses. The original book, issued in two volumes, contained beautiful hand-colored illustrations. The book was re-printed by the Faculty of Homœopathy in **1981**, as a limited edition, and has subsequently been reprinted in India.

1853: *NOUVELLE PHARMACOPÉE HOMŒOPATHIQUE, OU HISTOIRE NATULELLE ET PRÉPARATION DES MÉDICAMENTS HOMŒOPATHIQUES ET POSOLOGIE, OU DE L'ADMINSTRATION DES DOSES:* G. H. G. Jahr and A. Catellan.
J. B. Ballière, Paris; 436 pages.
"New homœopathic pharmacopœia, natural history and preparation of homœopathic remedies and posology, and administration of doses." The second edition of Jahr's 1840 work, "revised and extended" and included 135 pictures. Translated into Spanish in **1860** by D. Silverio Rodriguez Lopez; *NUEVA FARMACOPEA HOMEOPATICA*; 428 pages. A 3rd edition, of 436 pages and 144 pictures was published in **1862**.

1854: *CODEX DES MEDICAMENTS HOMŒOPATHIQUES OU PHARMACOPÉE PRATIQUE ET RAISONNÉE À L'USAGE DES MÉDECINS ET DES PHARMACIENS:* George P. F. Weber
J. B. Ballière, Paris; 440 pages.

1855: *HOMEOPATHIC PHARMACOPŒIA*: German Central Union of Homœopathic Physicians, edited by Carl Ernst Gruner
Arnold, Leipzig; 224 pages.
Authorized English edition. Translated from the second German edition.

1859: *BEKNOPTE HANDLEIDING, VOOR DE HOMEOPATHISCHE PHARMACIE*: F. Dorvault
J. Van Egrmond, Jr., Arnhem; 47 pages.

1860: *HOMÖOPATHISCHE PHARMACOPÖE*: Ludwig Deventer.
E. Gross, Berlin; 72 pages.
A second edition of 236 pages, was published by the author in **1876**.

1861: *MEDICAMENTA HOMOEOPATHICA ET ISOPATHICA OMNIA, AD ID TEMPUS A MEDICIS AUT EXAMINATA AUT USU RECEPTA*: Dr. H. Hagero.
Ernest Gunther, Lesnae; 192 pages.
"All homœopathic and isopathic remedies, in this time either proved or used." The first section on general preparations was translated into German by Edward Hahn, and is contained therein as an appendix.

1864: *REAL-LEXICON FÜR HOMÖOPATHISCHE ARZNEIMITTELLEHRE. Therapie und Arzneibereitungskunde. Nach seinen öffentlichen Vorlesungen an der Prager k. k. Universität und unter steter Angabe der neuern einfachen Heilmittel der physiologischen Schule*: Dr. med. Altschul
Fr. Aug. Eupel, Sondershausen; 450 pages.
"Real-Lexicon for the homœopathic Materia Medica. Therapy and preparation of remedies. From his public lectures at the university of Prague and by consequent listing of the recent simple remedies of the physiologic school: Dr. med. Altschul, editor."

1865: *HOMÖPATHISCHEN PHARMACOPOE AUFGENOMMENEN PFLANZEN*: Dr. H. Goullon.
W. Baensch, Leipzig; 443 pages. Full title: *Beschreibung der in der Homöpathischen Pharmacopoe aufgenommenen Pflanzen nebst dreihundert Tafeln naturgetreu colorirter Abbildungen, der Angabe ihrer Standorte, ihrer zur Verwendung kommenden Theile und ihrer Anwendungsweise sowie derjenigen ständigen Krankheitsformen, in denen sie sich heilkräftig erwiesen.*
"Description of the plants included in the homœopathic pharmacopœia with 300 pictures coloured according to nature, specification of their locations, their parts to be used and their ways of application as well as the constant forms of disease for which they have proven curative." A second volume included the 300 colored plates.

1870: *BRITISH HOMŒOPATHIC PHARMACOPŒIA.*
Published by the British Homœopathic Society, London; 336 pages.
Second edition (396 pages), printed in **1876**. Third edition (456 pages) was issued in **1882**.

1872: *PHARMACOPOEA HOMÖOPATHICA POLYGLOTTA*: Dr. Willmar Schwabe
Schwabe, Leipzig; 251 pages.
A pharmacopœia in several languages. Rendered into English by Suss-Hahnemann, MD, London. Adapted for France by Dr. Alphonse Noack, Lyons. Authorized by the homœopathic Central Union of Germany as the basic pharmacopœia. A second edition appeared in **1880** with further translations added by Dottore Tommaso Cigliano, Naples (Italian) and Spanish by Dr. Paz Alvarez, Madrid. The same year an English edition of 374 pages was printed by Boericke and Tafel.

1876: *UNITED STATES HOMŒOPATHIC PHARMACOPOEIA*
Chicago, Duncan Bros. 281 pages.

1878: *THREE LECTURES ON HOMŒOPATHIC PHARMACEUTICS*: Francis E. Boericke, MD
Boericke and Tafel; 50 pages.
The text of introductory lectures about homœopathic pharmacy, delivered to the students at

Hahnemann Medical College in Philadelphia. The author stated that these lectures were reprinted, not for pharmacists, but for the use of physicians.

Three wonderful lectures by a grand homœopath and pharmacist. They have oft been quoted and pieces reprinted in several of the old homœopathic journals.

1879: *LIST OF MEDICINES MENTIONED IN HOMŒOPATHIC LITERATURE*: Henry M. Smith
Smith's Homœopathic Pharmacy, New York; 160 pages.
A list of medicines, proven or unproven, that are mentioned in the homœopathic literature to date. It lists the natural order, synonyms, and official preparation. Although it is often listed as a source of provings, it is not.

c. 1880: *COMPANION TO BRITISH AND AMERICAN HOMŒOPATHIC PHARMACOPŒIAS, ARRANGED IN THE FORM OF A DICTIONARY*: Lawrence T. Ashwell
Keene and Ashwell, London; 200 pages.
A manual for chemists. The first *BRITISH HOMŒOPATHIC PHARMACOPOEIA* was issued in **1867**. In the preface to the 2nd edition, the author says that the first edition was sold out 12 months, and he waited for the 2nd edition of the *BRITISH HOMŒOPATHIC PHARMACOPOEIA* in **1883** to do his 2nd edition.

1882: *AMERICAN HOMŒOPATHIC PHARMACOPŒIA*
Boericke and Tafel; 523 pages.
The writing and printing was undertaken by Boericke and Tafel in an effort "to provide a reliable pharmacopœia to the profession." It went through 10 editions. The 2nd edition (511 pages) was edited by Joseph O'Connor, MD, and published in **1883**. The 3rd edition (521 pages) came in **1885**. The 4th in **1890**. The 5th (unknown date). The 6th (549 pages) in **1899**, the 7th in **1904**, the 8th in **1906**, the 9th in **1911**, and the 10th in **1928**.

1883: *MEDIZINAL PFLANZEN:* Hermann A. Köhler
Fr. Eugen Köhler and Nachf. Friedrich von Zezschwitz, Gera; 2000 pages. Full title: *Medizinal-Pflanzen in naturgetreuen Abbildungen mit kurzerläuterndem Texte. Atlas zur Pharmacopoea Germanica, Austriaca, Belgica, Danica, Helvetica, Hungarica, Rossica, Suevica, Nederlandica, British Pharmacopoeia, zum Codes Medicamentarius, sowie zur Pharmacopoeia of the United States of America.*
Edited by Gustav Pabst. Published from 1883-1898 as three volumes with 283 detailed illustrations by L. Müller and C.F. Schmidt, which were skillfully rendered by K. Gunther in chromolithography (the process of rendering images on stone or zinc plates, then inking them with color inks to yield color pictures). A review said, "From the botanical standpoint the finest and most useful series of illustrations of medicinal plants."

As pointed out by one of my proof-readers, this book "has nothing to do with homœopathy." It does, however contain excellent pictures of most of the plants used in the homœopathic materia medica, and has been a source of images for purposes of identification.

1884: *AMERICAN HOMŒOPATHIC DISPENSATORY:* Theo D. Williams, MD
Gross and Delbridge; 698 pages.

1884: *AMERICAN MEDICINAL PLANTS*: Charles F. Millspaugh, MD ✔
Boericke and Tafel; 806 pages.
First published in six parts by pre-paid subscription, it was published as a complete book in **1887**. This huge quarto-sized book was profusely illustrated with full size color plates of plants found in America, drawn *in situ*, by the author. The book details the botanical description of the plant, the method of tincture preparation, the chemical structure of the major active ingredients, and accounts of poisonings and cures. The book is inscribed to the author's father, "to whom I am

indebted for whatever I may possess of art in drawing and coloring," and to "Timothy F. Allen my honored professor and preceptor." The book was re-issued by Dover Publications in **1974**, in reduced dimensions and with only gray-scale illustrations.

In 1980 I found an original copy in good shape, but the boards were coming loose. I had it repaired. I paid $35 for it, and paid $15 for the repair. The last copy I saw for sale had a price of over $1,000. Needless to say this book sits in an honorable place in my library!

1893: *DIE PFLANZEN DES HOMÖOPATHICHEN ARZNEISCHATZES:* Dr. A. von Villers and F. von Thümen.
Wilhelm Baensch Königlich Sächsische Hofverlagbuchhandlung, Dresden.
"The plants of the homœopathic remedial treasure." Edited for medical content by Dr. A. von Villers, botanical illustrations by F. von Thümen. Three volumes, comprising 200 colored illustrations.

I found a copy of the book in poor repair in a used book store. It was only the third volume, but that was the one containing the illustrations. Water damage had caused the loss of a few of the colored plates at the beginning, but the majority of the plates were salvageable. The text portion of the book, sorry to say, was never located.

1897: *THE PHARMACOPŒIA OF THE AMERICAN INSTITUTE OF HOMEOPATHY*: The Committee on Pharmacopœia of the American Institute of Homœopathy
Otis Clapp; 674 pages.
The work of a committee to establish uniform standards with the *British Homœopathic Pharmacopœia*. The second edition was published in **1902**.

1898: *PHARMACOPÉE HOMŒOPATHIQUE FRANÇAISE:* Edited by Drs. Marc Jousset and Vincent Leon-Simon.
J. B. Baillière, Paris; 400 pages.

1901: *DEUTSCHES HOMÖOPATHISCHES ARZNEIBUCH*: Auf Veranlassung des Deutschen Apotheker-Vereins bearbeitet von einer Kommission von Hochschullehrern, Aerzten und Apothekern.
Berlin. 288 pages.
"At the insistance of the German Union of pharmacists, edited by a commission of teachers of universities, medical doctors and pharmacists." The German Homœopathic Pharmacopœia.

1914 : *THE HOMŒOPATHIC PHARMACOPŒIA OF THE UNITED STATES*: The Committee on Pharmacopœia of the American Institute of Homœopathy
Otis Clapp; 674 pages.
A re-naming of the *Pharmacopœia of the AIH*, of which this is the 3rd edition. The 4th edition, with 680 pages, was published in **1936**. With the passage of the Food, Drug, and Cosmetic Act in 1938, this book became the "sole authority" under the new law. The printing was sold out and the 5th edition was printed in **1938**. A 6th edition was printed in **1941**.

1964: *THE HOMŒOPATHIC PHARMACOPŒIA OF THE UNITED STATES*: The Committee on Pharmacopœia of the American Institute of Homœopathy
Boericke and Tafel and Ehrhart and Karl; 718 pages. The 7th edition.

1974: *COMPENDIUM OF HOMEOTHERAPEUTICS:* Wyrth Post Baker, MD, editor
American Institute of Homeopathy, Falls Church, VA; 117 pages.
An addendum to the *Homœopathic Pharmacopœia of the United States*. This spiral bound book was issued to provide a listing (and legitimacy) to a number of drugs which did not appear in the 7th edition of the *HPUS*. Note that in the introduction, the older use of preparation classes is maintained.

This is a very rare volume.

The Heritage of Homœopathic Literature

1979: *THE HOMŒOPATHIC PHARMACOPŒIA OF THE UNITED STATES*: The Committee on Pharmacopœia of the American Institute of Homœopathy
American Institute for Homeopathy, Falls Church, VA; 719 pages.
The 8th edition.

1982: *HPUS SUPPLEMENT A*
Homeopathic Pharmacopoeia Convention of the United States (HPCUS); 80 pages.
This was considered the first supplement to the 8th edition of the *HPUS*. It contained the bylaws of the organization and the general pharmacy procedures.

1990: *A FIELD GUIDE TO MEDICINAL PLANTS*: Steven Foster and James A. Duke
Houghton Mifflin Co., Boston; 366 pages.
One of the many "Peterson Field Guides," this work is devoted to the medicinal plants of the eastern/central states of the USA, an area where a goodly number of homœopathic sources are found.

Another book that isn't "homœopathic," yet it is an excellent modern reference work for use in the identification of medicinal plants.

1991: *THE HOMŒOPATHIC PHARMACOPŒIA OF THE UNITED STATES, REVISION SERVICE*:
Homeopathic Pharmacopoeia Convention of the United States ✔
HPCUS, Washington, DC.
The three prior texts (The *Compendium*, The *HPUS* 8th edition, and the *HPUS Supplement A*) have been combined into a single document that, for the purposes of law, supersedes them all. The official abbreviation is *HPRS*. Because it is continuously updated, it is offered in a loose-leaf format held in a ring binder. Updated pages are available on a subscription basis. The monographs consist of all the information needed to identify and manufacture the named remedy.

1994: *HPUS ABSTRACTS 1994*: Homeopathic Pharmacopoeia Convention of the United States
HPCUS; 78 pages.
This publication contains all the information in the HPRS minus the monographs: Criteria for eligibility, guidelines for drug provings, protocol for drug provings, guidelines for clinical verification, monograph review procedure, sample monograph, general pharmacy procedures, good manufacturing procedures, labeling guidelines, and a table of alcohol strength, manufacturing classes, and dispensing potencies for monographs recognized by the HPCUS. It was updated in **1997** when there were 1,261 monographs. "The Abstracts are provided only as a convenient and economic alternative to subscribers who do not require the complete Revision Service."

1995: *ENCYCLOPEDIA OF HOMEOPATHIC PHARMACOPOEIA* Volume 1: P. N. Verna ✔
Jain; 1103 pages. Volume 2, 909 pages, was printed in **1997**.
A "comprehensive book of standards." Includes the information from the US, Indian, and German Pharmacopœias.

While these books would not be sufficient for manufacturing purposes in the USA, the information they contain is otherwise useful, and the price is certainly right!

1997: *HOMEOPATHIC PHARMACY: AN INTRODUCTION AND HANDBOOK*:
Stephen Kayne, MRPharmS ✔
Churchill Livingston, New York; 236 pages.
"This book gives every pharmacist the broad information they need to be able to dispense and counter-prescribe homœopathic remedies with confidence."

A fascinating work that presents homœopathy to those with an allopathic-slant on things. It not only explains the pharmacy issues and defines all things like "nosodes" and "isodes," but it presents a good overview of prescribing methods (first-aid, acute, constitutional, complexist). It has a very good chapter on research.

Popular Books

Popular Books

These books are quite different from domestic manuals. They are aimed at an audience of people who know nothing of homœopathy (be they lay-folks or medical professionals), and thus are intended to offer a basic introduction. Although they usually give case examples and discuss the unique nature of homœopathic pharmacy and methods of dosing, they never give explicit instructions as to how to use the medicines. It is this lack of specific instruction that separates them from domestic manuals.

The first book published in English in the USA was a popular broadside. It is interesting to note that in Germany, after Bönninghausen assembled the first repertory, he authored the first full book aimed at the public. Sorry to say, it has never been translated into English.

While there were a number of domestic manuals issued during the 1800s, there were very few popular books issued at that time. The major book in this category, *Sharp's Tracts*, was issued continuously from its release in the early 1850s through a 14th edition by Boericke and Tafel in 1894.

It is only, it seems, when homœopathy was close to disappearing that books about its successes began to appear. There were very few offered during the 1950s, and it was not until the resurgence of homœopathy in the late 1970s that a new crop of popular books begin to blossom.

Popular books

1825: *THE CHARACTERISTICS OF HOMŒOPATHIA*: Hans Burch Gram, CML
Private printing, New York; 24 pages.
This was the first publication on homœopathy in the United States. It was a translation of Hahnemann's essay, "The Spirit of Homœopathy." Says Bradford, "It was written in such imperfect and obscure German-English that few were able to understand it."

This was distributed free. Bradford mentions that Dr. Smith has a copy in his library and "it is almost, if not quite, unique." I know of the existence of two copies of this work, one in a library in New York City, and another in the collection of William Kirtsos.

1834: *HOMŒOPATHY— A TEXT-BOOK FOR THE EDUCATED, NON-MEDICAL PUBLIC*:
C. von Bönninghausen
Coppenrath, Münster; 284 pages.
"Die Homöopathie— ein Lesebuch für das gebildete, nicht-ärztliche Publikum "
Never translated into English, this was the first book about homœopathy aimed at the public. It includes a biography of Hahnemann, the principles of the system, the smallness of the dose, using homœopathy to help intoxications, understanding the method and reason for case taking, and advice about the "homœopathic diet."

1835: *A POPULAR VIEW OF HOMŒOPATHY*: Rev. Thomas R. Everest
Academical Bookstore; 75 pages.
The first printing was done in England in **1834**. The book was again published by Radde in **1842**.

The Rev. Everest was a personal friend of Hahnemann, learned homœopathy from him, and was responsible for much of the spread of homœopathy in England. While F. F. H. Quin was working on bringing homœopathy to the medical profession, the good Reverend was introducing it to the lay community.

1842: *PRACTICAL ADVANTAGES OF HOMŒOPATHY, ILLUSTRATED BY NUMEROUS CASES*:
Harris Dunsford, MD
Pennington, Philadelphia; 201 pages.
Dedicated to Queen Adelaide, this is an early work outlining the advantages of the homœopathic system. Published simultaneously in England.

1845: *VIEWS ON HOMŒOPATHY; WITH REASONS FOR EXAMINING IT AND ADMITTING IT AS A PRINCIPLE IN MEDICAL SCIENCE*: Daniel Holt
J. H. Benham, New Haven, CT; 48 pages.

1852: *SHARP'S TRACTS ON HOMŒOPATHY*: William Sharp, MD
Radde; 232 pages.
These are a re-print of the London edition. There were 12 tracts offered at 5 cents each. They were used by physicians to educate their patients (or other physicians). The volumes were: 1. What is Homœopathy? 2. The Defense of Homœopathy. 3. The Truth of Homœopathy. 4. The Small Doses of Homœopathy. 5. The Difficulties of Homœopathy. 6. The Advantages of Homœopathy. 7. The Principles of Homœopathy. 8. Controversy on Homœopathy. 9. Remedies of Homœopathy. 10. Provings of Homœopathy. 11. Single Medicines of Homœopathy. 12. Common Sense of Homœopathy. The 14th edition was printed by Boericke and Tafel in **1894**. They were eventually bound into a single volume, "being worthy of a less ephemeral dress than that afforded in pamphlet form."

1863: *DIE THERAPIE UNSERER ZEIT*: Wilhelm Stens
Gupel, Sonderhausen, Germany; 283 pages.
Translated by Henry St. Clair Massiah, and published in England as *THERAPEUTICS OF THE DAY* by Wortheimer, London, **1863**, 344 pages. Stens was the physician to the Austrian Monarchy. The English edition was dedicated to William Leaf, a merchant who was an early pupil of Hahnemann.
The book is a comparison of the two systems of medicine that will show, as the translator says, "…the very foundations of Allopathy are rotten to the core."

1899: *HOMŒOPATHIC PAMPHLET SERIES*: F. M. Adams, MD
F. M. Adams, Boston, MA. Published later by Boericke and Tafel.
No. 1: What is Homœopathy. 2. Evidence of the Truth of Homœopathy. 3. (unknown) 4. Hahnemann. 5. What Homœopathy Has Accomplished.

1905: *HOMŒOPATHY EXPLAINED*: John H. Clarke, MD ✔
Homœopathic Publishing Co.; 212 pages.
"The object of this work is to put the facts of the case before the public, and before those members of the profession who have not closed their intelligence at the bidding of the goddess Authority."

1925: *HOMŒOPATHY: A PAMPHLET FOR THE PEOPLE*: American Foundation for Homeopathy
AFH, Baltimore, MD; 30 pages.
The American Foundation for Homeopathy was founded in 1922, and its bylaws called for it to "promote homœopathy." They supported a bureau of education (for physicians), a bureau of research, a bureau of publicity, and a bureau of publications. This small pamphlet was the first outreach they offered to stimulate interest in homœopathy.

1931: *MIRACLES OF HEALING AND HOW THEY ARE DONE: A NEW PATH TO HEALTH*:
J. Ellis Barker ✔
Homœopathic Publishing Co.; 401 pages.
Stories about homœopathy, its philosophy, and examples of cases taken from the literature.

1934: *NEW LIVES FOR OLD: HOW TO CURE THE INCURABLE*: J. Ellis Barker ✔
John Murray, London; 372 page.

1939: *MY TESTAMENT OF HEALING*: J. Ellis Barker ✔
John Murray, London; 344 pages.

J. Ellis Barker was a lay practitioner in Great Britain. A good friend of a number of homœopathic physicians, he assumed editorship of The Homœopathic World *when Clarke died, and changed its name to* Heal Thyself.

The three books above are all well worth reading. They contain much information gleaned from the work of others (Hahnemann, Kent, Farrington, Guernsey, and others are liberally quoted) and also a number of Barker's cases— all filled with clinical gems.

1946: *MAGIC OF THE MINIMUM DOSE*: Dorothy Shepherd, MD ✔
Homœopathic Publishing Co.; 269 pages.
Followed in **1949** by another 350 pages in *MORE MAGIC OF THE MINIMUM* DOSE.

Two wonderfully written, chatty narratives about the author's experiences with homœopathy. Although it is simply a group of stories about wonderful cures, buried within are some useful clinical tips.

c. 1945: *THE MIRACLE OF HOMŒOPATHY: A Live Explanation of What Homœopathy is and What it Means to Your Health*: C. Frazer McKenzie
Homœopathic Publishing Co.; 108 pages.

A very "British" ramble about homœopathy.

1946: *A QUALIFYING COURSE FOR LAYMEN*: American Foundation for Homeopathy (AFH)
AFH; 32 pages.
A small booklet discussing the principles of homœopathy and discussing why the homœopathic physician does what he does, and how one can determine how to select a good homœopathic physician.

The AFH always maintained that the practice of homœopathy (i.e., the giving of medicines) was a skill reserved for the physician. The job of the layman was to understand how to find a good homœopathic physician and how to cooperate with the physician to achieve the best homœopathic care. This small book was aimed as a study guide for study groups.

1949: *A PHILOSOPHY OF HEALING AND A PRACTICAL PRESENTATION OF HOMŒOPATHIC PRINCIPLES*: Frank Watt
C. W. Daniels; 61 pages.
"My purpose in writing this little book is to endeavour, so far as is in my power to do so, to place before the homœopathic public and others who may be interested that knowledge which will enlighten them a little in pure homœopathic philosophy."

1952: *THE PLACE OF HOMŒOPATHY IN MODERN MEDICINE*: Elinore Peebles
American Institute of Homeopathy, Falls Church, VA; 19 pages.
A short introduction to the principles written by a Boston lay person.

Elinore Peebles, along with Arthur M. Green, ran the Homœopathic Information Service, a group dedicated to spreading the word of homœopathy at a time when homœopathy was in decline. Peebles was one of the few non-physicians who was given an honorary membership in the AIH.

1955: *HOMŒOPATHY: A RATIONAL AND SCIENTIFIC METHOD*: A. Dwight Smith, MD ✔
Published by the author, Glendale, CA; 64 pages.

1958: *WHO IS YOUR DOCTOR AND WHY?*: Alonzo Shadman, MD
House of Edinboro, Boston; 440 pages.
The book included six of the nine books of Tyler's *POINTERS TO THE COMMON REMEDIES*. It was republished in paperback by Keats, New Cannan, CT in **1980**.

A magnificent journal written by a physician who graduated medical school as a homœopath in 1905, lived through the decline of homœopathy, and treated patients during the polio epidemic of 1955. A personal journey of 55 years of practice by a grand homœopath. A great read!

1971: *HOMEOPATHY: MEDICINE OF THE NEW MAN*: George Vithoulkas
Kouros Publishing, San Francisco; 117 pages.
Written, essentially, by Alain Naudé, from discussions he had with George Vithoulkas. It was republished by Avon in **1972**. It was re-edited by Bill Gray, MD in **1979** and published by Arco. In **2001** it was republished under the title *HOMEOPATHY: MEDICINE FOR THE NEW MILLENNIUM*.

This was the book that opened up homœopathy in the United States. It was generally available in many book-shops and health-food stores. It was the book that a number of now practicing homœopaths credit with being the one thing that turned on the light for them. I recall that as I read it (it was the first book I read also!) I wondered about some of the cases from Hahnemann from around 1800 and questioned why there weren't more modern cases offered. As a beginning book, it was a great one for the 1970s, but today we have much better works to share with the curious.

1972: *HOMŒOPATHIC MEDICINE*: Harris L. Coulter , PhD
Formur, St. Louis, MO; 73 pages.
A well written and researched essay on homœopathy that discusses the homœopathic model of health and disease in contrast to the allopathic model.

Coulter's first published work on homœopathy, written as he was completing his first volume of Divided Legacy. *A concise and scholarly essay. It was intended as an introduction to the materia medica/repertory by Baker, Young, and Neiswander (1974) but was thought to be too long, and was not used in that work, but published on its own.*

1975: *WHAT IS HOMŒOPATHY?*: Kay Vargo
NCH, Falls Church, VA; 10 pages.
A transcript of a talk by Kay Vargo, the Director of the Division of Laymen of the National Center for Homeopathy. This small pamphlet was one of the primary pieces of literature that the NCH mailed in their information package, and made available for distribution in physicians' offices.

1976: *THE PATIENT NOT THE CURE: THE CHALLENGE OF HOMŒOPATHY*: Margery Blackie, MD ✔
Macdonald and Jane's, London; 247 pages.
A solid introduction to the principles of homœopathy, by the physician who served Queen Elizabeth II for a number of years. It is one of the few places one can find the tables compiled by Dr. Boyd of Glasgow that list the remedies according to their electro-physical properties as measured by Boyd's "emanometer."

A chatty exposition of homœopathy by an experienced prescriber. Many stories about her experiences in the London Homœopathic Hospital with some of the greats (Weir, Wheeler, Borland, etc.).

1980: *HOMŒOPATHY: QUESTIONS AND ANSWERS*: Karl Robinson, MD
Private, Albuquerque, NM; 16 pages.
A small pamphlet that answers some basic questions about homœopathy. Written by a practicing homœopath for his patients.

1980: *HOMŒOPATHIC REASONING*: Richard Moskowitz, MD
Published by the author, Santa Fe, NM; 18 pages.
A delightful little tome that Dr. Moskowitz offered to his patients. It was republished in **1981** (22 pages) by the National Center for Homeopathy.

1982: *THE COMPLETE BOOK OF HOMEOPATHY*: Michael Weiner, PhD and Kathleen Goss ✔
Bantam Books, New York; 299 pages.
This was the first, broad-market book about homœopathy. It discusses the history (with a good biography of Hahnemann), the principles, the remedies, and the practice— through several case studies from Hahnemann, Kent, and others.

Although it contains some minor errors of fact, this was a wonderful book. At the time it was printed, it was the

best general book on the subject, a far clearer exposition of homœopathy than the earlier *Medicine of the New Man*. *It was reprinted a number of years ago, but it has been out of print for at least ten years, and deserves to be up-dated and re-issued. It was a classic.*

1987: *CATCHING GOOD HEALTH WITH HOMEOPATHIC MEDICINE*: Ray Garrett
Carleton Press, NY; 138 pages.
A testimonial by a long-time user of homœopathy.

1987: *HOMŒOPATHY FOR EVERYONE: WHAT IT IS, HOW IT DEVELOPED, HOW IT CAN HELP YOU, WHERE YOU CAN FIND TREATMENT*: Drs. Robin and Shelia Gibson ✔
Penguin Books, Middlesex, UK; 223 pages.
An interesting view of homœopathy by two consultant physicians at the Glasgow Homœopathic Hospital. A good overview, with an emphasis on the integration of the spiritual, mental, emotional, and physical plane. The end of the book contains a brief materia medica.

1988: *HOMEOPATHY: MEDICINE FOR THE 21ST CENTURY*: Dana Ullman ✔
North Atlantic Books; 271 pages. In **1991** it was re-titled, *DISCOVERING HOMEOPATHY: MEDICINE FOR THE 21ST CENTURY*.
An overview of homœopathy—the history, pharmacy, philosophy, the research, and a brief explanation of the uses of homœopathy in various ailments.

Twelve years after it was written, this book remains a best-seller. The information is accurate and it presents a synthesis of homœopathy, behavioral science, and allopathic medicine.

1991: *EVERYDAY MIRACLES: HOMEOPATHY IN ACTION*: Linda Johnston, MD ✔
Christine Kent Agency, Van Nuys, CA; 256 pages.
Written by a practicing homœopath, this work places homœopathy into the larger context of understanding health and disease. The explanations are helped by a number of excellent written and illustrated analogies.

A very clear book that will appeal to both auditory and visual learning styles. When I first read it I found myself using my highlighter to underline certain passages and I found that I wanted to highlight almost everything! The explanations are a sheer delight and the ideas are well grounded and never get lost in the "mumbo-jumbo" ether.

1993: *HOMEOPATHY: AN INTRODUCTION FOR SKEPTICS AND BEGINNERS*: Richard Grossinger ✔
North Atlantic Books; 162 pages.
Derived from Grossinger's chapter about homœopathy in his 1980 book, *PLANET MEDICINE*, it was reissued, with some added material, in **1999** as *HOMEOPATHY: THE GREAT RIDDLE*.

The best of the larger introductions. The author carefully places homœopathy into its historical context, and explains how it conceptually differs from conventional medicine. Well written and clear as a bell, it is the first book I recommend to someone who wishes to understand homœopathy in a bit more depth than that given in shorter works.

1994: *WHAT THE HELL IS HOMEOPATHY*: Jacob Mirman, MD ✔
New Hope Publishers, Minnesota; 36 pages.
Republished in **1995** as *DEMYSTIFYING HOMEOPATHY: A CONCISE GUIDE TO HOMEOPATHY*.

1994: *HOMŒOPATHY UNVEILED: AN EXPLANATION OF HOW IT REALLY WORKS*:
Giri Westcott , RSHom (NA) ✔
Satyam Publishing, Napa, CA; 66 pages.

An intriguing title, but no explanation of the "mechanism" of how homœopathy "works" is forthcoming. A simple introduction with illustrations of a number of substances from which the remedies are derived.

1995: *THE COMPLETE GUIDE TO HOMEOPATHY*: Andrew Lockie, MD and Nicola Geddes, MD ✔
Dorling Kindersley; 240 pages.
A full-color book with pictures of the remedy sources and the common conditions they treat.

A "coffee-table" book, that brings homœopathic concepts to such a basic level that it does not serve homœopathy well. Included are a number of pictures of people whose countenance describes a "remedy": the hard-working Calcarea, *the driving* Nux vomica *businessman, etc. It includes a "questionnaire" that will let the reader self-assess their "constitutional type." Bringing homœopathy to this simplistic level demeans the skill needed to properly assess a "constitutional case," and brings the book into the realm of a "do-it-yourself" sun-sign astrology book. While figuring out your astrological profile can be harmless fun, taking a dose of a remedy because you look like that "type" has the potential to be harmful. It is this type of book that, frankly, scares the hell out of me. Buy it, if you must, for the pictures of the remedy sources, the processes, and the many beautiful bottles. Forget about the rest.*

1995: *HOMEOPATHY: BEYOND FLAT EARTH MEDICINE*: Timothy Dooley, MD, ND ✔
Timing Publications, San Diego, CA; 111 pages.

This is my favorite "quick guide." Clearly written, it explains the idea and the method.

1995: *PATIENTS GUIDE TO HOMEOPATHIC MEDICINE*: Judyth Reichenberg-Ullman, ND and Robert Ullman, ND ✔
Picnic Point Press, Edmonds, WA; 111 pages.
Written by two homœopaths, based upon the answers to the most frequently asked questions they received from their patients. An easy to read guide that offers explanations along with illustrative cases from their practice.

1996: *RITALIN FREE KIDS*: Judyth Reichenberg-Ullman, ND, and Robert Ullman, ND ✔
Prima Publishing, Rocklin, CA; 300 pages
"Safe and Effective Homeopathic Medicine for ADD and Other Behavioral and Learning Problems." Almost one in every thirty children take medication to control their attention deficit disorder (ADD) or other behavioral problems. The book discusses the dangers of conventional medication, what homœopathy is, and presents a series of cases from the authors' practice illustrating the successful use of homœopathy in cases of behavioral difficulty.
The book was followed by two others, *PROZAC-FREE* (**1999**), and *RAGE FREE KIDS* (**2000**).

1997: *LET LIKE CURE LIKE: THE DEFINITIVE GUIDE TO THE HEALING PROPERTIES OF HOMEOPATHY*: Vinton McCabe ✔
St. Martin's Press, NY; 320 pages.
The original volume contained a number of historical errors that were corrected in the second edition, renamed: *HOMEOPATHY, HEALING, AND YOU.*

1999: *PROZAC FREE*: Judyth Reichenberg-Ullman, ND, and Robert Ullman, ND ✔
Prima Publishing, Rocklin, CA; 300 pages
"Homeopathic Medicine for Depression, Anxiety, and Other Mental and Emotional Problems." The use of Prozac has become endemic in our society. It is the "happy pill" and is readily prescribed by physicians for a wide variety of complaints. It has also been used in veterinary medicine. The book discusses the dangers of conventional medication, what homœopathy is, and presents a series of cases from the authors' practice illustrating the successful use of homœopathy in cases anxiety and depression.

Critical Works

Critical Works

Since the birth of homœopathy, articles and books have appeared attacking it. Bradford lists 68 works in this category, written by 44 different authors, and that is only those books and broadsides published from 1825 to 1892.

The attack on homœopathy has continued through the present day. The books in the 1900s have often attacked "alternatives" in general (chiropractic, herbalism, osteopathy, mesmerism, Christian Science) rather than homœopathy specifically. Several of the most recent attacks have come from the evangelical right, claiming that homœopathy is "occult" and "the work of the devil," linking Hahnemann's membership in the Masonic Order as proof of the "occult" nature of the system.

Critical Works

1835: *REMARKS ON THE ABRACADABRA OF THE NINETEENTH CENTURY:* William Leo-Wolf
Cary, Lea, and Blanchard, Philadelphia; 272 pages.
Says Bradford, "This is the book that was to entirely overthrow the Homœopathic System of Medicine."

```
        A
        AB
        ABR
        ABRA
        ABRAC
        ABRACA
        ABRACAD
        ABRACADA
        ABRACADAB
        ABRACADABR
        ABRACADABRA
```

An "abracadabra" was the word arranged in a triangular pattern that, when worn, was supposed to prevent the wearer from catching the plague. The author of the book obviously saw homœopathy as similar; a useless attempt to fend off disease.

1838: *HUMBUGS OF NEW YORK*: David Meredith Reese
J. S. Taylor, New York; 267 pages.
Chapter IV is devoted to the annihilation of homœopathy.

1842: *HOMŒOPATHY*: Thomas W. Blatchford, MD
Rensselaer County Medical Society, New York; 16 pages.
Delivered as an address before the Medical Society, it was subtitled, "The Homœopathic System: a Germanic Reverie of Transcendental Nonsense." The pamphlet was re-printed in **1843** and **1851**.

1842: *HOMŒOPATHY AND ITS KINDRED DELUSIONS*: Oliver Wendell Holmes, MD
William D. Ticknor, Boston; 72 pages. See 1861.
Holmes created the myth that high potency homœopathic medicines need more water to create them than exists on the face of the earth, and many people have since re-quoted him on this. It seems that they never asked a homœopathic pharmacy to describe the process of making homœopathic medicines.

This is the work usually cited when criticism is called for, primarily because of its noted author. Holmes was on the faculty of Harvard Medical School, and was known as a brilliant lecturer, essayist, and novelist. He was the father of Oliver Wendell Holmes, Jr, who went on to become the Chief Justice of the United States. Said his contemporary Ralph Waldo Emerson, "Holmes is the best example I have seen of a man of as much genius, who had entire control of his powers, so that he could always speak or write to order: partly from the abundance of the stream, which can fill indifferently any provided channel." His best known medical essay was on "Puerperal Fever" (1843) in which he suggested that the contagion is spread from patient to patient by the physicians. This four years before Semmelweiss published the similar conclusions in Europe. Holmes' wit and sarcasm found a place in his essays about homœopathy.

1846: *HOMŒOPATHY, ALLOPATHY, AND THE YOUNG PHYSIC*: John Forbes, MD.
Lindsay and Blakiston, Philadelphia; 121 pages.

1850: *LESSONS FROM THE HISTORY OF MEDICAL DELUSIONS*: Worthington Hooker, MD
Baker and Scribner, New York; 105 pages.

1851: HOMŒOPATHY. AN EXAMINATION OF ITS DOCTRINES AND EVIDENCES:
Worthington Hooker, MD
Charles Scribner, New York; 146 pages.

1852: *THE TREATMENT DUE FROM THE MEDICAL PROFESSION TO PHYSICIANS WHO BECOME HOMŒOPATHIC PRACTITIONERS*; Worthington Hooker, MD
J. G. Cooley, Norwich, CT; 11 pages.

1854: *HOMŒOPATHY; ITS TENETS AND TENDENCIES, THEORETICAL, THEOLOGICAL, AND THERAPEUTICAL*; James Y. Simpson
Lindsay and Blakiston, Philadelphia; 304 pages.
The first American edition from the 3rd Edinburgh edition.

1861: *CURRENTS AND COUNTERCURRENTS IN MEDICAL SCIENCE*: Oliver Wendell Holmes, MD
Ticknor and Fields, Boston; 406 pages.
A collection of essays, including "Currents and Counter Currents in Medical Science" (1860); "Homœopathy and its Kindred Delusions" (1842); "Some More Recent Views on Homœopathy" (1857); "Puerperal Fever as a Private Pestilence" (1843); "The Position and Prospects of the Medical Student" (1844); "Mechanism of Vital Action" (1857); and "Valedictory Address" (1858).

The "Recent Views on Homeopathy" begins with a magnificently erudite commentary about Pulte's Domestic Physician: "The book… lies before us with its valves open, helpless as an oyster on its shell, inviting the critical pungent, the professional acid, and the judicial impaling trident. We will be merciful. This fat little literary mollusk is well conditioned, of fair aspect, and seemingly good of its kind. Twenty-four thousand individuals,— we have its title page as authority,— more or less lineal descendants of Solomon, have become the fortunate possessors of this plethoric guide to earthly immortality. They could have done worse; for the work is well printed, well arranged, and typographically credible to the great publishing house which honors Cincinnati by its intelligent enterprise. The purchasers have done very wisely in buying a book that will not hurt their eyes…"
Holmes then discusses the desire of the patient to ask for help and the progression from the "specifics" of the past to the current "science" of medicine into which homœopathy has stepped and taken a giant leap backward, away from rationality.
"Most scientific men see through its deception at a glance. It may be practiced by shrewd men and by honest ones; rarely, it must be feared, by those who are both shrewd and honest. As a psychological experiment on the weakness of cultivated minds, it is the best trick of the century."

1880: *HOMŒOPATHY: WHAT IS IT?*: A. B. Palmer, MD
Davis, Detroit, MI; 109 pages.
Written by The Dean of Medicine and Surgery at the University of Michigan Medical School at Ann Arbor.

Says Dr. J. C. Wood, "We of the Homœopathic Department had our own chair for the theory and practice of medicine and did not therefore come under his teachings, thank God… Twice a year he delivered to his classes lectures on homœopathy in which he stressed what he believed to be its absurdities and incongruities; on each occasion he 'buried' it to his own satisfaction beyond resurrection… often for the fun of it, following his lectures, one of them [his own students] would hand down a written question touching upon homœopathy just to see the fireworks."

1887: *THE PAST, PRESENT, AND FUTURE TREATMENT OF HOMŒOPATHY, ECLECTICISM, AND KINDRED DELUSIONS*: Henry I. Bowditch, MD.
Cupples, Upham and Co., Boston; number of pages unknown.

1932: *FADS AND QUACKERY IN HEALING*: Morris Fishbein, MD
Blue Ribbon Books, New York; 382 pages.
"An analysis of the foibles of the various healing cults, with essays on various other peculiar notions in the health field." Fishbein was the editor of the *Journal of the American Medical Association*, and a leader in its fight against medical quackery.

The book, denouncing all forms of quackery, contains chapters on Christian Science, Chiropractic, Osteopathy, Naturopathy, "Physical Culture," Diet, and Psychoanalysis, among others. There is a 10-page section about homœopathy that sees it as a historical failure, and most homœopaths as using conventional medicine. "It came down to this: that a homœopath was just like any other physician, except that he gave essentially nothing but placebo in minor conditions."

1985: *HOMEOPATHY*: H. J. Bopp
Great Joy Publications, Belfast; 16 pages.
Describes homœopathy as the work of the devil.

The first of the works from the evangelical right to see homeopathy as an ultimate evil in medicine.

1992: *A CONSUMER'S GUIDE TO ALTERNATIVE MEDICINE*: Kurt Butler ✔
Prometheus Books, Buffalo, NY; 299 pages.
Contains a chapter critical of homœopathy.

1994: *THE VITAMIN PUSHERS: How the Health Food Industry is Selling America a Bill of Goods*:
Stephen Barrett, MD and Victor Herbert, MD ✔
Prometheus Books, Amherst, NY; 536 pages.
Written by two leading "quackbusters" in the United States, this book contains a chapter on homœopathy called "The Ultimate Fake." The chapter begins: "Homeopathic 'remedies' enjoy a unique status in the health marketplace: they are the only quack products legally marketable as drugs." The section about homœopathic theory is titled, "Basic mis-beliefs."

1995: *HOMŒOPATHY: SOME THINGS ARE NOT WHAT THEY SEEM*: Branson Hopkins ✔
Jubilee Publishers, Wellington, NZ; 28 pages.
This book has had word-wide distribution. In the introduction, Dr. Tony Hanne says, "He [the author] demonstrates very well why homœopathic medicine is more than useless water. It is frankly dangerous because of the essentially spiritual, but not Christian, nature of the movement."

1999: *HOMOEOPATHY: WHAT ARE WE SWALLOWING?*: Steven Ransom ✔
Credence Publications, Cathedral City, CA; 120 pages.
Written by a quackbuster in the UK, the book trots out the usual subjects: The building of homœopathy upon a faulty experiment (the Cinchona trial), the outgrown of homœopathy as occult science through Hahnemann's involvement in Freemasonry, the numbers of proving symptoms credited simply to imagination, the unlikely action of a sub-molecular dose, etc.

This book serves as an excellent summary of all the arguments put forth by all the other references.

History

History

To write critically about history, one has to view it from a timely distance. Dudgeon, in his *Lectures on Theory and Practice* (1854), could only give the barest outline of homœopathy. He was still too close to its beginnings.

The problem with homœopathic history, is that little source material is written about contemporary practices. By the time someone gets far enough back to write a "history," there is not much material from which to glean any information.

Bradford did a major service by documenting the literature, hospitals, pharmacies, state laws, etc. in 1892, and King and Bradford collaborated to further this service with the four-volume *History of Homœopathy in America* in 1905. But similar efforts were not made in other countries as homœopathy developed.

By the time people began to become interested in the history, the sources of information had long since vanished.

Bradford and King were only a generation removed from Hering, and just two generations from Hahnemann. It was possible for them to glean information from many primary sources, just by asking. But how does one extract information about times when no one could care less about homœopathy and all of the journals, books, and personal records were making their way to the junk-pile?

Fortunately, there has been a resurgence in interest in homœopathic history. One hopes it is not too late to uncover the information that can give us a snapshot of the times and allow us to put together an important historical record.

History

1854: *LECTURES ON THE THEORY AND PRACTICE OF HOMŒOPATHY*:
Robert Ellis Dudgeon, MD ✔
Henry Turner; 565 pages.
A record of the lectures Dudgeon delivered to the Hahnemann Hospital School in London, 1852-53. Although this is a book on "Theory and Practice," it contains a very good account of Hahnemann's life, as well as numerous details about the historical development of potentization, and about the development of homœopathy in general.

This is an invaluable read. Unfortunately, the original was small in size and in typeface, and the Indian reproductions are difficult to read because of poor copying and printing. However, it is well worth the effort to go through it. It gives a record of thought by one of the best writers in the field, and from a time which was just ten years after Hahnemann's death. It is the unvarnished beginning.

1870: *ANNUAL: RECORD OF HOMŒOPATHIC LITERATURE*: Charles G. Raue, MD, editor
Boericke and Tafel; 416 pages.
Editions were published each year through **1875**. Raue was assisted in the assembly of these works by a number of others, and these works are an invaluable historical resource as a record of cases and provings. In 1875, Boericke and Tafel said they would cease publication unless there were 500 subscribers. The number was not obtained, and no further volumes appeared.

Although the books contain no written "history" per se, the 1870 volume contained a listing of all the homœopaths practicing in the USA (and several other countries) at that time.

1876: *TRANSACTIONS OF THE WORLD'S HOMŒOPATHIC CONVENTION UNDER THE AUSPICES OF THE AMERICAN INSTITUTE OF HOMŒOPATHY. VOL. 2. HISTORY OF HOMŒOPATHY*
Sherman, Philadelphia, PA; 1117 pages.
Volume 1 was the transactions of the 1876 Congress; Volume 2 was a summary of the history of

The Heritage of Homœopathic Literature

homœopathy in a large number of countries plus details about the history of homœopathy in the USA.

Stiff reading and not very accessible, but filled with information. The first effort to weave it all together.

1884: REJECTED: An Address Delivered Before the Massachusetts Homœopathic Medical Society and Rejected by the Publication Committee: A. M. Cushing, MD
Published by the author; 22 pages.
"We find something that is called Homœopathy is increasing, but is it Homœopathy?… When they call for and expect homœopathic treatment, we have no right to substitute quackery."

The address presented by Cushing was rejected for publication because it was said, it might be used against the homœopaths. Cushing printed it and distributed it so others could read his words. It is an obscure dialogue which shows what the education and practice of homœopathy was like in 1884.

1885: HISTORY OF HOMŒOPATHY: ITS ORIGINS; ITS CONFLICTS: Wilhelm Ameke
E. Gould; 445 pages.
Translated from the German by Alfred E. Drysdale and Robert Ellis Dudgeon, MD
The first published source of many of Hahnemann's letters. Part I describes Hahnemann the man, the chemist, the physician. Part II discusses the opposition to this new school of medicine.

1888: SEMI-CENTENNIAL CELEBRATION OF THE INTRODUCTION OF HOMŒOPATHY WEST OF THE ALLEGHENY MOUNTAINS: J. C. Burgher, MD
Homœopathic Medical Society of Allegheny County, Pittsburgh, PA; 72 pages.
The history of the area with 10 portrait engravings.

Old men with long beards.

1888: ODIUM MEDICUM AND HOMŒOPATHY: THE "TIMES" CORRESPONDENCE:
edited by John Henry Clarke, MD
Homœopathic Publishing Co.; 126 pages.
In 1887, a surgeon was suspended from a hospital because he was known to be friendly toward homœopathy. He took the case to court where it was decided for him and on the appeal, against him. This action resulted in Lord Grimthorpe writing a letter about the situation to *The Times*. The letter was published on December 24, 1887. The letter was answered by a staunch supporter of conventional medicine, and the ensuing dialog became a wonderful history of homœopathy and the social fabric in which it fits. *The Times* finally stopped publishing the ongoing dialog on January 20, 1888.

1892: HOMŒOPATHIC BIBLIOGRAPHY OF THE UNITED STATES, FROM THE YEARS 1825 TO THE YEAR 1891, INCLUSIVE: Thomas Lindsley Bradford, MD
Boericke and Tafel; 596 pages.
The first 356 pages are devoted to the literature: a listing of all books, pamphlets, valedictory addresses and lectures ever published, and a listing of all the journals, publishers, and libraries in the USA at the time. The second part of the book is a complete record of hospitals, sanitariums, schools, societies, pharmacies, and dispensaries in the USA.

This book is an invaluable resource to anyone considering researching homœopathy in the USA. Unfortunately, it ends in 1891. A bit more information was developed by King, with the help of Bradford, for the four-volume classic The History of Homœopathy in America, *in 1905, but after that work little was recorded. The book contains enough hints (e.g., "Henry M. Smith has the largest private homœopathic library in the United States") to make one aware of how much has been lost. Many of the books and pamphlets mentioned have never been seen by most homœopathic historians and librarians. Sadly, they exist simply in the record.*

1898: *HISTORY OF THE HOMŒOPATHIC MEDICAL COLLEGE OF PENNSYLVANIA; THE HAHNEMANN MEDICAL COLLEGE AND HOSPITAL OF PHILADELPHIA*: Thomas Lindsley Bradford, MD
Boericke and Tafel; 904 pages.
The complete history of the school until that date. Well documented as only Bradford could do.

More details than one can ask for. The details of the split in 1867 and the merger in 1869 are especially interesting. It takes the history right up through the time when the education was becoming more and more allopathic.

1900: *AN HISTORIC SKETCH OF THE MONUMENT ERECTED IN WASHINGTON CITY (The History of the Hahnemann Monument)*: Rev. B. F. Bittinger
Putnam, Washington, DC; 153 pages.
A detailed record of the Hahnemann Monument at Scott Circle, from the beginning of the AIH Committee in 1893 to the dedication of the monument on June 21st, 1900.

The AIH was able to raise $75,000 in funds for the construction of the monument. The majority of the funding was raised in a four year period. This at a time when a good suit cost $5. The book lists the 2544 donors to the monument. Some donations were as little as ten cents. The largest donation came from Nancy T. Williams, MD of Augusta, Maine, who contributed $4,510— an impressive amount of money at the time. She said it all came from her income gained by putting the laws of Hahnemann into practice.

1900: *THE LOGIC OF FIGURES OR COMPARATIVE RESULTS OF HOMŒOPATHIC AND OTHER TREATMENTS*: Thomas Lindsley Bradford, MD
Boericke and Tafel; 212 pages.
A detailed comparison of mortality rates in hospitals and in medical practices throughout the world. The book discusses mortality figures in general, and specifically those for cholera, yellow fever, pneumonia, typhus, and diphtheria. The advantage of homœopathic treatment is clearly shown.

1904: *ARE WE TO HAVE A UNITED MEDICAL PROFESSION*: Charles S. Mack, MD
Private, La Porte, IN; 44 pages.
A vaguely written statement about the possibilities and benefits of uniting with the allopathic school.

1905: *HISTORY OF HOMŒOPATHY AND ITS INSTITUTIONS IN AMERICA*: William Harvey King, MD
Lewis Publishing Co., New York; 1670 pages in four volumes.
Volume I contains detailed histories of homœopathy in each state. Volume II and III present the history of each homœopathic school, including a listing of faculty for each term, and a full list of graduates up until 1905. The last 126 pages of Volume III, and all 409 pages of Volume IV are devoted to biographies of well over 1,600 homœopaths who were currently in practice.

This reference has it all, and in more detail than you might want to know. Much of it was written by T. L. Bradford. These volumes are rare and hard to find. The last set I saw for sale was in June, 2000, and the price was $900. These are invaluable works for the historian.

1910: *MEDICAL EDUCATION IN THE UNITED STATES AND CANADA: A REPORT TO THE CARNEGIE FOUNDATION FOR THE ADVANCEMENT OF TEACHING*: Abraham Flexner
The Carnegie Foundation, New York City, NY; 346 pages.
The "Flexner Report." The work many say was the cause for the closing of the homœopathic schools.

Although there is some anti-homœopathy bias, the level of reporting is very even and factual. It is a survey of ALL medical schools operating in the USA in 1909. Full details are provided on each school including the number of pupils, number of faculty, physical facilities, admission requirements, etc.

1913: *EDUCATIONAL REPORT OF THE COUNCIL ON MEDICAL EDUCATION:* AIH
AIH; 35 pages.
Another 13-page report was issued **1915**.

The Heritage of Homœopathic Literature

1916: *HOSPITALS AND SANITARIUMS OF THE HOMŒOPATHIC SCHOOL OF MEDICINES*
AIH; 128 pages.
Photographs of all homœopathic hospitals, with documentation as to number of beds, staff, etc.

An invaluable record of what we had.

1923: *AMERICAN HOMŒOPATHY IN THE WORLD WAR*: Frederick M. Dearborn, MD
AIH, Chicago, IL; 447 pages.
A record of the homœopathic doctors and nurses who were part of the armed forces during the First World War. Profusely illustrated with portraits and biographies of individuals, as well as a history of each unit.

More information in more detail than one could ask for. The biographies are brief, but there are a few pictures of homœopaths that can be seen nowhere else. There is a great portrait of H. A. Roberts in full uniform.

1927: *THE PRESENT-DAY ATTITUDE OF THE MEDICAL PROFESSION TOWARDS HOMŒOPATHY*: John Weir, MD
John Bale, Sons & Danielson, Ltd, London; 23 pages.
The Presidential Address of Weir to the British Homœopathic Society in 1926. An exposition of the history of the problems between allopathy and homœopathy.

1937: *THE METROPOLITAN HOSPITAL*: Frederick M. Dearborn, MD
Private; 351 pages.
A history of the Metropolitan Hospital on New York Ward's Island.

Metropolitan Hospital was the public hospital for the City of New York. It was an outgrowth of the Asylum for the Inebriated and the Charity Hospital on Ward's Island— an island in the East River between Manhattan and Queens. The Metropolitan Hospital was chartered as a homœopathic institution. Homœopathy ceased being used in the 1920s and today the island is home to a complex of buildings housing the New York Psychiatric Hospital.

1939: *GESCHICHTE DER HOMÖOPATHIE*: R. Tischner
Schwabe, Leipzig; 837 pages.
An extensive history of homœopathy, especially of German homœopathy. Includes many biographies.

1949: *ROYAL LONDON HOMŒOPATHIC HOSPITAL CENTENARY*
Royal London Homœopathic Hospital; 24 pages.

1965: *THE GIFT THAT GREW. THE HISTORY OF THE GENESEE HOSPITAL*: Anonymous
Rochester, NY; 84 pages.
The Rochester Homœopathic Hospital was incorporated in 1887. It was founded by Mrs. Hiram Sibley, wife of the founder of Western Union. It changed its name in 1926 to Genesee Hospital because "…any distinction between medical schools of thought no longer existed."

There is no mention of the Hahnemann Hospital in Rochester which was founded two years later (1889) by the Hahnemannian physicians who had seceded from the main body of Rochester's many homeopaths.

1967: *ONE HUNDRED YEARS OF MEDICAL PROGRESS: A HISTORY OF NY MEDICAL COLLEGE AND FLOWER HOSPITAL*: Leonard Paul Wershub
Charles C. Thomas, Springfield, IL; 259 pages.
The first half of the book traces the history of the New York Homœopathic Medical College and Flower Hospital. The second half is the history of the school after it abandoned the teaching of homœopathy in the late 1920s.

1971: *HOMEOPATHY IN AMERICA: THE RISE AND FALL OF A MEDICAL HERESY*:
Martin Kaufman, PhD
Johns Hopkins Press, Baltimore, MD; 205 pages.
The published doctoral thesis submitted for the author's PhD at Tulane University in 1969. It was the first published work on the history of homœopathy in the USA since the King books in 1905.

Although Kaufman claims to have no bias for or against homœopathy, his basic starting point was that homœopathy was a heresy. The book was written just before the homœopathic resurgence in the USA, and ends on a note of gloom, predicting the demise of homœopathy within a decade or two. The work is historically accurate and well-researched, but there is an underlying sense that it is not quite an unbiased view of things.

1973: *DIVIDED LEGACY: A HISTORY OF THE SCHISM IN MEDICAL THOUGHT: SCIENCE AND ETHICS IN AMERICAN MEDICINE, 1800-1914*: Harris L. Coulter, PhD ✔
McGrath, Washington, DC; 546 pages.
Reprinted in **1982** by North Atlantic Books as *Divided Legacy: The Conflict Between Homeopathy and the American Medical Association, 1800-1914*. The first of four volumes.
Written as a doctoral thesis, it is well documented, and provides a much deeper view than the Kaufman work, although it stops in 1914 and, therefore, does not cover the long slide of homœopathy toward its possible demise. Coulter is not an impartial observer. He presents the material as well as he does because he understands homœopathy and has a strong commitment to it.
This is *the* history book and, although dry and scholarly, it is a must read for those interested in history. It served to place Coulter in the position of *the* homœopathic historian in the late 20th century.

This was the first homœopathic history book I read. I discussed it with the author shortly after I finished reading it. One discussion lead to another, and we became close friends. I consult it regularly and I always find new tidbits or perspectives on particular events. His writing is convincing and masterful. Certainly an important book to have and to read.

1973: *HOMŒOPATHIC INFLUENCES IN 19TH CENTURY ALLOPATHIC MEDICINE*:
Harris L. Coulter, PhD ✔
AIH, Washington, DC; 83 pages.
Some material from Volume III of *Divided Legacy*, greatly expanded. Documentation of how homœopathy contributed toward allopathic medicine, and a discussion of how homœopathic methodology was not given due credit.

1975: *DIVIDED LEGACY: A HISTORY OF THE SCHISM IN MEDICAL THOUGHT: THE PATTERNS EMERGE; HIPPOCRATES TO PARACELSUS*: Harris L. Coulter, PhD ✔
Weehawken Press, Washington, DC; 537 pages.
When Coulter wrote *Divided Legacy* in 1973, he saw it as the third volume in a series. This is the second written, but the first volume of the series— covering the beginning of the split between empirical and rational thought in the history of medicine.

Nothing to do directly with homœopathy, but serves to fully describe the background of the empirical and rational schools from which the division between homœopathy and allopathy eventuated. Dense to read, packed with information.

1975: *HOMŒOPATHY; THE FIRST AUTHORITATIVE STUDY OF ITS PLACE IN MEDICINE TODAY*:
Dr. G. Ruthven Mitchel
W. H. Allen, London; 200 pages.
"A science, old in time but immature in development, succeeding at last in breaking away from superstition and ignorance." Described as a book "for the layman and the physician," the author attempts to describe all there is about homœopathy: a history of the movement, a biography of Hahnemann, the spread of homœopathy to different countries, the principles of the practice, and the place of homœopathy within the context of medical practice in the UK at the time.

This is a formless, rambling work that attempts to cover everything and the result is that it does none of it well. I try to steer clear of "authoritative" works. I have no idea where the author obtained the information about homœopathy in other countries, but some of the dates he offers are in error, and that can only cast doubt upon accuracy of the rest of the book. For example, Bradford gives the date of the first Dutch translation of the Organon *as 1827. The first homœopaths were practicing in Holland in 1834. Dr. Mitchel gives the date of homœopathy being introduced in Holland as 1861.*

1977: *DIVIDED LEGACY: A HISTORY OF THE SCHISM IN MEDICAL THOUGHT. PROGRESS AND REGRESS: J. B. VAN HELMONT TO CLAUDE BERNARD*: Harris L. Coulter, PhD ✔
Weehawken Press, Washington, DC; 785 pages.

A continuation in the series. The perpetual struggle between empiricism and rationalism as reflected in the development of "western" medicine in Europe.

1983: *SOME NOTES AND OBSERVATIONS*: Julian Winston
National Center for Homeopathy; 43 pages.
A report on the status of homœopathy in the USA after the author visited physicians, study groups, clinics, and pharmacies during 1981-1982.

I took a sabbatical from my University teaching in 1981-82 and spent six months driving across the USA, visiting homœopathic practitioners, pharmacies, and study groups. The first part of the report discusses those I visited. The second part is my personal observations based on my experiences. The issues I outlined in 1982 are the same ones facing the homœopathic community today. The more things change the more they stay the same!

1984: *THE TWO FACES OF HOMŒOPATHY*: Dr. Anthony Campbell ✔
Jill Norman, London; 158 pages.
An exposition of the rise of homœopathy in Great Britain, and the "split" which happened as they divided between those who followed Hughes' mechanistic models and those who were influenced by the more metaphysical approach of Kent.

An interesting volume, but flawed by many assumptions and inaccurate details. Dr. Campbell says, for example, that Margaret Tyler came to the USA to study with Kent. This is decidedly untrue. Tyler, according to an obituary she wrote of Kent, said she corresponded with Kent, but they never met. In another place the author says that "Hering's Laws" were developed on "theoretical a priori *grounds." Hering clearly wrote that they grew from his clinical observations. The author's stress on the mystical underpinning of homœopathy through the Society of the Golden Dawn and the work of Swedenborg, seems as though he has an axe to grind. The chapter "Homœopathy and the Occult" has been the primary stepping stone for other writers, mostly those of evangelical beliefs, to assert that homœopathy is "occult" and "work of Satan."*

1988: *OTHER HEALERS: UNORTHODOX MEDICINE IN AMERICA*: Norman Gevitz, Editor ✔
Johns Hopkins Press, Baltimore, MD; 302 pages.
Contains a number of essays about alternative therapies. Of particular interest is the 25-page essay on homœopathy by Martin Kaufman titled, "Homeopathy: The Rise and Fall and Persistence of a Medical Heresy." The first two-thirds of the essay is a summary of his 1971 book. The last third is a description of the resurgence of homœopathy between 1971 and 1986.

Probably the most concise history of homœopathy in the USA written— all in about 18 pages.

1988: *HOMŒOPATHY AND THE MEDICAL PROFESSION*: Philip A. Nicholls, PhD
Croom Helm, Ltd., Beckingham, UK; 298 pages.
This work began as a doctoral thesis submitted in 1984. It is a history of homœopathy in Great Britain.

1989: *HER PREFERENCE WAS TO HEAL: WOMEN'S CHOICE OF HOMEOPATHIC MEDICINE IN THE NINETEENTH CENTURY UNITED STATES*: Kristen M. Mitchel
Private; New Haven, CT; 73 pages.
An unpublished thesis from the Department of History at Yale University.

Although never published as a book, this thesis contains a valuable history of the involvement of women in the homœopathic movement in the United States. It is known to most homœopathic researchers.

1990: *THE MAGICAL STAFF; THE VITALIST TRADITION IN WESTERN MEDICINE*: Matthew Wood ✔
North Atlantic Books; 209 pages.
 Reprinted as *VITALISM: THE HISTORY OF HERBALISM, HOMEOPATHY, AND FLOWER ESSENCES*.
A fascinating and well researched work that describes the vitalistic tradition as seen through the work of Hahnemann, Kent, Clarke, Burnett, and others. The book has beautiful portraits of the characters involved, drawn by the author.

1991: *UN LIVRE SANS FRONTIERES, HISTOIRE ET METAMORPHOSES DE L'ORGANON DE HAHNEMANN*: Jaques Baur
Editions Boiron, Lyon; 311 pages.
A history of the development of the *Organon* through its various editions and publications, written by the preeminent French homœopathic bibliophile.

1994: *DIVIDED LEGACY: TWENTIETH CENTURY MEDICINE: THE BACTERIOLOGICAL ERA*:
Harris L. Coulter, PhD ✔
North Atlantic Books; 776 pages.
The final book in the series. Less about homœopathy, and more about the rise of the drug companies and the double-blind clinical trial as the "gold standard."

The model of the empiric/mechanistic split that Coulter proposed in his first book can now be clearly seen in this volume, and becomes the underpinning of understanding the development of medicine from Hippocrates through the modern era where the mechanistic model is in complete control. Aside from some very pointed commentary by Coulter, this last volume is, essentially, collected writings of others; carefully assembled to show the result of over–reliance on the mechanistic model. It is a fascinating work which clearly shows how orthodox medicine arrived at where it is.

1995: *HOMŒOPATHY IN THE IRISH POTATO FAMINE*: Francis Treuherz, FSHom. ✔
Samuel Press, London; 138 pages.
A delightful little work whose focus is on a single incident in history, with materia medica of *Solanum tuberosum aegrotans*, the diseased potato.

1996: *WELTGESCHICHTE DER HOMÖOPATHIE: LÄNDER—SCHULEN—HEILKUNDIGE*:
Martin Dinges ✔
C. H. Beck; Munich; 445 pages.
A series of essays, prepared for a conference on the History of Medicine held at Stuttgart in 1995, discussing the history of homœopathy in several countries including Germany, Austria, Switzerland, Poland, Denmark, Holland, Belgium, Spain, Italy, Romania, Great Britain, USA, Canada, Brazil, and India. Unfortunately, no English translation of the German is available.

1998: *AN ALTERNATIVE PATH: THE MAKING AND RE-MAKING OF HAHNEMANN MEDICAL COLLEGE AND HOSPITAL OF PHILADELPHIA*: Naomi Rogers, PhD ✔
Rutgers University Press, New Brunswick, NJ; 349 pages.
An exposition of the history of this magnificent institution, founded in 1848 by Constantine Hering.

A detailed study of how homœopathy was first put aside and then eventually abandoned at the first homœopathic college in the USA. One of the reservations I have about the work concerns the author's understanding of

homœopathy. Although Ms. Rogers is a fine historian, she is not a homœopath in her heart. Some of the inner workings of the school, especially the split of the school in the 1867-69 period, are well outlined but only as factual material. The depth of the split had much to do with philosophical homœopathic issues and the personalities of those involved, and these are not discussed in the work, leaving us knowing what happened but not much depth in understanding why.

1998: *CULTURE, KNOWLEDGE, AND HEALING: HISTORICAL PERSPECTIVES OF HOMEOPATHIC MEDICINE IN EUROPE AND NORTH AMERICA*: Robert Jütte, editor ✔
European Association for the History of Medicine, Sheffield, UK; 338 pages.
A collection of essays.

1999: *HOMŒOPATHY BEFORE HAHNEMANN: THE FORGOTTEN MEN*: Ian Oliver ✔
Midas Graphics, London; 35 pages.
An essay about those who discussed the principle of similars before Hahnemann and who had prepared the groundwork for him.

An unfortunate title, because there was no "homœopathy" before Hahnemann. Although there were a few who experimented with the idea of similia similibus, the system that is homœopathy came only from Hahnemann, as did the word itself.

1999: *A VITAL FORCE: WOMEN PHYSICIANS AND PATIENTS IN AMERICAN HOMEOPATHY: 1850-1930*: Anne Kirschmann, PhD
Private, Rochester, NY; 373 pages.
An unpublished doctoral thesis from the Department of History at the University of Rochester.

A well documented look at the place of women in the homœopathic movement in the USA. I hope it gets printed.

1999: *THE FACES OF HOMŒOPATHY: AN ILLUSTRATED HISTORY OF THE FIRST 200 YEARS*: Julian Winston ✔
Great Auk Publishing, Tawa, New Zealand; 656 pages.
The first illustrated history since 1905. A narrative, containing 137 biographies, 365 illustrations, numerous anecdotes, and many personal reflections. The primary focus is homœopathic history in the United States and England. An appendix offers brief histories of homœopathy in each state and in 67 countries.

What can I say? It is my effort to "walk the walk and talk the talk." I hope the book will urge others to take up the call to document the history of wherever they are. If not, it slowly goes away, and then we are all the losers.

Biographies

Biographies

Considering how many homœopaths there have been in the last 200 years, the number of available biographies is exceedingly small.

Of the 32 books I have listed (which are about all the homœopathic biographies that exist as books) ten are entirely about Hahnemann, and four concern Hering. Although many shorter biographies appear as memorials or obituaries in journals, full biographies of any homœopathic luminaries are rare. Occasionally, books do contain short biographies of the author (the biographies of E. A. Farrington and Carroll Dunham in their respective *Materia Medica* comes to mind), but when wondering about the life of someone as influential as Kent, we are left with a few short paragraphs from journals, and even these often contain conflicting information.

Biographies

1873: *CLEAVE'S BIOGRAPHICAL CYCLOPEDIA OF HOMŒOPATHIC PHYSICIANS AND SURGEONS*: Egbert Cleave
Galaxy Publishing; Philadelphia, PA; 512 pages.
Originally sold by subscription, it contains 705 short biographies and 65 steel-engraving portraits.

A rare and wonderful book. The steel-engravings are magnificent. Many of the biographies are not in great depth because the subjects were at the beginning of their homeopathic career, achieving further recognition of the profession in the 20 years after the book was published.

1881: *ECCE MEDICUS, OR HAHNEMANN AS A MAN AND AS A PHYSICIAN, AND THE LESSONS OF HIS LIFE*: James Compton Burnett, MD
Homœopathic Publishing Company; 164 pages.

1884: *A MEMORIAL TO CONSTANTINE HERING*; Charles G. Raue, MD
Private, Philadelphia, PA; 364 pages.
A collection of all the eulogies delivered at memorial services for Hering.

Reprinted in 1940 by Calvin Knerr in his Life of Hering, *these memorials to Hering offer many glimpses into the character of the man. Some wonderful tidbits within.*

1895: *THE LIFE AND LETTERS OF DR. SAMUEL HAHNEMANN*: Thomas Lindsley Bradford, MD
Boericke and Tafel; 513 pages.
"To let Hahnemann speak by the means of his writing." A narrative of Hahnemann's life, pieced together from the works of Ameke and Dudgeon, and punctuated by Hahnemann's letters which had appeared in journals, newspapers, and other sources.

Meticulously referenced, as only Bradford could do. It remained the most complete work on Hahnemann until Haehl gained access to Hahnemann's files and letters, and wrote his work 27 years later.

1896: *THE BIOGRAPHICAL CYCLOPEDIA OF HOMŒOPATHIC PHYSICIANS AND SURGEONS*: Temple Hoyne, MD
American Homœopathic Biographical Association, Chicago; 172 pages.
"Respectfully dedicated to the present and future historians of the Homœopathic School of Medicine." The American Homœopathic Biographical Association was formed in 1891 with Hoyne as president and W. A. Chatterton as secretary. The book contains 36 portraits and 181 biographies in the first 118 pages. From page 119 on is a Necrological Index of all homœopaths whose deaths were

The Heritage of Homœopathic Literature

reported through medical society transactions, and contains not only the date of death but a reference to the journal in which an obituary appeared.

This is a very rare book. I have seen only one, in the collection of William Kirtsos, and he reports that in his over 20 years of book dealing he has never come across another copy.

1897: *THE PIONEERS OF HOMŒOPATHY*: Thomas Lindsley Bradford, MD
Boericke and Tafel; 677 pages.
A major source of information. Short biographies gleaned from other sources, many from obituaries. The first section of the book contains biographies of those who directly assisted Hahnemann. The rest of the book is for the others who were instrumental in building the foundations of homœopathy: the first generation.

A book I could not be without. Sorry to say, like most of Bradford's works, it is as rare as hen's teeth.

1898: *THE PORCELAIN PAINTER'S SON: A FANTASY*: Samuel A. Jones, MD
Boericke and Tafel; 126 pages.
"You will see that I have formed the web of fact in Hahnemann's life, the woof of fancy alone is mine… the fantasy is a 'projection' not at all difficult when a deep reverence inspires the attempt to people the dead past…"

*We are aware of biographical films that take literary license (*Amadeus *and* Armistad *spring to mind), Here is a book that could serve as the beginning of a wonderful script. It is the flowing pen of Jones at his best.*

1904: *LIFE AND WORK OF JAMES COMPTON BURNETT*: John Henry Clarke, MD
Homœopathic Publishing Company; 142 pages.

1904: *THOMAS SKINNER, MD*: John Henry Clarke, MD
Homœopathic Publishing Company; 90 pages.

Two magnificent biographies written by a dear friend of both men.

1905: *HISTORY OF HOMŒOPATHY AND ITS INSTITUTIONS IN AMERICA*: William Harvey King, MD
Lewis Publishing Co., New York; 1670 pages in four volumes.
The last 126 pages of Volume III, and all 409 pages of Volume IV are devoted to biographies of over 1,600 homœopaths who were currently in practice. For more comments see the "History" section.

1915: *CONSTANTINE HERING, MD: A BIOGRAPHICAL SKETCH*: Herman Faber
AIH, Philadelphia, PA; 28 pages.
Faber, an artist, was a friend of Hering's and spent much time at the Hering house.

1917: *REMINISCENCES OF CONSTANTINE HERING*: Arthur M. Eastman, MD
Private; 26 pages.
Eastman was a pupil of Hering and spent much time in the Hering household.

1918: *CHRONOLOGY OF EVENTS IN THE LIFE OF CONSTANTINE HERING, MD*; Carl Hering
Transactions of the International Hahnemannian Association, 1918; pages 11-38.
A very detailed biography of Constantine Hering, assembled by his son.

1919: *CONSTANTINE HERING— AN APPRECIATION*: Rudolph Hering
Journal of the American Institute of Homeopathy, Vol. 11 number 8, February 1919; pages 853-856.

A fascinating short account of Hering by his eldest son. Hering, says his son, had been searching for something

"exceedingly small" that could be seen as the "cause of disease," and Rudolph implies that Hering might have been a supporter of the germ theory and the use of anti-toxins, had he lived longer— something the very allopathically inclined AIH loved to hear.

1922: *SAMUEL HAHNEMANN, HIS LIFE AND WORK*: Richard Haehl, MD ✔
Homœopathic Publishing Company; Vol. 1, 443 pages, vol. 2, 515 pages.
Translated from the German by Marie Wheeler and W. H. R. Grundy, and edited by F. E. Wheeler and John Henry Clarke.
The major work on Hahnemann's life. All later work stems from this. The first volume is the chronological story, documented with quotes from letters to and from Hahnemann and from other sources. The second volume is the record of the sources used. If a paragraph is quoted from a letter in Volume 1, the whole letter appears in volume 2.

All other books are but popular efforts, akin to Reader's Digest excerpts. If you are interested in Hahnemann's life, therapeutical developments, the development of potencies and the arguments he had with the medical profession, then this is an essential reference.

1926: *FORTY-ONE YEARS OF HOMEOPATHY:* Alfred Pulford, MD
Private, Toledo OH; 8 pages.

A brief autobiography by one of homœopathy's grand word-crafters.

1933: *LIFE OF CHRISTIAN SAMUEL HAHNEMANN, FOUNDER OF HOMŒOPATHY*:
Rosa Waugh Hobhouse ✔
C. W. Daniel; 288 pages.
A literary narrative of Hahnemann's life based upon the work of Haehl. The author corresponded with Haehl during the writing of the manuscript, and used impressions of Köthen, gleaned from letters from her husband (who went there to do research), to bring life to her story.

The book contains portraits of some of the major characters, including the only portrait of Charlotte Hahnemann I have ever seen. The book is well written and has recently been reprinted in India.

1935: *LIFE OF MAHENDRA LAL SIRCAR*: Dr. Sarat Chandra Ghose
Homœopathic Publishing Company, Calcutta; 412 pages.
A well written biography of the person who is known as "the Hering of India."

1938: *CARROLL DUNHAM HIS LIFE AND WORKS*: E. Wallace MacAdam, MD
reprinted from the July 1938 *Homœopathic Recorder*; 8 pages.

1939: *GESCHICHTE DER HOMÖOPATHIE*: Rudolf Tischner
Schwabe, Leipzig; 837 pages.
An extensive history of homeopathy, especially of German homeopathy. Includes many biographies.

1940: *LIFE OF HERING*: Calvin B. Knerr, MD ✔
Magee Press, Philadelphia, PA; 347 pages.
In the late 1930s, Calvin Knerr found the journals he kept while he was a medical student and living in Hering's house. The first part of the book is a transcription of those journals, giving a "feel" of what Hering was like. The second part of the book is Hering's own narrative about leaving Germany and going to Parimaribo. The third section is a list of Hering's literary works, and the fourth section is a reprint of Raue's *HERING MEMORIAL*.

There is not much clinical information in the book, but there are an untold number of glimpses into the private

The Heritage of Homœopathic Literature

life of this fascinating man. Buried in the book are all sorts of answers to things homœopathic. We've heard that Hahnemann's father locked him in the room to contemplate difficult problems. Nowhere in Haehl's work is this mentioned. Where does it come from? From Hering— who heard the story from a friend who had worked at the same porcelain factory as Hahnemann's father.

Through this book we find Hering's personal opinions on many things— flavorful cheese, the science of astronomy, the health dangers of using a swing and, of course, his opinion of other homœopaths. A direct record of conversations around the dinner-table and a glimpse into the Hering household.

1942: *AN OLD DOCTOR OF THE NEW SCHOOL*: James Craven Wood, MD
Caxton Printers, Ltd., Caldwell, OH; 393 pages.
An autobiography. Educated at Ann Arbor, Wood was the President of the AIH in 1902. Wood never quite understood the depth of homœopathy and practiced as a gynecological surgeon. The book is a journey into the education of a homœopath in the late 1880s and the internal conflicts between someone who never quite believed in it all, and the lure of conventional medicine.

A pedantic, self indulgent, and often boring story of Dr. Wood's interface with homœopathy. There are interesting moments, especially those concerning his student years at Ann Arbor, but much of it might be lost upon a reader who was not fully conversant with the major players along the way.

1945: *HAHNEMANN; THE ADVENTUROUS CAREER OF A MEDICAL REBEL*: Dr. Martin Gumpert
L. B. Fischer, New York; 251 pages.
Translated from the German by Claud W. Sykes. "The study of an individual who would have been a rebel in any era in any profession." Originally published in German, the author was a medical advisor to *Time Magazine*.

circa 1945: *WHY I BECAME A HOMŒOPATH*; Assorted authors
Homœopathic Publishing Company, Boston, MA; 17 pages.
First person experiences related by Dorothy Shepherd, Roger Schmidt, T. K. Moore, Eugene Underhill, and C. V. Bryant.

1981: *SAMUEL HAHNEMANN: THE FOUNDER OF HOMEOPATHIC MEDICINE*: Trevor Cook ✔
Thorsens; 192 pages.
The author "attempted to weave into the text other momentous events of his time which influenced Hahnemann's life and work which were to shape the world's history up to the present day."

1985: *BRASS TACKS: THE ORAL BIOGRAPHY OF A 20TH CENTURY PHYSICIAN*: Adelaide Suits
Halyburton Press, Ann Arbor, MI; 138 pages.
A biography of John Renner, MD, based on interviews conducted before he died, at the age of 99, in 1989. Renner had been a pupil of Grimmer at the Hahnemann Medical College (Chicago) shortly after Kent's death. An interesting personal exposition by someone very opposed to the use of high potencies.

1986: *CHAMPION OF HOMŒOPATHY; THE LIFE OF MARGERY BLACKIE*: Constance Babington Smith
John Murray, London; 185 pages.
Written after Blackie's death by an admirer who pieced together Blackie's story from memoirs, letters, and interviews with those who knew her.

A somewhat pedantic work that has an occasional jewel buried within— which keeps one reading to look for more.

1990: *A HOMEOPATHIC LOVE STORY: THE STORY OF SAMUEL AND MELANIE HAHNEMANN*:
Rima Handley ✔
North Atlantic Books; 251 pages.
Most of the information we have of Hahnemann's second wife, Melanie, comes from the extensive

letters found in Haehl's work, but Haehl's description of her was flavored by the prevailing opinion at the time: that Hahnemann had been dragged away by a younger woman who was after fame and fortune and treated him poorly, even though the letters contradict this view. Before these letters came to light in Haehl's book, Hering reported hearing that Melanie had kept Hahnemann on a mattress in a back room and did not allow him out.
This book is a narrative, with some poetic license, of the life of Samuel and Melanie, as derived from their letters.

A wonderful synopsis of the life of Hahnemann, and more about Melanie than has been generally known. I would love to have an illustration of the scene described in the book of Sam and Melanie strolling arm in arm along the river in Paris, eating ice cream. What a wonderful image!

1991: *IKONOGRAPHIE SAMMLUNG, DOKUMENTATION, HISTORIE, UND LEGENDEN DER BILDER DES HOFRATES, DR. MED. HABIL. C. F. S. HAHNEMANN*: Wolfgang Schweitzer
Haug Verlag; 164 pages.
A visual journey of Hahnemann's life. 159 pictures of all known visual material relating to Hahnemann: the houses he lived in, the statues erected in his honor, all known portraits of him and his wives, including a photo of him on his deathbed.

1993: *DIRECTORY OF DECEASED AMERICAN PHYSICIANS 1804-1929*: Arthur W. Hafner, PhD, editor ✔
American Medical Association, Chicago, IL; 1823 pages
This two-volume set contains brief biographies of almost 150,000 medical practitioners. Buried within these are biographies of 7,625 practitioners who were "Self Designated Homeopaths."
Although the books themselves are out of print, the database file is available as a CD-ROM, published by Broderbund under their "Family Tree Maker" series.

The information included date and place of birth; date, place, and cause of death, places of practice, schools attended, licensure, and society affiliations.
The American Medical Association maintained complete records of all practitioners, regardless of affiliation, taken from state medical society records. The records were kept on file cards, and were finally transferred to a database.

1997: *IN SEARCH OF THE LATER HAHNEMANN*: Rima Handley ✔
Beaconsfield; 235 pages.
An exposition of Hahnemann's life and practice in Paris, with an emphasis on the development of his Fiftieth millesimal potencies and the cases he saw in his practice with his wife Melanie.

1999: *THE FACES OF HOMŒOPATHY: AN ILLUSTRATED HISTORY OF THE FIRST 200 YEARS*: Julian Winston ✔
Great Auk Publishing, New Zealand; 634 pages.
Gleaned from journals, books, and through personal interviews, 157 short biographies are presented, most accompanied by a likeness of the subject.

Other Books

Other Books

After all the books are sorted into neat piles, there is always a "left over" stack. How can these other books be categorized? Where do you put the book of poems by the grand homœopathic surgeon William Tod Helmuth? Or the short futuristic fantasy from homœopathic historian William Harvey King? Or Yasgur's magnificent *Dictionary* of homœopathic terminology? Or books of collected writings, containing a bit of everything?

The books here are like many of the others. Some are historical curiosities, some are tangentially related to homœopathic issues, and some are on your desk and usable every day. None (at least in my thinking) fit into the other categories.

Other books

1837: *ORGANON DER SPECIFISCHEN HEILKUNST*: Gottlieb Ludwig Rau, MD
Schumann, Leipzig; 392 pages.
Translated by Hempel and published by Radde in **1847** as *ORGANON OF THE SPECIFIC HEALING ART*. Rau was a contemporary of Hahnemann, who "looked for salvation in medicine through a discriminating, rational empiricism… he felt himself necessarily attracted by the teachings of Hahnemann, although he had reached through a different and more scientific path a similar position to that from which Hahnemann started out empirically." He thought that the ideal medicine would treat all diseases specifically, and he saw homœopathy as extending in that direction. The book is an effort to place homœopathy on a more "scientific" basis. Although Rau wrote his first work on homœopathy in 1824, he was still very interested in the methods of conventional medicine, which he believed were still of use if properly studied.

1846: *A MANUAL OF HOMŒOPATHIC COOKERY*: Anonymous
Radde; 176 pages.
"Designed chiefly for the use of such persons as are under homœopathic treatment."
"By the wife of a homœopathic physician, with annotations by the wife of an American homœopathic physician." Apparently first published in England.

1850: *HAHNEMANN AND SWEDENBORG*: Rev. Richard De Charms
New Jerusalem Print; 8 pages.
"The Affinities Between the Fundamental Principles of Homœopathia, and the Doctrine of the New Church."

The first work which attempts to weave the philosophical constructs of the Swedish philosopher with those of Hahnemann.

1853: *DR. J. T. TEMPLE'S REPLY TO PROF. PALLEN'S ATTACK ON HOMŒOPATHY IN HIS VALEDICTORY ADDRESS BEFORE THE ST. LOUIS UNIVERSITY*: John Taylor Temple, MD
T. W. Ustick, St. Louis, MO; 16 pages.

One of many such works. Few were printed as books or pamphlets. Most that Bradford reports were simply letters that were published by the author and distributed to those interested.

1854: *HOMEOPATHY FAIRLY REPRESENTED*: William Henderson, MD
Lindsay and Blakiston, Philadelphia; 302 pages.
"A reply to Professor Simpson's 'Homœopathy Misrepresented." James Simpson, of Edinburgh, was a critic of homeopathy. This book is a reply to one of his essays. It is interesting to note that the publishers, Lindsay and Blakiston, were one of America's oldest allopathic publishing houses. They had published Simpson's original work.

1854: *ORGANON OF SPECIFIC HOMŒOPATHY*: Charles J. Hempel, MD
Rademacher and Sheek; 216 pages
"An inductive exposition of the principles of the homœopathic healing art, addressed to physicians and intelligent laymen." Beginning with "12 Golden Rules about Diet," the book follows in three parts: "Homœopathy Proper: The Homœopathy of Symptoms"; "A Critical Review of the Doctrines of Homœopathy as Apparently Taught in the Organon"; and "Formula of the Homœopathic Law as Suggested By the Union of Pharmacodynamics and Therapeutics upon a Physiologico-Pathological Basis."
Hempel throws himself into the camp of those who believed that homœopathy as expounded by Hahnemann was too abstract and the materia medica was next to useless. He questions the usefulness of many remedies, and suggest refining the materia medica to understand the physiological action of the remedy and develop specific remedies for specific diseases.
"Some of these remedies when testing their therapeutic value by the specific method are found to be of very little, or at any rate, of only limited use in practice; among them we may mention such remedies as Alumina, Natrum muriaticum, Agaricus, Carbo vegetabilis, Lycopodium, Sulphuric and Nitric acid, the north and south pole of the magnet, and a number of other drugs more particularly among the recent additions to our Materia Medica. I am fully aware that cures are pretended to be effected with all these drugs; but I doubt the correctness of many of the observations…
"Aconite possesses a higher degree of medicinal power than Natrum muriaticum, for this reason, that the former is a drug in an absolute sense, whereas, the latter fulfils mixed uses, among which its properties as a culinary agent are much more remarkable than its remedial virtues. Indeed it is highly questionable whether its sphere of its remedial action is at all as extensive as it is supposed to be, and whether the boasted richness of its symptoms is not on a par with the pathogenesis of fluoric acid, bromine, lachesis, and the like, all grandeloquent sounds and moonshine."

A work written in a flowery, obtuse manner, common to much of the work of the time. Hempel's objection to the materia medica seems to be almost a contemporary rant about the newer provings and the tendency to report such trivial things that the information becomes useless for prescribing. "It is to be hoped that the time is fast approaching when the minds of homeopathic practitioners will be emancipated from the degrading thraldom of childish symptom hunters; when homeopathy will cease to be a science of inglorious illusions, and when the living, unerring truths of experience and reason will be substituted in their stead."
The second part of the book suggests that if one were to follow Hahnemann's ideas about taking a case, then one would have so many symptoms that it would be impossible to select the correct remedy. Hempel obviously did not understand the concept of "characteristic symptoms." Part three is a flowery essay on the meaning of symptoms, the meaning of life, and man's relationship to God, all couched in Swedenborgian terms. It ends by suggesting the need to study the materia medica to understand which remedies are specific for which diseases (using Aconite and Mercurius as examples) so as to make the job of the physician easier.

1857: *THE UNCERTAINTY OF HUMAN TESTIMONY. CONCLUSIONS NOT JUDGMENT.*
A LETTER TO THE HONORABLE WILLIAM KENT: Federal Vandenburgh, MD
J. F. Trow, New York; 77 pages.

Vandenburgh was the third practicing homœopath in New York City. Who was William Kent? What testimony did he give?

1865: *THE GEOMETRY OF VITAL FORCES*: Federal Vandenburgh, MD
C. T. Hurlbert; 94 pages.

Another mystery title from Bradford. What is in those 94 pages? What was Vandenburgh's thesis?
Vanderburgh was hailed by his contemporaries as a great prescriber. He has five entries in Bradford's Bibliography. The other three are public letters and/or addresses. These are his only "books."

1868: HINTS FOR THE PRACTICAL STUDY OF THE HOMŒOPATHIC METHOD, IN THE ABSENCE OF ORAL INSTRUCTION WITH CASES FOR CLINICAL COMMENT:
Edward D. Chepmell, MD
Simpkin, Marshall, London; 194 pages.
35 cases are presented and analyzed.

An interesting effort to show the homeopathic method through cases. The cases, from a vantage point of time, are questionable. In one case of Rheumatic Fever from June 8, 1846 to July 15, 1846, the patient was given seven different remedies in potencies from the 3rd to the 800th.

1871: *THE REJECTED ADDRESS. MAN'S TRUE RELATION TO NATURE; HIS ORIGIN, CHARACTER AND DESTINY*: Thomas P. Wilson, MD
L. H. Witte, Cleveland, OH; 26 pages.
Says Bradford, "This address was repudiated by the American Institute of Homœopathy before which it was delivered [June 6, 1871], on account of its liberal scientific bias. It was delivered in the Academy of Music, Philadelphia, and the writer of this well remembers the excitement that ensued for some minutes at its close. Various members rose excitedly, each trying to speak, some upholding and some denouncing the lecture. On the following day, the Institute rejected it. Dr. Wilson published it in the above form and it was widely circulated."

T. P. Wilson was one of those, just nine years later, that left the AIH Meeting in Milwaukee and became a founding member of the International Hahnemannian Association. He was the editor of the Cincinnati Medical Advance *from 1873 to 1885. I would love to know what he said on that night in Philadelphia!*

1873: *INSTRUCTIONS FOR THE USE OF N. F. COOKE'S FAMILY MEDICINES*: Nicholas Francis Cooke
Private; 84 pages.
"An oddly shaped book. When open it is two and a half by ten and three fourths inches; when shut, it's length is the same but its diameter is but five eighths of an inch."

Diameter? I saw this one in Bradford's and because of the uniqueness decided to include it here.

1873: *OPHIDIANS; ZOOLOGICAL ARRANGEMENT OF THE DIFFERENT GENERA*: S. B. Higgins
Boericke and Tafel; 239 pages.
Information about snakes and their poisons.

1877: *ON THE APPLICATION OF ELECTRICITY AS A THERAPEUTIC AGENT*: Julius H. Rae
Boericke and Tafel; 132 pages.

The use of electricity for medical therapy was in vogue from the 1880s through the early 1900s. Electricity was usually applied using batteries and subjecting one part of the person to the negative pole while attaching the positive pole to another. Kent talked about using "Faradisation" where the patient sat on a wetted sponge containing the negative pole, while the positive pole was massaged up and down the spine.
Many of the homœopathic schools had a "Department of Electro-therapeutics" and W. H. King, who wrote the four volume history, was the professor of Electro-therapeutics at the New York Homœopathic Medical College.
As a therapeutic modality where the "thing itself" was unseen, it fell naturally to the homœopathic side of medicine. A good number of the books on the subject were published by "homœopathic" publishers, and many of the practitioners of electro-therapeutics were also homœopaths.

1877: *THE KABBALA; OR THE TRUE SCIENCE OF LIGHT*: Seth Pancoast, MD
J. M. Stoddard; 312 pages.
"An introduction to the Philosophy and Theosophy of the Ancient Sages. Together with a Chapter on Light in the Vegetable Kingdom."

"Light is nature's own and only remedy for disease; and explaining how to apply the red and blue rays in curing the Sick and Feeble."
Say Bradford, "This curious book is printed in red and blue ink."

Dr. Pancoast is said to have possessed the most complete library on the subject of mysticism, in the United States. His earlier works were mostly home health guides aimed at young men and women.

1878: *TERATOLOGY, OR THE SCIENCE OF MONSTERS*: Mahlon Walker, MD
Sherman and Co.; 15 pages.

Teratology is the study of abnormalities, malformations or deviations from normal growing patterns. Another book from Bradford that has not been recently seen.

1878: *HOW TO BE PLUMP:* Thomas Cation Duncan, MD
Duncan Brothers; 60 pages.

The title says it all. An essay on "Leanness as a Disease" and "The necessity for starchy foods and sweets." A book of the times, written by a corpulent author, whose other books were about homœopathic practice.

1879: *SCRATCHES OF A SURGEON*: William Tod Helmuth, MD
W. A. Chatterton: 120 pages.
The grand surgeon's first dip into publishing his verse.

1879: SEXUAL NEUROSES: James Tyler Kent, MD
Maynard and Tetford, St. Louis; 144 pages.
The very first book by Kent. It came out just before he began to explore homœopathy.

Although listed in Bradford, I have seen only one copy of this little work. Filled with Kent's dogmatic view on sex, and eclectic treatment of disorders. It is NOT about homœopathy, but is placed here simply to mark the first book by Kent. For an excerpt of the book, see page 158-159 in The Faces of Homœopathy.

1880: *ELECTRICITY: ITS NATURE AND FORMS, WITH A STUDY ON ELECTRO-THERAPEUTICS*:
Captain William Boyce, MD
W. A. Chatterton; 85 pages.

1882: *ELECTRICITY IN SURGERY*: John Butler, MD
Boericke and Tafel; 108 pages.
"Based on the author's own experience." The introduction says that 20 years earlier the use of electricity as a therapeutic means was considered quackery but at the present time "…electricity is honorably enrolled among our list of therapeutic agents… one of the most potent weapons we possess, in combating many forms of disease."

1882: *PLAIN TALKS ON AVOIDED SUBJECTS*: Henry Newell Guernsey, MD
F. A. Davis; 120 pages.
"Causes which commonly produce sexual impressions on young children are: allowing them to repose playfully on their belly, to slide down banisters, to go too long without urinating, constipation or straining at stool, cutaneous affection, and worms… The sliding down banisters produces a titillation which is agreeable to the sexual organs. Children of both sexes will constantly repeat this act until they learn to become inveterate masturbators, even at a very early age."

Written by a prominent homœopath, the book offers domestic advice on how to raise your children to be completely innocent about sexual matters. An interesting view of the times. See page 55 in The Faces of Homœopathy.

1888: *CATALOGUE OF MORBIFIC PRODUCTS, NOSODES, AND OTHER REMEDIES, IN HIGH POTENCIES*: Samuel Swan, MD
Pusey & Co., New York; 32 pages.
A catalogue of the remedies made by Dr. Swan. Says Bradford, "The articles potentized are very remarkable."

Remarkable indeed! Buttermilk, the blue ray of the sun (and the other primary colors), Fuligo splendens *(chimney soot where hardwood is burned), diabetic sugar,* Scomber scomber *(Mackerel),* Vomito *(blood from a yellow fever patient when moribind,* Lachryma filia *(the tears of a young girl in great grief and suffering), and many more! Dr. Swan was the first to prepare* Tuberculinum *and* Medorrhinum.

1891: *THE POCKET MEDICAL DICTIONARY*: Charles Gatchell, MD
Era Publishing Co., Chicago; 303 pages.
"For the use of the students of medicine, containing ten-thousand words, including all the essential terms used in Medicine and the Allied Sciences."

1892: *WITH THE "POUSSE CAFÉ;" BEING A COLLECTION OF POST-PRANDIAL VERSES*:
William Tod Helmuth, MD
Boericke and Tafel; 141 pages.
A second collection of verse including the impressive (and amusing) "How I became a Surgeon."

1895: *PRESCRIPTION CARD:* Stacy Jones, MD
Boericke and Tafel; 16 pages.
Certainly one of the stranger contributions to our literature. This little pamphlet contained a listing of symptoms, followed by an anagram of the abbreviated name of the remedy (reversing the first and second letter). The intent was to have the patient underline their symptoms, and then the prescriber could look at them and see the remedies without consulting a repertory. As an example: "Never Warm enough— Lau Rgap Isl." (Alumina, Graphites, Silica)

1901: *INDEX TO PROVINGS*: Thomas Lindsley Bradford, MD ✔
Boericke and Tafel; 305 pages.
An index that references the source of every proving conducted until 1901.

An invaluable resource when trying to locate information on when a remedy was first proven and where to find more detailed information. Unfortunately many of the sources quoted are homœopathic journals that are rare and/or difficult to access.

1904: *MEDICAL UNION NUMBER SIX*: William Harvey King, MD
Monograph Press, New York; 60 pages.
A fantasy. The author is shipwrecked and is found some 30 years later. He returns to New York in October, 1940 to find that the doctors have unionized into specialties and it is illegal for a "throat man" to treat a cough— which must be referred to a "chest man." Needless to say an emergency arises…

A strange little story, and so close to the truth! The physicians were the last to unionize. Even the clergy unionized before them!

1907: *THE ELEMENTS OF HOMŒOPATHIC THEORY, MATERIA MEDICA, PRACTICE, AND PHARMACY*:
Felix A. Boericke and Edward Pollock Anshutz
Boericke and Tafel; 218 pages
A small book that has history, philosophy, pharmacy, materia medica, and a therapeutic index all in one.

It was claimed that hundreds were sold to doctors of other schools of medicine. This little book give a taste of the whole thing, and includes a reading list of books.

1907: *HOW TO TAKE THE CASE AND FIND THE SIMILLIMUM*: E. B. Nash, MD ✔
Boericke and Tafel; 54 pages.
"I have been questioned as to my method of selecting the remedy. This little book is the answer."

Excellent advice from a master prescriber.

1909: *HYDROTHERAPY*: William Diffenbach, MD
Rebman, New York; 267 pages.
An excellent manual concerning the use of "water cures" by a professor at the New York Homœopathic Medical College, and a member of the IHA.

Diffenbach was the prover of Radium bromide.

1915: *HOW TO USE THE REPERTORY*: Glenn Irving Bidwell, MD ✔
Boericke and Tafel; 156 pages.
An excellent little book to guide the student through the intricacies of Kent's *Repertory*.

Written by someone who learned it first-hand from Kent.

1915: *CATALOGUE OF THE HOMŒOPATHIC BOOKS OF BOERICKE AND TAFEL*
Boericke and Tafel; 127 pages.
An invaluable resource in compiling this book. Many of the reviews I have quoted are derived from this wonderful little catalogue.

1955: *HOMEOPATHY AND HOMEOPATHIC PRESCRIBING*: Harvey Farrington, MD ✔
AIH, Philadelphia, PA; 264 pages.
A plastic-spiral-bound collection of 43 lessons, "Prepared for and Offered Only to Graduate Physicians." Lesson six through 42 concern materia medica. After lesson 43 there is a 16 page section concerning the use of the repertory.

This was the prime instruction book in the American Foundation for Homœopathy Post-graduate Courses. The material is reliable, although not the easiest to use by itself, as it really needs to have another level of explanation.

1968: ESSAYS ON HOMEOPATHY: B. K. Sarkar
Hahnemann Publishing, Calcutta; 1043 pages.
A collection of articles, editorials, presidential address, and more from one of India's greatest homœopaths.

1974: *WINE IS THE BEST MEDICINE*: E. A. Maury, MD
Editions Du jour (France); 1978 Corgi Books; 127 pages.
Translated by M. L. Monferran-Parker.
Written by a prominent French homœopath. Beginning with a discussion of the composition of the soils needed for grape production, and defining how each section in France differs, the author then suggests which specific wines are useful for a number of "maladies." For example, for "cystitis" one should look to the sweet or semi-sweet white wines from Anjou.

1980: *A SCIENTIFIC APPROACH TO HOMEOPATHY*: George Russell Henshaw, MD
Exposition Press, Hicksville, NY; 199 pages.
A collection of previously published (in the *Journal of the American Institute of Homeopathy*) articles concerning the use of the serum flocculation test for determining the choice of remedy. A number of cases are presented.

Serum flocculation is a complex and labor intensive test that can determine an appropriate remedy in a case. The serum of the patient's blood is separated and placed into a series of test tubes. A number of remedies are

selected and, using a low potency trituration, are dissolved in saline and then carefully placed over the serum in the test tubes. A different remedy is placed in each tube. After about an hour or so, the remedy that is most indicated in the case will have shown a flocculation at the boundary between the serum and the saline/remedy. This is seen as a series of "fingers" extending from the two components into the other.
I have seen this test used with good results. Unfortunately, it is very time intensive and requires a good laboratory to work in as well as a good supply of lower potency (under 3X) triturates.

1983: *THE ENCYCLOPEDIA OF HOMŒOPATHY*: Trevor Smith, MFHom, BChir. ✔
Insight Editions, Worthington, Sussex; 283 pages.
"A comprehensive reference book and survey of the subject from its beginnings to the present day." Unfortunately, this edition contained many errors in the bibliographic references— wrong dates, wrong connections. The biggest *gaffe* was having Sir Henry Tyler (father of Margaret Tyler) born in 1849 in Woodhull, NY— the date and place of James *Tyler* Kent. Unfortunately, other books relied on this information without checking it, and errors were multiplied. A second edition was printed in **1994** with 317 pages, with most of the glaring errors corrected.

1984: *MEDICINE FOR BEGINNERS*: Tony Pinchuck and Richard Clark
Writers and Readers, New York; 173 pages.
A history of medicine, advertised as "a first rate guide to the ailments of modern medicine." A "Writers and Readers Documentary Comic Book," it traces the history of medicine thorough its empirical/rational split, through the philosophical works of Bacon, Harvey, Descartes, Hobbes, and many others, through Hahnemann and the rise of the British Medical Association and the AMA. Almost a comic book style with original illustrations and creative use of collage created from other illustrations, it is filled with insights into history and our current medical system on almost every page.

A magnificent book that deserves to be reprinted. It should be required reading for all persons in the medical field.

1984: *BIBLIOTHECA HOMŒOPATHICA*: Jacques Baur, Klaus-Henning Gypser, Georg von Keller, Philip W. Thomas
Aude Sapere Publishers, Germany; 121 pages.
An index of all the known journals that were published in every country.

An invaluable resource for the homœopathic historian. Every known journal is listed by name (with an abbreviated code). Journals which changed name or went through a series of different editors, are clearly delineated.

1985: *THE BIBLE AND HOMEOPATHY: A DEFENCE OF PURIST HOMEOPATHIC MEDICINE*:
Ronald Male
Missionary School of Medicine, London; 12 pages.
The Missionary School was started in London in 1903 to train Christian Missionaries in basic medical sciences. It was connected with the Faculty of Homeopathy and trained missionaries in the use of homœopathy. The book was written to help counter the rise of fundamentalist thought which associated homœopathy with "occultism" and the work of the devil.

1986: *CLASSICAL HOMEOPATHY*: Margery Blackie, MD ✔
Beaconsfield; 312 pages.
Edited by Charles Elliot, MFHom and Frank Johnson, FFHom.
A collection of assorted essays by Blackie, mostly concerning materia medica. 33 of the essays are about "constitutional remedies" and the materia medicæ of 111 other remedies is discussed in shorter essays.

1986: *TUTORIALS ON HOMŒOPATHY*: Donald Foubister, MD ✔
Beaconsfield; 202 pages.
Materia medica, and therapeutic insights by a renowned British homœopath. Detailed chapters on casetaking, pediatrics, and *Carcinosin* are included.

1989: *THE HOMEOPATHIC RECORDER AND PROCEEDINGS OF THE INTERNATIONAL HAHNEMANNIAN ASSOCIATION, CUMULATIVE INDICES 1881-1958*: Maesimund B. Panos, MD, and Della P. Desrosiers
The Woodward Foundation, Tipp City, Ohio; 330 pages.
177 page author index, 90 page title index, 63 page remedy index.

A flawed attempt at a much needed work. In 1927, the IHA took over the Homœopathic Recorder *from Boericke and Tafel. Dr. Panos had a full set of the* IHA Journals and Transactions. *She did not realize the heritage of the* Recorder. *Therefore, the index is NOT a complete index to the* Homœopathic Recorder *(which was first published in 1886), but only to those issues of the* Recorder *that were published under the auspices of the IHA.*
In the attempt to create an index of authors, titles, and remedies, a few pieces that were integral to the journal and important to researchers, were left out. An index to the many obituaries of prominent homœopaths was not made, nor was an index of the portraits that often graced the first internal page of the journal.
Of secondary importance was the lack of an index for the "Carriwidget" column or the "Question and Answer" column, both filled with valuable information about the practice of homœopathy.
Furthermore, a number of articles have not been indexed. This I found out only after looking for specific articles, finding them in *the journals through looking at each issue, and then finding they were not in the index.*
It is, therefore, a somewhat useful work, but far from as complete as it could be.

1989: *ENCYCLOPEDIA OF REPERTORIES*: Dr. J. Benedict D'Castro
B. Jain; 250 pages
More of a discussion about casetaking than about Repertories *per se*. The text has many misspellings of names and places, and contradictory dates (i.e., Kent did his repertory in 1877/1897). It contains a glossary of words used in Kent's *Repertory* and their definitions.

A rambling discourse about the use of repertories, and very little about the repertories themselves. The history of Kent's work is given short shrift, perhaps because the author was not aware of the details. A great deal of emphasis on case-taking and how to get the information which one then uses in the repertory to find a suitable remedy. There is useful information in the book, but it must be winnowed from the rest.

1990: *INSIGHTS INTO HOMEOPATHY*: Frank Bodman, MD ✔
Beaconsfield; 119 pages.
Edited by Anita Davies, FFHom and Robin Pinsert, MFHom.
Based on lectures given at the Faculty of Homœopathy in London, this work primarily discusses therapeutics, with some materia medica and a small amount of philosophy.

1990: *A MODERN GUIDE AND INDEX TO THE MENTAL RUBRICS IN KENT'S REPERTORY*:
David Sault ✔
Emryss bv Pub., Haarlem, Holland; 248 pages (2nd edition).

1990: *A DICTIONARY OF HOMEOPATHIC MEDICAL TERMINOLOGY*: Jay Yasgur ✔
Van Hoy Publishers, Greenville, PA; 92 pages.
2nd edition **1992** (180 pages), 3rd edition **1995** (240 pages). The 4th edition in **1998** was called *YASGUR'S HOMEOPATHIC DICTIONARY, AND HOLISTIC HEALTH REFERENCE* and had grown to 422 pages.

One of the best references one can have. It contains definitions of all those unusual words in Kent's Repertory *that you always wondered about, plus definitions of all the antiquated medical terminology that you come across in all those old books. Furthermore, it contains definitions of almost every aspect of homœopathy including over 400 mini-biographies. The author also briefly defines a great number of holistic health modalities now in vogue. The information is accurate and can be trusted. A must have.*

1991: *HOMŒOPATHY IN THE UNITED STATES: A BIBLIOGRAPHY OF HOMŒOPATHIC MEDICAL IMPRINTS, 1825-1925*: Francisco Cordasco ✔
Junius Vaughn Press, Fairview, NJ; 231 pages.
Divided into 3 periods: Beginnings and Growth: 1825-1859; The Heroic Years: 1860-1889; Twilight and Decline: 1890-1925. Essentially, a bibliographic listing containing all that is in Bradford's *Bibliography* in reference to books, and expanded upon to include publications through 1925.

This is an example of a good idea, poorly executed. The author says "Outside of the National Library of Medicine, there is no large extant collection of homeopathic literature." Unfortunately, the author never contacted the National Center for Homeopathy (which has 2000+ volumes), nor any of the other private collections, nor the collections at the University of Michigan at Ann Arbor, the Ohio State University at Columbus, the University of California at San Francisco, or the National College of Naturopathic Medicine, all which have large collections. By failing to take those steps, he excluded important books by many of the "classic authors" of the early 1900s. Boger, Nash, Clarke, and others are missing. It has some value, but misses so much after Bradford that the section from 1890-1925 is almost worthless.

1991: *THORSONS ENCYCLOPAEDIC DICTIONARY OF HOMEOPATHY*: Harald Gaier, ND, DO, DHomM
Thorsons; 601 pages.
"The definitive resource to all aspects of homœopathy." The book "…attempts to explain in some detail those technical and other terms that are encountered in reading or during conversation about… homeopathy." The author says that the "sources were diligently checked" but many of the biographies come from Smith's 1983 *Encyclopedia*, and repeat all the errors found therein.

A mysterious book. One reviewer said it was filled with "neologisms"— new words whose meaning is not obvious to the reader. In it, there are many words that I, for one, have never come across in homœopathy: pathotropism, trivial names, xenomania, nutritional equipoise, etc. Explanations of homœopathic processes are excessively long, and drawn out. Although the author claims to have diligently checked his sources, the errors that crept into the biographies do not give one confidence about the accuracy of this work. A cumbersome and inflated work.

1991: *KRANKENJOURNAL*: Samuel Hahnemann, MD ✔
Haug Verlag, Heidelberg.
Hahnemann's Casebooks. Transcribed from his handwritten case books. Three volumes are now in print: D2 (1801-1802), published in 1993, 136 pages; D3 (1802), published in 1995, 248 pages; D4 (1802-1803), published in 1997, 257 pages; D5 (1803-1806) published in 1991, 407 pages; D34 (1830) published in 1998, Two volumes. Commentary by Fishback-Sabel (290 pages) and the Casebooks (999 pages); DF5 (1837-1842) published in 1992, 1205 pages.

These are transcription of Hahnemann's case-books. The hope is that ALL the books will eventually be transcribed and published. The notes in German are in German, the notes in French are in French. No explanation is offered as to Hahnemann's abbreviations of doses or potencies— the work is simply a transcription from the hand-written notes. The D34 volume has a separate commentary.

1992: *HOMŒOPATHIC IMPRINTS, 1825-1925*: Christopher Ellithorp and Julian Winston
Homœopathic Archives, Philadelphia, PA; 20 pages.
A listing of 208 books that did not appear in the Cordasco volume, but were found in the private libraries of the National Center for Homeopathy, Boericke and Tafel, Chris Ellithorp, and Julian Winston.

1992: *THE CONTROLLED CLINICAL TRIAL: AN ANALYSIS*: Harris L. Coulter, PhD
Center for Empirical Medicine, Washington DC; 165 pages.
A masterful exposition of the history of the double-blind, controlled clinical trial, and an analysis of why it is not only meaningless for general research, but useless for studying homœopathic therapeutics.

Coulter at his penetrating best. The book is online, at <http://www.empiricaltherapies.com/CCT1web.html>

1993: *CHRISTIAN COMMON SENSE AND MEDICAL CONTROVERSY*: Richard Culp, DO
Christian Printing Mission; 60 pages.
A reply, from a Christian and a homœopath, to those who accuse homœopathy of being "evil" and "satanic."

1994: *THE COLLECTED WRITINGS OF C. M. BOGER:* Edited by Robert Bannan, RSHom ✔
Churchill Livingstone, Edinburgh; 365 pages.
All of Boger's writings, gleaned from a number of older homœopathic journals. Essays on philosophy, practice, and materia medica.

Boger was a great scholar and homœopathic thinker. A contemporary of Kent, his work is equally insightful. This book is filled with treasures which, until its publication, remained buried in hard to find journals. Robert Bannan did a great service in assembling this work and having it published.

1994: *THE DYNAMICS AND METHODOLOGY OF HOMOEOPATHIC PROVINGS*: Jeremy Sherr
Dynamis; 136 pages.
The first modern text to discuss the concept of provings and establish a methodology to follow which is consistent with the instructions outlined by Hahnemann in the *Organon*.

If only all provings were done with this methodology... Sherr clearly outlines the need for supervision, the time-frame needed, the extraction of the symptoms from the mass of information, and the uselessness of trying to force onto the proving remedy any "essence" or "theme." He sees it all very clearly and simply as a compilation, with extreme care and judgment, of the reactions of a group of people to an ingested substance.
A very valuable book that, unfortunately, too few read and heed.

1994: *A TUTORIAL AND WORKBOOK FOR THE HOMEOPATHIC REPERTORY*: Karen B. Allen ✔
Homeopathic Tutorials, Redmond, WA; 115 pages.
A quarto-sized spiral bound volume that comes with an 85 page "solution guide." An introduction, through a series of exercises, to the complexities and use of the Kent *Repertory*.

Probably the best guide offered. The lessons are concise, and take one through the use of the book in easy steps.

1995: *HOMEOPATHY: A FRONTIER IN MEDICAL SCIENCE*: Paolo Bellavite, MD and
Andrea Signorini, MD ✔
North Atlantic Books; 335 pages.
The first of the books to explain the science behind the concept of the microdose. A new edition is coming in early 2002 that will bring the research up to date.

This is the only book on homœopathy ever reviewed by the British medical journal, The Lancet.

1996: *A CHRISTIAN'S GUIDE TO HOMŒOPATHY*: Alan Crook, MA, RSHom ✔
Winter Press, London; 85 pages.
Written by a registered homœopath who has been a "local preacher of the Methodist Church since 1964," the book is aimed at Christians who wish to obtain accurate information and an "analysis of the main Christian objections to it [homœopathy]."

1996: *GUIDE TO KENT'S REPERTORY*: Ahmed N. Currim, PhD, MD ✔
Hahnemann International Institute of Homeopathic Documentation, Norwalk, CT; 250 pages.
A guide to the intricacies of Kent's major work.

It is overly complex, and while it is probably useful for someone who has used the repertory for a number of years and is looking for something "more," it is not a beginner's book in any sense.

Even with Repertory in hand, I found the explanations overly confusing, with too many cross references, footnotes, and personal codes. The author is undoubtedly a master of the work, but has internalized much of his information, so in trying to explain it something is getting lost along the way.

1996: *THE COLLECTED WORKS OF ARTHUR HILL GRIMMER*: Arthur H. Grimmer, MD ✔
Hahnemann International Institute of Homeopathic Documentation, Norwalk, CT; 890 pages.
Edited by Ahmed N. Currim, PhD, MD.
A complete collection of all the writings by A. H. Grimmer, a pupil of Kent, and one of the leaders in homœopathy through the 1930s and 1940s. The book contains all his essays on Materia Medica, Philosophy, Therapeutics (including a large section on the therapeutics of Cancer), and all of his other lectures to various homœopathic organizations.

A treasure trove. Elizabeth Wright Hubbard said of Grimmer, "Unfortunately he never published a book. Some people write it and others live it." Happily, his writings were collected and finally published. Where else would one find any information about the materia medica of remedies like Toxicophus *and* Congo red*?*

1996: *THE ELEMENTS OF HOMŒOPATHY:* Dr. Pichiah Sankaran, edited by Rajan Sankaran ✔
Homœopathic Medical Publishers; 430 pages vol. 1, 310 pages volume 2.
Two volumes of compiled writings by a prolific author and master homœopath. Volume 1, Part II contains a narrative materia medica of 51 remedies and an essay on the Bowel Nosodes.

All of Sankaran's useful little pamphlets are assembled within this book. They contain untold treasures. My favorite is the one on "The Potency Question" where half the essay has testimonials gleaned from the literature saying "I saw no result with the low potency, so I went high and cured the patient," and the second half has testimonials that said, "I saw no result with the high potency, so I went low and cured the patient."

1996: *THE VACCINE GUIDE: MAKING AN INFORMED CHOICE*: Randall Neustaedter, OMD ✔
North Atlantic Books; 260 pages.
The question of vaccines has been an issue within homœopathy since Burnett noted the multitude of reactions to the smallpox vaccine and the cure of the symptoms with homœopathy. This book grew out of a previous work , *THE IMMUNIZATION DECISION: A GUIDE FOR PARENTS* (North Atlantic Books, **1990**; 114 pages). The book discusses each vaccine, what it contains, why it was developed, and the pros and cons of its use. An important reference for all parents facing the question of immunizations for their children.

Probably the best book available on the subject.

1996: *CUMULATIVE INDEX TO THE HOMŒOPATHIC PHYSICIAN*: Jay Yasgur ✔
Van Hoy Publishing, Tempe, AZ; 304 pages.
Looseleaf bound in a ring-binder, pages printed on one side only.
A complete index divided in many ways: by author, by title, by topic, by remedy. A full listing of all the obituaries contained in the journal. The collection includes a 65-page excerpt of cases and articles from the journal.

The Homeopathic Physician was one of the best "Hahnemannian" journals ever published. The usefulness of the index might be a moot point, in that there are not many copies of the journals, especially a full run, in collections.

1996: *QUICK REMEDY INDEX TO THE HOMEOPATHIC MATERIA MEDICA*: Bart Hiusmans. Edited by Rene Otter ✔
Lutra, Eindhoven Holland; 144 pages.
A listing of where remedy information can be found in the classic works of Hahnemann, Hering, etc., as well as more recent references from Vithoulkas, Ghegas, and others.

1997: *NATURAL RELATIONSHIP OF REMEDIES:* Jorg Wichmann and Anglica Bolte ✔
Wichmann, Refrath, Germany; 208 pages.
Noting that the Materia Medica is always arranged alphabetically, and rarely provides us with the understanding of *what* the remedy is, this book outlines the biological remedies (plants and animals) in the order of their species and phyllum. It is written in both German and English.

1997: *REMEDY RELATIONSHIPS:* Abdur Rehman ✔
Haug Verlag; 362 pages.
Commenting that prior information was scattered through many sources, the author has pulled together all the information from the "reliable record of verified facts" and presented a complete survey that will "give the reader a clearer picture of the more or less extensive sphere of action of these remedies with their manifold healing powers."

A very useful reference book, and well bound as well!

1997: *SIGNALS AND IMAGES:* Madeleine Bastide, MD ✔
Kluwer Academic Publishers, Dordrecht; 299 pages.
The latest European research which supports an understanding of the mechanism of homœopathy.

1998: *FUNDAMENTAL RESEARCH ON ULTRA HIGH DILUTIONS*: assorted authors ✔
Kluwer Academic Publishers, Dordrecht; 261 pages.
A collection of scientific papers, all discussing the concept of the ultra-molecular dilution.

1998: *HERINGS MEDIZINISCHE SCHRIFTEN*: Klaus-Henning Gypser, MD, editor.
Göttingen; 1658 pages.
Includes all articles written by Hering in German, and placed in chronological order. It includes a biographical sketch of Hering and a list of all his publications. Provings done by Hering are not included in the book.

2000: *INTERNATIONAL HOMEOPATHIC DICTIONARY*: Jeremy Swayne, editor. ✔
Churchill Livingstone, Edinburgh; 251 pages.
A book designed to be used by health professionals who are interested in understanding homœopathic terminology.

It contains some biographic and pharmacy errors, which easily could have been avoided by consulting Yasgur's latest work. A good book for the non-homœopath, the writer or physician who is trying to understand what it is all about. The practicing homœopath would find Yasgur's book much more serviceable.

Journals

The Journals

When Bradford issued his *Homœopathic Bibliography* in 1892, he cited 174 journals that had been in publication until that date. Some, like the *Homœopathic Recorder*, were "current." Others, like *The Record*, from Boston, was published "irregularly and for only a short time." Many lasted no more than a year or two.

In 1984, a fairly complete bibliography of all known journals, world-wide, was compiled by the team of Jacques Baur (France), Klaus-Henning Gypser (Germany), George Von Keller (Germany), and Philip W. Thomas (Glasgow). This rare volume, *Bibliotheca Homœopathica*, is a treasure trove of information about the journals published until that date. In the introduction, the compilers say:

"Three years after the publication of the second edition of the *Organon*, the first homœopathic journal— *Archiv für die homöopathische Heilkunst*— was published in Leipzig in 1822… In all, 682 periodicals have been identified, of which 240 originated in the USA, which took the leadership. They were followed by France (76), Germany (73), India (53), Great Britain (45), Spain (34) and Italy (32)."

When articles of worth appeared in foreign publications, they were invariably translated and republished in the American journals. As with the books, this brief listing of journals will focus mainly on those published in the English language.

When homœopathy was first introduced to the USA, it came, primarily, through German speakers who learned it through the only works available— all in German and all by Hahnemann. It was not until 1836, eleven years after the introduction of the system by Gram in New York, that works began to be issued in English through the Academical Bookstore (Constantine Hering) in Allentown, PA. It was two years later, in 1838, that the first original book written in English on homœopathy was published.

As the number of practitioners grew the need to share information was paramount and this task was assumed by the publication of journals. But to have a successful journal, one needs to maintain a large enough subscription base to support the printing costs, and one needs to have enough of a base to have a regular flow of articles, cases, and other materials to make a journal viable.

The first English language journal, *The American Journal of Homœopathia*, was edited by John Gray, MD and A. G. Hull, MD, both pupils of Gram in New York. Issued in 1835, it was published bi-monthly. It lasted but four issues.

In 1835, Hering established the *Correspondenzblatt*, a slim 4-page "newspaper" of homœopathic information that was related to the Allentown Academy. It was in existence for just two years.

In 1838, the *American Journal of Homœopathy* was published in Philadelphia.

In 1840, the call was again taken up by Hull with *The Homœopathic Examiner*. A monthly, 48-page journal, it lasted three years. Two years later it was started again by John Gray and Charles Hempel and published by William Radde. It lasted another two years.

Within a few years there appeared to be enough interest among homœopaths to maintain a journal, and in 1846 *The New York Journal of Homœopathy* was issued. By the second issue its name was changed to *The American Journal of Homœopathy*, and was a semi-monthly 12-page journal. Edited by Dr. S. R. Kirby and R. A. Snow, it was enlarged to a 16-page monthly with the second volume. It continued until 1854. By the time it ceased publication, the first of the journals which were to become "well-established" had appeared. Homœopathy had reached its "critical mass."

These early journals give a good picture of the development of homœopathic practice in the early days. They often reflect the amazement which seasoned allopaths had when they made the move to homœopathy and discovered they could cure "difficult" conditions with a few granules of something as simple as *Rhus toxicodendron*. They make fascinating reading.

The list that follows highlights the major journals of the time. Many change editorship, publishers, and titles frequently. For example, *The Medical Advance*, a major journal of Hahnemannian homœopathy, went through four substantial changes of ownership during its 42 years of publication.

I have endeavored to list those that were dedicated to "pure" homœopathy, because those are the ones which contained information we find most useful today.

It should be kept in mind that these were journals. They were, in some sense, designed to be ephemeral. They were not always printed on the best paper, and the tendency to deteriorate was almost built in. Many of those that have survived have done so primarily because someone took the time to have the volumes bound, converting them into valuable books and not pamphlets to be thrown away.

With two exceptions— *The Transactions of the AIH* and the *Transactions of the IHA*— I have not included any transactions or proceedings in this list. *Bibliotheca Homœopathica* cites 21 yearly published transactions and 12 regularly published proceedings of state or local homœopathic societies.

Most of the quotes about the early journals come from an unsigned review of journals that appeared in the *American Homœopathic Review*, June/July, 1866.

Journals

1838: *THE AMERICAN JOURNAL OF HOMŒOPATHY*
Published in Philadelphia, it was edited by Hering, Lingen, and Neidhard, although their names do not appear on the title page. It lasted but six issues. The content of these six issues was then published as *MISCELLANIES ON HOMŒOPATHY*, (216 pages). Dr. Metcalf, in his work, referred to this as *THE PHILADELPHIA HOMŒOPATHIC JOURNAL*.

1840: *THE HOMŒOPATHIC EXAMINER*
Edited by A. G. Hull, and then by John Gray and Charles Hempel, only five volumes were ever published. It contained two very important works as appendices: Ruekert's *Therapeutics* and Bönninghausen's *Intermittent Fever*.

1843: *BRITISH JOURNAL OF HOMŒOPATHY*
Edited by Drysdale and Dudgeon, it was formally imported to the USA by Radde in 1851, and remained an important contributor to the homœopathic profession on both sides of the Atlantic. It was published until **1884**.

1846: *THE AMERICAN JOURNAL OF HOMŒOPATHY*
Edited by S. R. Kirby, MD, and R. A. Snow, MD, it published its first issue as *THE NEW YORK JOURNAL OF HOMŒOPATHY*, and then changed its name. It was published through 1854 (volume. 9) and contains an excellent historical record of what was transpiring in the homœopathic movement.

1848: *THE NORTH-WESTERN JOURNAL OF HOMŒOPATHY*
Edited by George Shipman, MD, "No journal has done more to disseminate homœopathy among the Western physicians than this." Published monthly, it lasted four years. It was reestablished in **1858**.

1849: *QUARTERLY HOMŒOPATHIC JOURNAL*
Published by Clapp in Boston, this 144 page journal had as its purpose "to lay before the American reader, scientific and practically useful articles, selected from the current homœopathic literature of the day in Germany and France." It was one of the main sources of information from the homœopaths in Europe. It lasted four volumes.

1851: *THE NORTH AMERICAN HOMŒOPATHIC JOURNAL*
Edited by Constantine Hering, MD, E. E. Marcy, MD, and J. W. Metcalf, MD. It was discontinued at the end of Volume 3 in 1853, and resumed in **1855**, edited by Marcy, John C. Peters, MD, and William H. Holcombe, MD, under the title *The North American Journal of Homœopathy*. Over the years it had a number of well-known editors, Hale, Bayard, Snelling, Neidhard, to name a few. With Volume 20, the editorship was assumed by Samuel Lilienthal, MD, who remained as editor until Volume 33 in 1885. From 1887 on it was issued as a monthly with 64 pages. It continued publication until **1923**.

This journal was eventually merged with the "Pan Therapist" and contained a lot of information about "autohemic" therapy— the potentization of one's own blood. There was very little homœopathy discussed in its pages in the last few years of publication.

1852: *THE PHILADELPHIA JOURNAL OF HOMŒOPATHY*
Edited by William A. Gardiner, and later by J. F. Geary and A. E. Small, it was published by Rademacher and Sheek. It lasted but four volumes. Within its pages were articles by B. F. Joslin, Carroll Dunham, A. E. Small, Samuel Dubs, James Kitchen, and P. P. Wells— the "cream of the crop" at that time. The first three volumes contained many clinical articles, provings, and materia medica. The fourth volume "was filled with personalities, attacks, and rejoinder" and "did not sustain the character of the preceding." Subscriptions fell off and publishing was discontinued.

1854: *THE HOMŒOPATHIC NEWS*
Edited by Hering and Lippe, it was an eight page paper published by Boericke and Tafel as an "independent advertising sheet" and gave two pages over to homœopathic news. They contained all the "mistakes" found in *Jahr's Manual* and also made mention of many of the "new remedies."

1856: *THE TRANSACTIONS OF THE AMERICAN INSTITUTE OF HOMŒOPATHY*
The first of the yearly transactions. Although not a true "journal," it contained the records of the annual meetings, and transcripts of all papers presented. It was continued until **1909**.

Filled with historical information and fascinating cases. The earlier volumes are the most interesting in terms of "Hahnemannian homœopathy." By 1870, Dunham had suggested the "opening" of the organization, and by 1880, very little "pure" homœopathy was discussed within its pages. The Transactions *were discontinued in 1909, when the* Journal of the AIH *began publication. After that date, the transactions of the meetings were incorporated into the* JAIH.

1858: *THE AMERICAN HOMŒOPATHIC REVIEW*
First published between 1858 and 1860, it ceased publication because of "The breaking out of the rebellion." In **1862** it was re-started under the editorship of Carroll Dunham, MD, P. P. Wells, MD, and H. M. Smith, MD. It ceased publication in 1866. During the time of its publication it became a primary source for the information about new provings. The first provings of *Apis*, *Aloes*, and *Allium cepa* were published as a supplement.

1860: *THE UNITED STATES JOURNAL OF HOMŒOPATHY*
Drs. Marcy and Preston, withdrawing from editorship of the *NORTH AMERICAN JOURNAL OF HOMŒOPATHY*, began a new journal. It lasted two years and was then merged again with the *NAJH*.

1860: *THE MEDICAL INVESTIGATOR*
Published by Halsey Brothers in Chicago. It went through a number of editors, before it was edited by E. M. Hale, MD, R. Ludlam, MD, and G. Shipman, MD in 1867. The editorship eventually passed to T. C. Duncan, MD. In 1875 the Duncan Brothers took over as publishers, and the name changed to *The United States Medical Investigator*. It continued until 1892.

1864: *THE AMERICAN HOMŒOPATHIC OBSERVER*
"A monthly journal devoted to the interest of homœopathic physicians" began publication under the auspices of E. A. Lodge, MD, in Detroit, Michigan. Although it had a number of exemplary editors (Lilienthal, S. A. Jones, E. M. Hale, H. C. Houghton, Samuel Worcester) it always remained under the firm control of Dr. Lodge. The journal ceased publication in **1885** when Dr. Lodge died.

1865: *THE UNITED STATES MEDICAL AND SURGICAL JOURNAL*
Published by C. S. Halsey, Chicago, with George Shipman as editor. Several other (Dunham, Wells, Wesselhoeft, T. F. Allen) served on the editorial board. In **1875** it was merged with *The Medical Investigator*.

1865: *THE HAHNEMANNIAN MONTHLY*
Founded by J. H. P. Frost and Adolph Lippe. It was to be one the most sought after of the

"Hahnemannian" journals. It was published by the Faculty of the Homœopathic Medical College of Pennsylvania. It was eventually acquired by Boericke and Tafel and later by the "Hahnemann Club" of Philadelphia. In 1880, E. A. Farrington, MD, became the editor. After Farrington's death, the editorship passed to Pemberton Dudley, MD, and then to Clarence Bartlett, MD, and W. B. Van Lennep, MD. After Farrington, the content ceased to be "pure." The ownership passed back to the Hahnemann Medical College, and it continued publication as a quasi–homœopathic/allopathic journal until **1948**, the year Hahnemann Medical College abandoned homœopathy.

During its "glory years" it published Berridge's *Repertory of Eye and Head Symptoms*, and a master work by Lilienthal on Diseases of the Skin.

When it ceased publication as an organ of Hahnemann Medical College, it resumed publication as *The Hahnemannian*, under the aegis of the Homœopathic Medical Society of the State of Pennsylvania. It was published, in one form or another, until late **1990**.

1866: *THE NEW ENGLAND MEDICAL GAZETTE*
Published under the auspices of Otis Clapp, Boston. "A journal exceedingly well got up, of great promise, and intended for the professional reader," it was continued until **1918**.

1866: *THE HOMŒOPATHIC WORLD*
Originally edited by E. Harris Ruddock in the UK, this small journal was in continuous publication for over 100 years. When Ruddock died in 1875, the editorship was assumed by Edward B. Shuldham, MD, who passed it to James Compton Burnett, MD in 1879. In 1886 John Henry Clarke, MD assumed editorship and continued until 1898 when it was assumed by Charles E. Wheeler, MD. Clarke resumed editorship in 1923 and edited the journal until his death in 1931.

The magazine was taken over by J. Ellis Barker, a friend of Clarke's. The name was changed to *Heal Thyself*. When Barker died in 1948 the editorship was assumed by S. Phillip Clements. In 1952, publication was assumed by Health Science Press and the name was changed to *Health and You*. Clements was joined by Eric Powell and Phyllis Speight as editors. In 1958, Phyllis Speight assumed sole editorship and the name was changed back to *The Homœopathic World*. It ceased publication in 1967. In June, **1979** it was re–issued as *The Homœopathic World* (new series), edited by Phyllis Speight. It ceased publication just three years later in March **1982**.

Under the editorship of Clarke, it was always an "unorthodox" publication, often "baiting" the establishment as Clarke was wont to do. When Barker took over in 1931, it became even more-so, and contained blistering attacks on medical orthodoxy— all based on Barker's belief that conventional medicine had failed, yet homœopathy had not been allowed a fair trial by the medical establishment. The magazine was strongly supported by the growing lay movement in the UK.

1867: *THE AMERICAN JOURNAL OF HOMŒOPATHIC MATERIA MEDICA*
Edited by Constantine Hering, MD and Henry Noah Martin, MD. Although it was only published for nine years, it contained much valuable information. It was in these pages that H. N. Guernsey first published his "Lectures on Key-Notes" and E. A. Farrington published his supplement to *Gross's Materia Medica*. In 1869, the complete volumes 1 and 2 were bound together into a single volume called *THE JOURNAL OF HOMŒOPATHIC CLINICS*. The title was continued through Volume 4. With Volume 5 (1871) it became *THE AMERICAN JOURNAL OF MATERIA MEDICA AND RECORD OF MEDICAL SCIENCE*. It was published through nine Volumes, the last appearing in 1876.

In 1990, Paul Herscu, ND, republished a facsimile of Volume 1 and 2. The original had belonged to William Boericke, and contains many of his hand-written notes in the margins. The book is still in publication through the New England Journal of Homeopathy.

1873: *THE CINCINNATI MEDICAL ADVANCE*
Owned and edited by T. P. Wilson, MD. In 1882, H. C. Allen, MD, took it over and moved the publishing to Ann Arbor, Michigan; the name changing to *Ann Arbor Medical Advance*. In 1884 the name was changed simply to *The Medical Advance* and published under that name until 1894, when the name

was changed to *The Hahnemannian Advocate*. It continued until 1907, when the name was changed back to *The Medical Advance*. It ceased publication in 1915.

The pages of this journal contained writings by the guiding lights of Hahnemannian homœopathy. H. C. Allen published an extensive series on Comparative Materia Medica. Hahnemann's *Chronic Diseases* (theoretical part) appeared as an appendix. Articles by Adolph Lippe were common.

1877: THE AMERICAN HOMŒOPATHIST
Published by A. L. Chatterton in Chicago, and later, New York. The name was changed to *The American Homœopath* in 1881, and then changed back to the original in 1885. In 1888, the editorship was assumed by Frank Kraft, MD, with its motto being: "Hew to the line; let the chips fall where they may." It was published until the end of **1891**. See **1994**.

1878: THE ORGANON
"A quarterly Anglo-American Journal of Homœopathic Medicine and Progressive Collateral Science." An outgrowth of a meeting of like minds at the 1876 International Homœopathic Congress in Philadelphia. The journal was edited by Adolph Lippe, MD and Samuel Swan, MD in the USA and Thomas Skinner, MD and Edward Berridge, MD in the UK. The last issue was Number 1, Volume 4 in 1881.

In the three years of publication this journal contained more valuable information than almost all the others combined. Every issue has cases or commentary by Lippe. Several of Swan's provings appear within the pages. A magnificent series, authored by Lippe called "Fatal Errors," is filled with gems and insights into homœopathic methodology. The "Skinner Machine" and the Boericke Potentizer" are both illustrated and discussed. It remains a hard-to-find journal, and is especially sought after because of the inherent value of almost everything that appeared within its pages.

1881: THE HOMŒOPATHIC PHYSICIAN
Devoted to "Hahnemannian Homœopathy," it was edited by E. J. Lee, MD, and then Walter James, MD, and G. H. Clark, MD. It ceased publication in 1899. Over its 19 years of publication it printed a number of invaluable small repertories. In **1996** Jay Yasgur produced an index using the set at the National Center for Homeopathy library as the prime source.

An invaluable homœopathic resource. Always Hahnemannian in outlook and approach. There are very few collections that include all the volumes.

1881: THE TRANSACTIONS OF THE INTERNATIONAL HAHNEMANNIAN ASSOCIATION
Although not a "journal," these yearly volumes contain the proceedings of the IHA and transcripts of all the papers presented and discussions held. The individual transactions were printed until **1926**. The proceedings were then printed in THE HOMŒOPATHIC RECORDER starting in 1927.

Where would homœopathy be without these? A full record of the thinking of the greatest homœopaths of the time. Always "Hahnemannian" in its outlook, the papers printed were often followed by discussions which followed the presentations, and it is in these discussions that off-the-cuff remarks are made by stalwarts such as Kent, Boger, Fincke, Wells, Case, Close, and others.

1882: THE CALIFORNIA HOMŒOPATH
"A Bi-Monthly journal, devoted to the Interests of Homœopathy on the Pacific Coast." Edited by William Boericke. It continued until 1892, when it was replaced with THE PACIFIC COAST JOURNAL OF HOMŒOPATHY. The latter ceased publication in 1941 and was replaced by the PACIFIC COAST HOMŒOPATHIC BULLETIN, which continued until **1974** when A. Dwight Smith, the editor, stepped down. It then became HOMŒOTHERAPY.

During the 1930s, until it became the BULLETIN in 1941, this journal contained exemplary articles about homœopathy.

1886: *THE HOMŒOPATHIC RECORDER*
"A bi-monthly journal Devoted Chiefly to Presenting Interesting Excerpts from Foreign Homœopathic Literature, to the Introduction of New Remedies, and to Advancing our Knowledge of the Older Ones." Published by Boericke and Tafel, this took the place of the *Quarterly Bulletin* that had been published by Boericke and Tafel since 1871. Originally edited by J. T. O'Connor, MD, the editorship passed to C. F. Millspaugh, MD, in 1889, and then to E. P. Anshutz in 1890. Anshutz remained editor until his death in 1918, when editorship was assumed by Rudolph Rabe, MD.
In **1927**, the publication was assumed by the International Hahnemannian Association, and it became the journal of that association. It was continued until **1959** when it merged with the *Journal of the American Institute of Homœopathy*.

The only record of "pure" homœopathy through homœopathy's "lean years." Papers by Roberts, Dixon, Hayes, Grimmer, Green, Wright-Hubbard, and others. Buried within is a column called "Carriwidgets"— which is filled with all kinds of practical advice. A very valuable resource.

1889: *THE JOURNAL OF HOMŒOPATHICS*
Says Bradford, "This was devoted to the more abstruse theories in connection with the Hahnemann Method of Healing." It contained the first part of the translation of the *Organon* by Fincke. The journal lasted but two issues.

1890: *THE HOMŒOPATHIC ENVOY*
Edited by E. P. Anshutz. Bradford says, "…this is really a homœopathic campaign magazine, and is conducted with the unanswerable logic that so grandly characterizes the older journals." It was published until **1918**.

1893: *JOURNAL OF THE BRITISH HOMŒOPATHIC SOCIETY*
Published from 1893 to 1910, when it was superseded by THE BRITISH HOMŒOPATHIC JOURNAL.

1894: *THE DENVER JOURNAL OF HOMŒOPATHY*
Published until 1896. Became THE CRITIQUE.

1897: *THE CRITIQUE*
Took over after Volume 3 of the *DENVER JOURNAL*. Published Volumes 4-20, ceasing publication in 1913.

Contained excellent materia medica articles by J. H. Allen, and some writings by Kent when he was "between journals."

1898: *THE JOURNAL OF HOMŒOPATHICS*
Edited by James Tyler Kent, MD and later by Alexander Villers, MD (Dresden) and Hugh Cameron, MD (Philadelphia). Originally the "voice" of Kent's School of Homœopathics, it contained much of his writing on materia medica and other pieces which were compiled in *Kent's Lesser Writings*, by W. W. Sherwood in 1926. It ceased publication in **1904**.

1901: *JOTTINGS*
A house publication of Boericke and Tafel. "Published occasionally," it appeared at irregular intervals. It was filled with ads for B&T products, testimonials, book reviews, and commentaries. It gives an interesting (and informative) view of homœopathy through the 1920s and 1930s. The last known issue, Number 90, appeared in February, 1949.

1909: *THE JOURNAL OF THE AMERICAN INSTITUTE OF HOMEOPATHY* ✔
This took the place of the *AIH Transactions*. It continues until the present day.

The journal of homœopathy for medical doctors in the USA. At the time it began publication, homœopathy was in its decline. Through the years there were always a few articles of homœopathic interest, but the majority of the

content was quite allopathic in nature. It changed its format size several times along the way, seemingly unable to decide upon a standard. It struggled through the 1950s and absorbed the Homœopathic Recorder in 1959. During homœopathy's lean years between 1968 and 1977, the editorship was ostensibly in the hands of Allen Neiswander, MD of Alhambra, CA, but the actual editing was being done by Allen's wife Georgiana, who could not be recognized because she was not a medical doctor.

In late 1977, Alain Naudé assumed the editorship of the journal. In December 1978 he questioned the "lack of motivation" on the part of the physician members, and suggested that if they did not take the initiative to begin homœopathic schools, it would be done by the laymen, and control of homœopathy would be removed from the hands of the physician. Naudé, for his comments, was removed as editor, and Neiswander returned until 1982, when the editorship was assumed by Karl Robinson, MD. The journal was revived, and continues to this day.

1911: THE BRITISH HOMŒOPATHIC JOURNAL ✔
It was preceded by the *Journal of the British Homœopathic Society*, which was published from 1893 to 1910. It is still published by the Faculty of Homœopathy in London. It is probably the best source for information about current homœopathic research.

1912: THE HOMŒOPATHICIAN
Edited by James Tyler Kent, MD and Julia Loos, MD. It contained much of Kent's later writing which was subsequently compiled in his *Lesser Writings*. Originally published bi-monthly, it became a 100-page quarterly in 1916. It published but two issues when Kent died, and the journal ceased publication.

It was reprinted, by subscription only, in the late 1970s. Sad to say, only 25 people world-wide chose to subscribe.

1926: HOMŒOPATHIC SURVEY
Published by the American Foundation for Homœopathy. This is a very rare publication. Little information about this journal is known. The last extant issue known was Number 2 in 1930.

This journal contains a few articles by Boger, Gladwin, and Green. The extant issues give a good overview of the position of homœopathy in the USA at the time, and the battles it was fighting for recognition.

1947: THE LAYMAN SPEAKS
Formed as the "publication" of the Bureau of Layman of the American Foundation for Homeopathy, this small pamphlet–sized journal was edited by Arthur B. Green, the brother of Julia M. Green, MD, the guiding light of the AFH. It contained many articles taken from previous issues of *Heal Thyself* (from the UK) and from The *Homœopathic Recorder*. There were also some original articles, and always an editorial or two by Arthur B. Green. Green retired in 1974, and the editorship passed to Richard Dykeman. Then in 1977 Alain Naudé assumed editorship. Always run at a loss by the Foundation, the magazine ceased publication in mid-1977. See 1978.

1957: ZEITSCHRIFT FÜR KLASSISCHE HOMÖOPATHIE ✔
Published until 1968 when the name was changed to *Acta Homoeopathica* for 2 years, and then back to *Zeitschrift für Klassische Homöopathie*. For a short period of time between 1988 and 1992 while under the editorship of K-H. Gypser, an English edition, *The Classical Homeopathic Quarterly*, was issued by the publisher, Haug Verlag (Heidelberg). The German edition continues. Current.

A wonderful resource. The English translations were done by Hela Michot-Dietrich, and were filled with valuable material; clinical cases, repertory corrections, philosophical issues, etc. They remain a source of excellent information. It is unfortunate that the journal was never supported enough by the homœopathic community to ensure further publication of the English edition.

1974: HOMŒOTHERAPY
A continuation of the *Pacific Coast Homœopathic Bulletin*, Originally edited by Alain Naudé, the editorship passed to Robert Schore in **1980**. The journal continued with many magnificent original and

re-printed articles, but the homœopathic community was too small to sustain it, and it ceased publication in 1985.

Another magnificent resource. The Aphorisms of Hippocrates by Bönninghausen appeared in these pages, as well as many articles gleaned from the best of the literature. The reprints were selected by Christopher Ellithorp. It was edited with extreme integrity and there was never a wasted word in its pages. It was the crème de la crème.

1978: *THE JOURNAL OF HOMŒOPATHIC PRACTICE*
A premature attempt to start a journal, it was an outgrowth of the Bay Area Homeopathic Study Group. Published for only four issues, this was a well put together 116-page journal edited by Stephen Cummings and Randall Neustaedter.

The four issues contain some wonderful material. It was too good at a time when the community was not large enough to support it.

1978: *HOMŒOPATHIC HEARTBEAT*
A six-page newsletter published by the National Center for Homeopathy, meant to take the place of *The Layman Speaks*. It continued until 1981, when it was replaced with *Homeopathy Today*. See **1981**.

1979: *IFPH NEWSLETTER*
The International Foundation for the Promotion of Homeopathy was formed in California in 1978 by George Vithoulkas, Bill Gray, and others. Their first newsletter came out in 1979. In 1981 the name of the organization was changed to the International Foundation for Homeopathy. In 1985 the base of operations was moved to Seattle, and the newsletter name changed to *Resonance*. Published bi-monthly, it continued until the IFH ceased operations in **1998**.

1980: *THE HOMŒOPATH* ✔
Published by the Society of Homœopaths in the UK. Current.

1981: *HOMEOPATHY TODAY* ✔
The monthly newsletter of the National Center for Homeopathy in the USA. Starting as a six page fold-out, it is currently a 40-page magazine with a full color cover. It has been edited by Julian Winston since 1984. Current.

1981: *AMERICAN HOMEOPATHY*
Published by the "Homeopathic Headquarters of America" who then became the "United States Homeopathic Association," it grew out of the split between the American Foundation and the National Center for Homeopathy. Toward the end of its publication it seemed to be in the hands of electro-acupuncturists. It ceased publication in **1985** when the USHA closed its operation.

1987: *HOMEOPATHIC LINKS* ✔
Begun by Beat Spring, MD in Switzerland, the base of operations moved to Holland in 1995. Current.

Seeing itself as an international magazine, there have been a number of guest editors from different countries, where the content focuses on homœopaths from that country. Much of the work is on the "leading edge" of homœopathy— new provings including meditative and dream provings, an emphasis on smaller, rare remedies, and many articles about doctrine of signatures and kingdom analysis, etc.

1987: *SIMILLIMUM* ✔
The journal of the Homeopathic Academy of Naturopathic Physicians. Published quarterly. Current. Conceived as a journal to spread communication between naturopaths who were using homœopathy, it began to devote itself to publishing cases shortly after the HANP began to present yearly case conferences. Over the years it drifted slowly toward an empathic approach until the editorship

was assumed in early 2001 by Barbara Osawa, RSHom (NA), who brought the focus back to solid case taking and the inductive method of Hahnemann.

The recent change of editorship bodes well for the journal. May it continue to flourish!

1988: CLASSICAL HOMEOPATHIC QUARTERLY
Haug Verlag, Heidelberg. See 1957.

1989: PROCEEDINGS OF THE PROFESSIONAL CASE CONFERENCE
Published yearly by the International Foundation for Homeopathy from 1989 through 1996. Subtitled, "Small Remedies and Interesting Cases."

Not quite a "journal" but where else does it fit? These volumes contain much information about "small" remedies such as Cyclamen, Origanum, Aristolochia, *and present strong cases with clear methodology. It is of interest to note that the early volumes were using the sub-title above, but the last volume switched the sub-title with the main title— the "Small Remedies" had overwhelmed the Professional Case Conference.*
A subtle shift had taken place in about 1995 and the presentations began to be less concerned with the rational inductive method of Hahnemann and more to discussion of remedy themes and newer provings, thus drifting toward the empathic edge of homœopathy and away from the inductive method. It was certainly a harbinger of the next few years where the "small remedy" gained god-like ascendency and strict methodology was apparently bypassed.

1991: THE NEW ENGLAND JOURNAL OF HOMEOPATHY ✔
Edited by Paul Herscu, ND and Amy Rothenberg, ND. "…only by combining our efforts can we advance our empirically derived knowledge of the art and cure through homeopathy." A peer–reviewed journal for cases and articles. Much of the material has begun to reflect Herscu's teaching of "Cycles and Segments." Current.

1995: THE EUROPEAN JOURNAL OF CLASSICAL HOMEOPATHY
Published quarterly by the International Academy of Classical Homeopathy. Edited by George Vithoulkas. Designed to support "classical" homœopathy, the magazine contained in the first issue a veritable broadside by Vithoulkas attacking the "artistic distortions" found in the work of many contemporary homœopaths, singling out the work of Rajan Sankaran as a prime example. Although the journal contained many other articles, this broadside took up much of the energy of the magazine. The invective continued through the remaining issues. The magazine received little financial support from the community, and ceased publication after four issues.

1994: JOURNAL OF THE LMHI
A journal from the Liga Medicorum Homeopathica Internationalis.

A beautiful full color, glossy magazine. To my knowledge only a single issue was published.

1994: THE AMERICAN HOMEOPATH ✔
The newsletter of the North American Society of Homeopaths. First edited by Greg Bedayn, it is a large, yearly journal filled with interviews, case studies, and historical material. It is presently edited by Melanie Grimes. Current.

When first conceived, Greg Bedayn went back to the first American Homœopath *(see 1877), edited by Frank Kraft, and adopted the motto: "Hew to the line; let the chips fall where they may." The first issue was about Hering, the second issue about Kent, the third issue about women in homeopathy with a beautiful color portrait of Melanie Hahnemann gracing the cover. It is a magnificent magazine, that comes out once a year.*

Appendices

The Literary Armamentarium: or Books that the Homœopathic Physician Cannot do Without, and Something About Them

by Benjamin Woodbury, MD

*Read before the Connecticut Homœopathic Medical Society, Derby, Conn., October 20, 1931.

The request of the Executive Committee of the Connecticut Homœopathic Medical Society for me to present a paper on the subject of "Books That the Homœopathic Physician Cannot Do Without, and Something About Them," reminds me that there is after all no subject that is more important from the standpoint of the homeopathic physician than his literary equipment.

What is meant, briefly, by this literary armamentarium? In the first place, it must be taken for granted that the homeopathic physician, like any other physician, must have had at the outset of his career, a well-rounded training in the classics or their equivalent, one or more modern languages, a good knowledge of the general sciences, of chemistry and physics particularly, and, if he is destined to succeed, a certain inborn or indwelling love of his fellowmen and the innate desire to become to the fullest extent in his power, a healer of the sick. He must, either consciously or unconsciously, embody in his cosmos, or more specifically perhaps within his ego, that divine purpose so well set forth by our immortal Hahnemann in the first paragraph of the *Organon*, namely: "The first and sole duty of the physician is to restore health to the sick. This is the true art of healing." The edition just quoted is the First American, from the British Translation of the Fourth German Edition, by Stratten, of Dublin. There is another version by Dudgeon that is much better known, that reads thus: "The physician's high and only mission is to restore the sick to health, to cure, as it is termed." The late Conrad Wesselhoeft of Boston renders it thus: "The physician's highest and only calling is to restore health to the sick, which is called healing." And Fincke, one of the most profound thinkers of the Hahnemannian wing of the profession, in an unpublished translation of the Fifth edition transcribes this same passage as follows: "The physician's highest and only calling is to make sick people well, which is called healing."

However we may translate this remarkable aphorism of Hahnemann's, we are brought face to face with the dignity of the physician, his superior worth in the world of men, and the high calling to which the God, All-Heal has called him. I am reminded here of the story of a small boy who was asked by someone who had called at his father's office, and was about to turn away in disappointment, if he knew where his father, who was a physician, could be found. "I do not know," replied the sturdy little fellow, "where my daddy can be just now, but wherever he is, I am sure he is helping somebody." If this be the end and aim of the student of medicine, and of the homeopathic physician, I am sure his future career will be a successful one. Thus to heal the sick, to make sick folk well, is the be-all and the end-all of the physician.

It is to the wisdom of Bacon that we are indebted for the observation that of the making of many books there is no end; and John Milton has remarked that "a good book is the precious life blood of a master spirit, embalmed and treasured up on purpose to a life beyond life." Richard le Gallienne has said in one of his exquisite romances that "books are the good Samaritans that find us robbed of all our dreams by the roadside of life, bleeding and weeping and desolate; and such is their skill and wealth and goodness of heart, that they not only heal up our wounds, but restore to us the lost property of our dreams..." and "a library is a better world, built by the brains and hearts of poets and dreamers; as a refuge from the real world outside; and in it alone is to be found the land of milk and honey which it promises." If this sort of works obtains in the secular, why should it not apply likewise to the scientific or medical shelves? I believe there is a world of romance hidden within the mighty tomes of all ages, and who shall say that there is not a divine afflatus in the man of science or the man of medical learning as well as in the poet or the dilettante?

Before entering into more details respecting our subject, let me call your attention to the general opinions of some literary minds concerning books. If we are, first of all, as interested in books for their own sake as the late Dr. Crothers' Old Librarian (Among Friends, p. 96) we can never allow them to suffer from lack of care. For there is much neglect that may befall a book, especially an old one. But here again modern ingenuity has devised ways and means for the permanent preservation of a library of books that are well worthy of the collector's notice. In the antiquarian's "convention of books" cited by Dr. Crothers, the books themselves assume the responsibility for the care not of themselves but of their readers, and arrange them carefully in order and groupings, and decide upon their various merits. For books in their own way set great store by their readers, and when a book misplaces its readers, or loses them, it is looked upon as an especial *faux pas*. It is no small achievement for a work to look after a large collection of miscellaneous readers, and to select those that are worthy of cultivation. It has not perhaps occurred to some of us that there is a specificity among readers as well as among books. Yet such, Dr. Crothers would have us believe. This gifted author and critic also wrote another essay entitled "The Hundred Worst Books" in which he says that: "Like all the lower organisms, poor books multiply prodigiously, though the total number is kept down by a corresponding mortality… The worst books sink speedily into the depths of oblivion. It is in these black waters that we must dredge for our specimens."

Fortunately, homeopathy boasts of a multitude of good books, and of a comparatively small number of bad ones, even applying all the strictures that the critic of general literature would unfeelingly employ. Certainly the works of Hahnemann, Jahr, Bönninghausen, Hempel, Hering, Kent and Allen, (to mention only a few of the earlier compilers of homeopathic literature) measure up to a high literary value.

Let us examine some of the treasures to be found in the literary armamentarium of the homeopathic physician:

First, let us go back to the fountain head, and see what contributions were made by Hahnemann himself that are still worthy of a place in modern times. Hahnemann's chief works include, as is well known, *The Organon, The Materia Medica Pura* and *The Chronic Diseases*. There is much, however, in his *Lesser Writings* that is worthy of the consideration of every physician of whatever method of practice.

In his monumental volumes, *Samuel Hahnemann: His Life and Work,* Dr. Richard Haehl of Stuttgart has included a list of the Essays and Works of Hahnemann. By actual count, this list embraces no less than twenty-two extensive volumes of Translations and Revisions of the leading medical writers of the times, from the year 1777 to 1800. Of Hahnemann's own works and essays, there are sixty listed from the year 1779 to 1810 which marks the publication of the first edition of the *Organon*, and from this time on until 1833 there are various editions of *The Materia Medica Pura* and *The Chronic Diseases*, with such epoch-making papers as "The Spirit of the Homeopathic Doctrine of Medicine," which, though imperfectly rendered into English, formed the medium for the introduction of homeopathy into America by Hans Burch Gram, in the year 1825; "Dissertation on the Helleborism of the Ancients," his thesis to the Faculty of Leipsic; "On the Preparation and Dispensing of Medicines by Homeopathic Physicians;" "Allopathy, a Word of Warning to Sick People;" "The Cure of Cholera;" and his papers on the Antipsorics; and Bönninghausen's writings in general. This list includes some twenty-two or more essays, also introductions by Leber and Lich and Kammerer of Ulm. And finally, his sixth and last edition of the *Organon*, with his own annotations, as presented to the profession through the energies of Drs. James W. Ward and the late William Boericke of San Francisco. What ones of these works can the homeopathic physician do without? Certainly not the great triad—*The Organon, The Materia Medica Pura* and *The Chronic Diseases*.

I have long conceived the idea of formulating a list of homeopathic works to occupy a similar place in the library of the homeopathic physician as that so popularly known at one time as "Dr. Eliot's Five Foot Shelf of Books." This the great educator set forth in his Harvard Classics (Collier, NY, 1910). This collection consisted of fifty selected volumes which, when one had carefully familiarized himself with them, would enable him to become a man or woman of culture. Dr. Crothers naively remarked of this Five Foot Shelf that: "There are little jealousies among books, and it is impossible to please any of them. The old Librarian was conscious of this when, in a corner of the hall, he saw a number of books chosen for their especial serviceableness being seated on a divan five feet long. Each as his name was called came forward with a look of modest merit, while betraying a momentary surprise at his neighbor."

In the above-mentioned essay, Doctor Crothers makes reference to between ninety and one hundred authors. Let us see how comprehensive a list of homeopathic works one could select for a five foot shelf. Hahnemann, we are told by Bradford, gives in his article on "Arsenical Poisoning" no less than 861 quotations from 389 different authors and books, in different languages and belonging to different ages, and gives these references "accurately both volume and page" and Haehl informs us that in his "Dissertation on the Helleborism of the Ancients" he was "able to quote verbatim (and give the location of the passages concerned) from manifold German, French, English, Italian, Latin, Greek, Hebrew and Arabic medical writers and he could examine their views—either in disagreement or in extension. He quoted from more than fifty more or less known doctors, philosophers and naturalists." Such was the wisdom of Hahnemann!

To return to our own homeopathic classics. As the director of the Bureau of Publication of the American Foundation for Homeopathy, I have frequently been asked to compile lists of homeopathic reference books which can be recommended for the use of the laity, for beginners in homeopathy and for more advanced study. A partial list of such works was published in the *Homeopathic Survey* for January, 1928, and in the *Homeopathic Recorder* for April, 1931 will be found a paper read before the Foundation Post-Graduate Summer School on "The Homeopathic Library and How to Profit by It," which outlines in a general way the fundamentals of homeopathic literature and their uses in the library of the homeopathic physician.

In the lists of reference works on homeopathy suggested for library and home study the textbooks were arranged in four groups as follows: Some forty to fifty or more works were listed on materia medica in Group I; Group II consisted of fifty works on homeopathic philosophy; Group III, of some ninety or more works on the repertory; and Group IV, of some eighty or more works on therapeutics and homeopathic practice. If we were to select from this list of three hundred or more works fifty volumes for our five foot shelf of homeopathic classics we might well condense the above groupings about thus:

GROUP I—MATERIA MEDICA

H. C. Allen's *Keynotes*
Hahnemann's *Materia Medica Pura*
Hering's *Condensed Materia Medica*
T. F. Allen's *Hand Book*
Boericke's *Pocket Manual of Materia Medica*
Boger's *Synoptic Key*
Clarke's *Dictionary of Practical Materia Medica* (3 vols.)
Farrington's *Clinical Materia Medica*
Gross' *Comparative Materia Medica*
Kent's *Lectures on Materia Medica*
Guernsey's *Keynotes to Materia Medica*
Hughes' *Manual of Pharmacodynamics*
Wheeler's *Introduction to the Principles and Practice of Homœopathy*
Choudhuri's *Repertory* (with the Materia Medica)

GROUP II—HOMŒOPATHIC PHILOSOPHY

Bönninghausen's *Lesser Writings*
Clarke's *Homeopathy Explained*
Close's *Genius of Homeopathy*
Dunham's *Homeopathy, the Science of Therapeutics*
Dudgeon's *Lectures on the Theory and Practice of Homœopathy*
Fincke's *On High Potencies and Homœopathics*
Gram's *Characteristics of Homœopathia*
Hahnemann's *Organon* (1st Edition, Everyman's Library Edition and 6th Short Edition, Boericke)
Hahnemann's *Chronic Diseases* (Theoretical Part only) (translated by Prof. L. H. Tafel)
Hahnemann's *Lesser Writings*
Joslin's *Principles of Homœopathy*
Kent's *Lectures on Homeopathic Philosophy*

The Heritage of Homœopathic Literature

Kent's *Lesser Writings*
R. Gibson Miller's *Outlines of Homeopathic Philosophy*
Wheeler's *The Case for Homœopathy*

GROUP III—REPERTORIES

Allen's *Bönninghausen's Therapeutic Pocket Book*
Bell's *Repertory of Diarrhoea*
Boger's *Bönninghausen's Characteristics and Repertory*
Field's *Symptom-Register*
Gentry's *Concordance Repertory*
Hering's *Analytical Therapeutics* (Vol. 1 only one published)
Jahr's *Repertory and the New Manual*
Kent's *Repertory of the Materia Medica*
Knerr's *Repertory to Hering's Guiding Symptoms*
Lippe's *Repertory to the More Characteristic Symptoms of the Materia Medica*
Lee and Clark's *Cough and Expectoration*
Shedd's *Clinical Repertory*
Worcester's *Repertory to the Modalities*
Lilienthal's *Homeopathic Therapeutics*

GROUP IV—THERAPEUTICS AND HOMŒOPATHIC PRACTICE

Arndt's *System of Medicine*
Baehr's *Science of Therapeutics*
Burnett's *New Cure for Consumption*
Carleton's *Homeopathy in Medicine and Surgery*
Cowperthwaite's *Text-Book of the Practice of Medicine*
Dewey's *Practical Homeopathic Therapeutics*
Guernsey's *Application of the Principles and Practice of Homœopathy to Obstetrics*
Jahr's *Forty years' Practice*
Nash's *Leaders in Homeopathic Therapeutics*
Pulford's *Leaders in Pneumonia*
Raue's *Special Pathology and Diagnostics*
Royal's *Textbook of Homeopathic Theory and Practice of Medicine*
Schuessler' *Tissue remedies*

It will be observed that in compiling even a five foot shelf of homeopathic books, many well-known works must needs be omitted, owing to their bulk; as, for example, Allen's *Encyclopedia*, of ten volumes, and Hering's *Guiding Symptoms*, likewise of ten volumes. Of the latter sets of books it might well be said that no library could be considered complete without them. Yet here we have listed only *The Handbook* and the *Condensed Materia Medica*. Bartlett's three-volume work on Practice might well be included, as this is the latest work of its kind from the pen of a living author, and contains an up-to-date resume of the general field of medicine, including homeopathic therapeutics. There are countless smaller works, such as Burnett's classic monographs, Dudgeon's Essays, bound volumes of Skinner's *Organon*, Kent's *Journal of Homœopathics*, many of the essays of Clarke, Wheeler, Weir, Tyler, and other modern writers, which should find a place in the library of every homeopathic physician. The above list and many not here mentioned are books which the homeopathic physician cannot well do without. In case-taking, such works as Boger, Close, Kent, Nash's *How to Take the Case and Find the Similimum*, Bidwell's *How to Use the Repertory*, Margaret Tyler's *Repertorizing and How Not to Do It*, are of inestimable value. In the study of philosophy one should familiarize himself with all of Hahnemann's works. He should know Kent from cover to cover, and he can read with profit Joslin and Carroll Dunham, many of the essays and introductions of Hempel, and the lectures of Stuart Close. He must have read the *Lesser Writings of Bönninghausen* and the latter's translation of the *Aphorisms of Hippocrates*. He should know materia medica thoroughly, the materia medica of no fewer than one hundred remedies, should have a comprehensive knowledge of the thousand more which comprise the complete materia medica. He must have read such comprehensive works as Bradford's *Life of Hahnemann*, Haehl's *Samuel Hahnemann, His Life and Work*, Ameke's *History of Homeopathy*, and be familiar with Bradford's *Pioneers*. He must be more or less conversant with homeopathic bibliography, he must be familiar with the Bönninghausen Method, the Kent Method, and with the use of different types of card-index repertories. He must be familiar with, and have in his possession, if possible, a varied collection of the works of the old masters, and bound volumes of early homeopathic journals. Such an array, transcending to an immeasurable degree any five foot shelf of collected works, would constitute a comprehensive library for the studious and conscientious homeopathic practitioner. The student of homeopathic classics, the bibliophile, the true connoisseur of Hahnemanniana could never cease to wander amid the fascinating highways and byways of homeopathic literature. The libraries of the pioneers of our art consisted of such an *omnium gatherum*. Many of these libraries have been in recent years bequeathed to our generation. Happy indeed is he, and fortunate, who is the possessor of such a literary armamentarium. Whenever possible, may each and every one of us gather together these literary treasures. For what a priceless treasure is a book, of whose possessor it has been so well said:

He ate and drank the precious words,
His spirit grew robust;
He knew no more that he was poor,
Nor that his frame was dust.
He danced along the dingy days,
And this bequest of wings
Was but a book. What liberty
A loosened spirit brings!

And today?

As this works attests, there have been a good number of books published in the 70 years since Dr. Woodbury compiled his list. Given these more recent additions, would I change Woodbury's selection?

In attempting to answer that question, I asked 40 practising homeopaths to give me a list of "the books you think a practitioner cannot be without."

Only 25 replied to my question. The Materia Medicæ quoted were-- Clarke (19), Allen (16), Kent (13), Boericke (12), Hering (12), Hahnemann's Chronic Diseases (12), Hahnemann's Materia Medica (8), Nash (6), Dunham (4), Farrington (4), Lippe (5), Allen's Keynotes (3), Boger's *Synoptic Key* (2). Six included the *Synthesis* Repertory, 13 included the *Complete* Repertory. Five did not even mention any repertory. Lilienthal's *Therapeutics* was mentioned by two, as was Clarke's *Prescriber*. For philosophy, there were Kent (11) and Close (5). Of the group, only 14 mentioned the *Organon*. Six mentioned Boenninghausen's *Lesser Writings*, and four mentioned Hahnemann's *Lesser Writings*.

The newer works that were most frequently included were Phatak's *Materia Medica* (11), Vermeulen's *Synoptic Materia Medica* and *Concordant* (10), Morrison's *Desktop Guide* (9), Sankaran (7), Scholten (6), Vithoulkas' *Science of Homeopathy* (5), the newer provings of Sherr (4), Tyler's *Drug Pictures* (4), Retzik's *Materia Medica of the Mind* (3), Vithoulkas' *Materia Medica Viva* (3), Mirelli's *Thematic Repertory* (2), and one each to Murphy's *Lotus Materia Medica*, Herscu's *Children*, Shinghal's *Bedside Prescriber*, Eizayaga's *Treatise*, Dhawale's *Principles*, Julian's *Materia Medica*, Stephenson's *Provings*, and Logan's *Eczema*.

Several mentioned that they accessed the repertory through a computer program as well as accessing the books with a program like *ReferenceWorks* or *Encyclopedia Homeopathica*.

When did we stop reading? I suggest that with the near demise of homeopathy in the 1950s and 1960s, most of the larger libraries held by the first and second generation practitioners were dispersed. There were few homœopaths around to take the books. (see "The Treasures that were Lost," pg. 478, *Faces of Homeopathy*).

Then, in the 1970s, there was a resurgence led by Vithoulkas. He did not spend much time discussing the *Organon*. How well did he instill in his pupils the understanding of the richness of the heritage of literature? Says one of his pupils: "What he said was, 'Go home, study Kent, read the old materia medicae. On top of that I will give some information' — that is what became his essences.

"However, many of his students just skipped part one, wanting only his info. There's the problem in a nutshell. They had a little bit of information floating around not grounded in anything real. So if one happened to see or feel or perceive an 'essence' great, but if one did not, there was no philosophy, no tool, no way to move forward and try to help the patient. This also was/is a tremendous problem with the issue of follow up because without a strong philosophy and understanding of where things are going, it is difficult, if not impossible, to follow a person over time."

It is the teachers who have the responsibility of passing on the awareness of our literary heritage. When the teachers of today don't have that awareness, or worse, see no need for it, what happens?

Few understand what is buried in our "homeopathic pile." Few even use the primary literature to verify the selection from the repertory.

The risk is that when one uses a program like *ReferenceWorks* or *Encyclopedia Homeopathica* to search for a phrase or symptom in all available materia medicæ, the "book" is lost. The context is lost.

For example, if you look in a literature database for the phrase "Alas, poor Yorick," you will find it is in Shakespeare's *Hamlet*, but that tells you nothing of the context in which it is used.

Similarly, finding that *this* symptom is in the proving of *Nux vomica* and *that* symptom is in the proving of *Nux* does not mean that the remedy needed is *Nux*. One needs to get a larger grasp of what the proving of *Nux vomica* was about— and this can come only from reading the primary literature.

The best homeopaths I know are those who read the books. They read, read, and read. They search out the old journals. They read Dunham's words *in* his books rather than from summaries of Dunham's books, or snatches found when searching for a remedy.

Everything is now being pre-digested. All the wonderful little repertories have been absorbed into the larger ones, all the materia medica from Boericke, Phatak, Boger, Clarke, Hering has been absorbed into a single volume by Vermeulen, and all the books (often without introductions or annotations) have been assembled into *ReferenceWorks*.

We have reduced our five foot shelf to a one-foot shelf and a laptop. In combining it all we have lost the individual pieces. By doing so, we have turned our back on our vast literary heritage, and are slowly losing the ability to use our "necktop computer."

Homœopathic Publishers

The name of the publisher and location is given. The dates of operation are given, if known. A date of 1892 given as a termination indicates the company was still operating when Bradford published his *Bibliography*.

A good number of the publishers were also homeopathic pharmacies.

American Homœopathic Publishing Society (J. M. Stoddard & Co.)
Philadelphia, PA. 1879 to 1885
It published the first four volumes of Hering's Guiding Symptoms *and then disbanded.*

Academical Bookstore
Allentown, PA 1833 to 1836
Published material from the Allentown Academy.

Arnoldischen Buchhandlung
Dresden, Germany
Published most of Hahnemann's works.

H. Balliere
London. mid-1800s.

J. B. Ballière
Paris. mid-1800s

F. E. Boericke
Philadelphia, PA. 1867 to 1869.
Run by Francie E. Boericke, it also published under the imprint of **Hahnemann Publishing House**, 1883-1890.
The business was sold, in 1890, to Boericke and Tafel

Boericke and Tafel
Philadelphia, PA and New York, NY. 1869 to 1883.
F. E. Boericke retired from the pharmacy to form the Hahnemann Publishing House *in 1883.*

Boericke and Tafel
Philadelphia, PA. 1883 through the 1950s.
Boericke (F. L. and then Felix) and Tafel (A. J. and then A. L.)

Boericke and Runyon
San Francisco and New York
A branch of Boericke and Tafel that published a number of books for them.

Editions Boiron
Lyons, France. Current.
The publishing division of Boiron Pharmacy.

British Homœopathic Association
London
Published from the 1920s through the 1990s.

Otis Clapp
Boston, MA. 1842 to 1873.

Otis Clapp & Son
Boston MA. 1873 through the 1950s

A. L. Chatterton & Co.
New York, NY. 1884-1892
Traded also as the Homeopathic Publishing Company.

W. A. Chatterton & Co.
Chicago, IL 1876-1892

C. W. Daniel, Ltd.
Saffron Walden, UK. Current.
(see Homeopathic Publishing Co.)

F. A. Davis
Philadelphia, PA. 1885 to 1892

Duncan Brothers
Chicago, IL. 1876 to 1892
Formed by Thomas Cation Duncan and his brother David

H. B. Drake
Detroit, MI. 1879 to 1892

Judah Dobson
Philadelphia, PA. 1841 to 1847

H. W. Derby & Co.
Cincinnati, OH. 1850

Dynamis
Northampton, UK. Current.
The publishing arm of Jeremy Sherr and the Dynamis School.

James Epps
London, England (circa 1839 to 1911)

Formur
St. Louis, MO. Current
The publishing arm of Luyties Pharmacal

E. Gould
London, England (circa 1870 to 1917)

Gross and Delbridge
Chicago, IL. 1877 to 1892

Globe Printing House
Philadelphia, PA. 1881 to 1892
Printing company owned by Walter Hering, son of Constantine Hering.

Hahnemann Clinic Publishing
Nevada City, CA. Current.

Halsey & King
Chicago, IL 1860 to 1861

C. S. Halsey
Chicago, IL. 1861 to 1871

Halsey Brothers
Chicago, IL. 1871 to 1892

Karl F. Haug Verlag
Heidelberg, Germany. Current.

Health Science Press
Holsworthy, Devon (see Homeopathic Publishing Co.) 1950 to 1985

Homeopathic Medical Publishers
Bombay, India. Current.

Homœopathic Publishing Company
London.
Started by John Henry Clarke in about 1879 to publish his own books. It was sold to Leslie Speight in about 1950 and became Health Science Press, *which in turn was sold in 1985 to* C. W. Daniel Co. Ltd.

C. T. Hurlburt
New York, NY 1858 to 1892

Indian Book and Periodical Syndicate (IBPS)
New Delhi, India. Current.

IRHIS
Leidschendam, Holland. Current.

B. Jain
New Delhi, India. Founded 1965. Current

Leath and Ross
London, England (circa 1842 to 1902)

E. A. Lodge
Detroit, MI. 1862 to 1886

Matthews & Houard
Philadelphia, PA. 1852

Merlijn Publishers
Haarlem, Holland. Current.

New Jerusalem Print
Philadelphia, PA. 1850

North Atlantic Books
Berkeley, CA. Founded 1979. Current.

Pankaj Publications
Delhi, India.

Quality Medical Publishing
St. Louis, MO. Current.

William Radde
New York, NY. 1839 to 1869

Charles L. Rademacher
Philadelphia, PA. 1846 to 1848

Rademacher & Sheek
Philadelphia, PA. 1848 to 1855

Lewis Sherman
Milwaukee, WI. 1874 to 1892

Sherman and Co.
Philadelphia, PA. Circa 1880

G. W. Smith
Cincinnati, OH. 1888 to 1892

Henry M. Smith & Brother
New York, NY. 1869 to 1872

Henry M. Smith
New York, NY. 1872 to 1892

Stiching Alonnissos
Utrecht, Holland. Current.

Adolph Tafel
Philadelphia, PA 1865 to 1869

Jeremy Tarcher
New York and Los Angeles, USA. Current.

Thorsens Publishers Ltd.
Wellingborough, Northamptonshire, UK. Current.

Henry Turner
London and Manchester, England (circa 1854 to 1877)

J. G. Wesselhoeft
Philadelphia, PA. 1833 to 1842

World Homeopathic Links
New Delhi, India. Current.

The Book in Chronological Order

Key:
Materia Medica (MM); Repertory (R); Therapeutics (T); Anatomy and Physiology (AP); Domestic (D); Popular (P); Veterinary (V); Pharmacy (PH); Principles (PR); History (H); Biography (B); Other (O); Critical (CR). All *Organon* are in the first setion of that name.

1810: ORGANON DER RATIONELLEN HEILKUNDE: Samuel Hahnemann, MD (first edition)
1811-1821: THE MATERIA MEDICA PURA: Samuel Hahnemann, MD (MM)
1817: THE SYMPTOM DICTIONARY: Samuel Hahnemann, MD (handwritten) (R)
1819: ORGANON DER HEILKUNST: Samuel Hahnemann, MD (second edition)
1824: ORGANON DER HEILKUNST: Samuel Hahnemann, MD (third edition)
1825: HOMÖOPATHISCHES DISPENSATORIUM FÜR AERZTE UND APOTHEKER: C. Caspari (PH)
1825: THE CHARACTERISTICS OF HOMŒOPATHIA: Hans Burch Gram, CML (P)
1826: HOMÖOPATHISCHER HAUS-UND REISEARZT: Carl Caspari (D)
1826: SYSTEMATIC DESCRIPTION OF THE PURE EFFECTS OF REMEDIES): C. G. C. Hartlaub (R)
1828: THE CHRONIC DISEASES; THEIR PECULIAR NATURE AND THEIR HOMŒOPATHIC CURE: Samuel Hahnemann, MD (MM)
1829: DISPENSATORIUM HOMŒOPATHICUM (in Latin): Dr. C. Caspari (PH)
1829: ELEMENTI DI FARMACOIPEA OMIOPATICA ESTRATTI DALLA MATERIA MEDICA DI S. HAHNEMANN: Dr. Vincenzo la Raja (PH)
1829: HOMÖOPATHISCHE PHARMAKOPÖE FÜR AERZTE UND APOTHEKER: Franz Hartmann (PH)
1829: ORGANON DER HEILKUNST: Samuel Hahnemann, MD (fourth edition)
1830: MEDICAMENTORUM HOMŒOPATHICIS; Dr. G. Widenmann (PH)
1830: SYSTEMATIC DESCRIPTION OF ANTIPSORIC REMEDIES: Georg Adolph Weber (R)
1831: SPECIAL THERAPY OF ACUTE AND CHRONIC DISEASES: Franz Hartmann, MD (T)
1831: SYSTEMATIC PRESENTATION OF ALL HOMŒOPATHIC MEDICINES: Ernst Ferdinand Ruckert (R)
1832: REPERTORY OF ANTIPSORIC MEDICINES C. von Bönninghausen (R)
1833: ORGANON DER HEILKUNST: Samuel Hahnemann, MD (fifth edition)
1833: THE HOMŒOPATHIC MEDICAL DOCTRINE OR THE ORGANON OF THE HEALING ART: Samuel Hahnemann, MD (first English)
1833: DIE DYNAMIK DER ZAHNHEILKUNDE BEARBEITET NACH DEN GRUNDSÄTZEN DEN HOMÖOPATHIE (The Dynamics of Dentistry According to the Principles of Homœopathy): Salomo Gutmann (T)
1834: HOMŒOPATHY— A TEXT-BOOK FOR THE EDUCATED, NON-MEDICAL PUBLIC: C. von Bönninghausen (P)
1834: JAHR'S MANUAL: George Heinrich Gottlieb Jahr (R)
1834: MANUAL OF HOMEOPATHIC MEDICINE: George Heinrich Gottlieb Jahr (MM)
1834: PHARMACOPŒIA HOMŒOPATHICA: Frederick Foster Hervey Quin, MD (PH)
1835: A POPULAR VIEW OF HOMŒOPATHY: Rev. Thomas R. Everest (P)
1835: PHARMACOPÉE HOMŒOPATHIQUE: L. Noirot and Ph. Mouzin (PH)
1835: REMARKS ON THE ABRACADABRA OF THE NINETEENTH CENTURY: William Leo-Wolf (CR)
1835: THE HOMŒOPATHIST OR DOMESTIC PHYSICIAN: Constantine Hering, MD (D)
1836: ABBILDUNGEN DER ARZNEIGEWÄCHSE WELCHE HOMÖOPATISCH GEPRÜFT WORDEN SIND UND ANGEWENDET WERDEN: Eduard Winkler (PH)
1836: AUSFÜHRLICHE BESCHREIBUNG SÄMMTLICHER ARZNEIGEWÄCHSE, WELCHE HOMÖOPATHISCH GEPRÜFT WORDEN SIND UND ANGEWENDET WERDEN. FUR HOMÖOPATHIKER ZUR BENUTZUNG BEIM EINSAMMELN DER ARZNEIKÖRPER AUS DEM PFLANZENREICHE; Eduard Winkler (PH)
1836: HOMÖOPATHISCHE PHARMACOPÖE: Von Dr. A. Rollink (PH)
1836: JAHR'S MANUAL OF HOMEOPATHIC MEDICINE: George Heinrich Gottlieb Jahr (MM)
1836: REPERTORY OF MEDICINES THAT ARE NOT ANTIPSORIC: C. von Bönninghausen (R)
1836: THE ORGANON OF HOMŒOPATHIC MEDICINE: Samuel Hahnemann (first American)

1837: HOMOEOPATHIC MATERIA MEDICA FOR VETERINARIANS: Carl Ludwig Genzke (V)
1837: ZOOIASIS, OR HOMŒOPATHY IN ITS APPLICATION TO THE DISEASES OF ANIMALS: Wilhelm Lux (V)
1837: ORGANON DER SPECIFISCHEN HEILKUNST: Gottlieb Ludwig Rau, MD (O)
1838: HOMŒOPATHIC PRACTICE OF MEDICINE: Jacob Jeanes, MD (T)
1838: HUMBUGS OF NEW YORK: David Meredith Reese (CR)
1838: PHARMACOPOEA UNIVERSALIS (PH)
1838: REPERTORY TO THE MANUAL: Edited by Constantine Hering, MD (R)
1838: THE PATHOGENIC EFFECTS OF SOME OF THE PRINCIPAL HOMŒOPATHIC REMEDIES: Harris Dunsford, MD (MM)
1838: REPERTORIUM FÜR DIE HOMÖOPATHISCHE PRAXIS: A. Joseph Fredericus Ruoff (R)
1839: DOMESTIC HOMŒOPATHY: John Epps, MD (D)
1839: DOMESTIC HOMŒOPATHY: Paul F. Curie, MD (D)
1839: PERCEPTION AND CURE OF THE MOST IMPORTANT DISEASES OF THE HORSE: Ernst Ferdinand Rueckert (V)
1840: THEORY AND PRACTICE OF HOMŒOPATHY: I. G. Rosenstein, MD (PR)
1840: HOMOOPATHISCHE ARZNEIBEREITUNGSLEHRE: Joseph Benedict Buchner (PH)
1840: NOUVELLE PHARMACOPÉE ET POSOLOGIE HOMOEOPATHIQUE: G. H. G. Jahr (PH)
1840: REPERTORY OF HOMŒOPATHIC MATERIA MEDICA: A. Joseph Fredericus Ruoff (R)
1841: DISEASES OF THE ALIMENTARY CANAL AND CONSTIPATION, TREATED HOMŒOPATHICALLY: W. Broackes (T)
1841: HOMOEOPATHIC DOMESTIC MEDICINE: Joseph Laurie, MD (D)
1841: HULL'S JAHR; A NEW MANUAL OF HOMŒOPATHIC PRACTICE: A. Gerald Hull, MD (R)
1841: PRACTICAL OBSERVATIONS ON SOME OF THE CHIEF HOMEOPATHIC REMEDIES: Franz Hartmann, MD (MM)
1842: HOMŒOPATHY AND ITS KINDRED DELUSIONS: Oliver Wendell Holmes, MD (CR)
1842: HOMŒOPATHY: Thomas W. Blatchford, MD (CR)
1842: NEW HOMŒOPATHIC PHARMACOPOEIA AND POSOLOGY: G. H. G. Jahr (PH)
1842: PURE SYMPTOMATOLOGY OR SYNOPTIC PATTERN OF ALL THE MATERIA MEDICA PURA: P. J. Lafitte (R)
1842: PRACTICAL ADVANTAGES OF HOMŒOPATHY, ILLUSTRATED BY NUMEROUS CASES: Harris Dunsford, MD (P)
1843: MANUAL OF HOMŒOPATHIC MATERIA MEDICA: Alphons Noack, MD and Carl Freidrich Gottfried Trinks, MD (MM)
1843: THE ORGANON OF HOMŒOPATHIC MEDICINE: Samuel Hahnemann (second American)
1845: HOMÖOPATHISCHE PHARMACOPOE Carl Ernest Gruner (PH)
1845: HOMÖOPATHISCHE PHARMACOPOE: De Horatiis (PH)
1845: VIEWS ON HOMŒOPATHY: Daniel Holt (P)
1846: ADDITIONS TO THE MATERIA MEDICA PURA: Ernst Stapf, MD (MM)
1846: HOMŒOPATHY, ALLOPATHY, AND THE YOUNG PHYSIC: John Forbes, MD (CR)
1846: HOMOOPATHISCHE ARZNEILBEREITUNG UND GABENGRÖSSE: Dr. Georg Schmid (PH)
1846: THE HOMEOPATHIC DOMESTIC PHYSICIAN: Charles Hempel, MD (D)
1846: THE HOMŒOPATHIC FARRIER: Christian Bush (V)
1846: THE THERAPEUTIC POCKET BOOK: C. von Bönninghausen (R)
1846: A MANUAL OF HOMŒOPATHIC COOKERY: Anonymous (O)
1846: THE TRANSACTIONS OF THE AMERICAN INSTITUTE OF HOMŒOPATHY: AIH (MM)
1847: DISEASES OF THE EYE TREATED HOMŒOPATHICALLY: Alexander C. Becker (T)
1847: NEUVA FARMACOPEA Y POSOLOGIA HOMEOPATICA, O MODO DE PREPARAR LOS MEDICAMENTOS HOMEOPATICOS Y DE ADMINISTRAR LAS DOSIS: G. H. G. Jahr (PH)
1847: NEW MANUAL OF HOMOEPATHIC VETERINARY MEDICINE: Günther, F. A. (V)
1849: ORGANON OF MEDICINE: Samuel Hahnemann (Dudgeon translation)
1849: THE HOMŒOPATHIC TREATMENT OF CHOLERA: Benjamin Franklin Joslin, MD (T)
1849: THE POCKET HOMEOPATHIST AND FAMILY GUIDE: John A. Tarbell, MD (D)
1850: ALPHABETICAL REPERTORY OF THE SKIN SYMPTOMS: G. H. G. Jahr (R)

1850: HAHNEMANN AND SWEDENBORG: Rev. Richard De Charms (O)
1850: LESSONS FROM THE HISTORY OF MEDICAL DELUSIONS: Worthington Hooker, MD (CR)
1850: NEW HOMŒOPATHIC PHARMACOPOEIA AND POSOLOGY: G. H. G. Jahr & C. E. Gruner (PH)
1850: PATHOGENIC CYCLOPEDIA: Robert Ellis Dudgeon, MD (R)
1850: THE HOMOEOPATHIC DOMESTIC PHYSICIAN: Joseph Hypolyte Pulte, MD (D)
1850: THE PRINCIPLES OF HOMŒOPATHY IN FIVE LECTURES: Benjamin Franklin Joslin, MD (PR)
1850: JAHR'S CLINICAL GUIDE OR POCKET REPERTORY: G. H. G. Jahr (T)
1851: A POCKET MANUAL: Joel Bryant, MD (D) (R)
1851: HOMŒOPATHY. AN EXAMINATION OF ITS DOCTRINES AND EVIDENCES: Worthington Hooker, MD (CR)
1852: ELEMENTS OF HOMŒOPATHIC PRACTICE OF PHYSIC: Joseph Laurie, MD (T)
1852: FAMILY GUIDE TO THE ADMINISTRATION OF HOMOEOPATHIC REMEDIES: H. V. Malan, MD (D)
1852: FLORA HOMŒOPATHICA: Edward Hamilton, MD (MM) (PH)
1852: HOMŒOPATHIC DOMESTIC PHYSICIAN: Carl Caspari, MD (D)
1852: SHARP'S TRACTS ON HOMŒOPATHY: William Sharp, MD (P)
1852: THE LESSER WRITINGS OF SAMUEL HAHNEMANN: Samuel Hahnemann (PR)
1852: THE TREATMENT DUE FROM THE MEDICAL PROFESSION TO PHYSICIANS WHO BECOME HOMŒOPATHIC PRACTITIONERS: Worthington Hooker, MD (CR)
1853: DISEASES OF CHILDREN AND THEIR HOMŒOPATHIC TREATMENT: Franz Hartmann, MD (T)
1853: HOMEOPATHIC DOMESTIC PRACTICE: Egbert Guernsey, MD (D)
1853: HOMEOPATHIC PROVINGS: James W. Metcalf, MD (MM)
1853: HOMŒOPATHIC TREATMENT OF INTERMITTENT FEVER: James S. Douglas, MD (T)
1853: JAHR AND POSSART'S NEW MANUAL OF HOMŒOPATHIC MATERIA MEDICA, ACCOMPANIED BY AN ALPHABETIC REPERTORY: G. H. G. Jahr. (R)
1853: NOUVELLE PHARMACOPÉE HOMŒOPATHIQUE: G. H. G. Jahr and A. Catellan (PH)
1853: PROVINGS OF THE PRINCIPAL ANIMAL AND VEGETABLE POISONS OF THE BRAZILIAN EMPIRE: Benoit Mure, MD (MM)
1853: THE COMPLETE REPERTORY: Charles J. Hempel, MD (R)
1853: THE HOMEOPATHIC MATERIA MEDICA, ARRANGED SYSTEMATICALLY AND PRACTICALLY: Alphonse Teste, MD (MM)
1853: DR. J. T. TEMPLE'S REPLY TO PROF. PALLEN'S ATTACK ON HOMŒOPATHY IN HIS VALEDICTORY ADDRESS BEFORE THE ST. LOUIS UNIVERSITY: John Taylor Temple, MD (O)
1853: THE HOMŒOPATHIC PRACTICE OF MEDICINE: Martin Freligh, MD (D)
1853: WOMAN'S MEDICAL GUIDE: Joseph Hypolyte Pulte, MD (D)
1854: CODEX DES MEDICAMENTS HOMŒOPATHIQUES OU PHARMACOPÉE: George P. F. Weber (PH)
1854: ORGANON OF SPECIFIC HOMEOPATHY: Charles J. Hempel, MD (O)
1854: HOMŒOPATHY; ITS TENETS AND TENDENCIES, THEORETICAL, THEOLOGICAL, AND THERAPEUTICAL: James Y. Simpson (CR)
1854: LECTURES ON THE THEORY AND PRACTICE OF HOMŒOPATHY: Robert Ellis Dudgeon, MD (H) (PR)
1854: MANUAL OF HOMEOPATHIC PRACTICE FOR THE USE OF FAMILIES AND PRIVATE INDIVIDUALS: Alvan Edward Small, MD (D)
1854: THE HANDBOOK OF VETERINARY HOMŒOPATHY: John Rush (V)
1854: THE SIDES OF THE BODY AND DRUG AFFINITIES: C. M. Bönninghausen (R)
1854: HOMEOPATHY FAIRLY REPRESENTED: William Henderson, MD (O)
1854: KEY TO THE MATERIA MEDICA OR COMPARATIVE PHARMACODYNAMICS: Adolph Lippe, MD (MM)
1855: GENTLEMAN'S HANDBOOK OF HOMEOPATHY: Egbert Guernsey, MD (D)
1855: HOMEOPATHIC PHARMACOPŒIA: German Central Union of Homœopathic Physicians (PH)
1855: SURGERY, AND ITS ADAPTATION TO HOMŒOPATHIC PRACTICE: William Tod Helmuth, MD (AP)

1855: THE HOMŒOPATHIC GUIDE IN ALL DISEASES OF THE URINARY AND SEXUAL ORGANS, INCLUDING THE DERANGEMENTS CAUSED BY ONANISM AND SEXUAL EXCESSES: William Gollman, MD (T)
1855: THE HOMŒOPATHIC PRACTICE OF SURGERY AND OPERATIVE SURGERY: B. L. Hill, MD (AP)
1856: HOMŒOPATHY SIMPLIFIED: John A. Tarbell, MD (D)
1856: HUMPHREYS' MANUAL OF SPECIFIC HOMEOPATHY: Frederick Humphreys, MD (D)
1856: NEW MANUAL OF HOMŒOPATHIC VETERINARY MEDICINE: J. C. Schaeffer (V)
1856: THE HOMOEOPATHIC POCKET COMPANION: Martin Freligh, MD (D)
1856: THE HOMŒOPATHIC TREATMENT OF DISEASES OF FEMALES, AND INFANTS AT THE BREAST: G. H. G. Jahr (T)
1856: HOMÖOPATHISCHEN HAUS UND SCHIFFSARZT (The Home and Ship doctor/Physician): Ludwig Reichenbach (D)
1857: PROFESSOR REMSEN'S HOMŒOPATHIC FAMILY GUIDE FOR TRAVELLERS, ETC.: J. B. F. Remsen (D)
1857: THE UNCERTAINTY OF HUMAN TESTIMONY. CONCLUSIONS NOT JUDGMENT. A LETTER TO THE HONORABLE WILLIAM KENT: Federal Vandenburgh, MD (O)
1857: MEDICAL REFORM: BEING AN EXAMINATION INTO THE PREVAILING SYSTEMS OF MEDICINE: Samuel Cockburn, MD (PR)
1857: OUTLINES IN VETERINARY HOMŒOPATHY: James Moore (V)
1857: SPECIAL THERAPEUTICS ACCORDING TO HOMŒOPATHIC PRINCIPLES: VOLUME 3: MENTAL DISEASES: Franz Hartmann, MD (T)
1857: THE HOMOEOPATHIC CATTLE DOCTOR: Carl Ludwig Bœhm (V)
1859: A NEW AND COMPREHENSIVE SYSTEM OF MATERIA MEDICA AND THERAPEUTICS: Charles Hempel, MD (MM)
1859: ACUTE DISEASES AND THEIR HOMEOPATHIC TREATMENT: Jabez P. Dake, MD (D)
1859: BEKNOPTE HANDLEIDING, VOOR DE HOMEOPATHISCHE PHARMACIE: F. Dorvault (PH)
1859: CONFERENCES UPON HOMŒOPATHY: Dr. Michel Granier (PR)
1859: HOMŒOPATHIC MATERIA MEDICA: Martin Freligh, MD (MM)
1859: REPERTORY OF THE HOMŒOPATHIC MATERIA MEDICA (CYPHER REPERTORY): Robert Ellis Dudgeon, MD (R)
1859: THE HOMŒOPATHIC SURGICAL ADVISOR AND TRAVELLER'S COMPANION: "A. Z." (D)
1860: HOMÖOPATHISCHE PHARMACOPÖE: Ludwig Deventer (PH)
1860: MANUAL OF VETERINARY SPECIFIC HOMŒOPATHY: Frederick Humphreys (V)
1860: ON THE EFFICACY OF CROTALUS HORRIDUS IN YELLOW FEVER, ALSO IN MALIGNANT, BILIOUS, AND REMITTENT FEVERS: Charles Neidhard, MD (T)
1860: PRACTICAL HOMEOPATHY: James S. Douglas, MD (D)
1861: CURRENTS AND COUNTERCURRENTS IN MEDICAL SCIENCE: Oliver Wendell Holmes, MD (CR)
1861: HULL'S JAHR: revised and edited by Frederick Snelling, MD (R)
1861: MEDICAMENTA HOMEOPATHICA ET ISOPATHICA OMNIA, AD ID TEMPUS A MEDICIS AUT EXAMINATA AUT USU RECEPTA: Dr. H. Hagero (PH)
1861: REPERTORY OF THE VETERINARY HEALING ART ACCORDING TO PRINCIPLES: Carl Ludwig Bœhm (V)
1862: A MONOGRAPH ON GELSEMIUM: Edwin M. Hale, MD (MM)
1862: MANUAL OF HOMEOPATHIC THEORY AND PRACTICE DESIGNED FOR THE USE OF PHYSICIANS AND FAMILIES: Arthur Lutze (D)
1863: A GUIDE FOR EMERGENCIES: Henry B. Millard, MD (D)
1863: THE DISEASES OF DOGS AND THEIR HOMŒOPATHIC TREATMENT: James Moore (V)
1863: DIE THERAPIE UNSERER ZEIT: Wilhelm Stens (P)
1864: HOMŒOPATHY IN VENEREAL DISEASES: Stephen Yeldham, MD (T)
1864: NEW REMEDIES: Edwin M. Hale, MD (MM)
1864: REAL-LEXICON: Dr. med. Altschul (PH)
c. 1864: STEPPING STONES TO HOMEOPATHY AND HEALTH: E. Harris Ruddock, MD (D)

1865: CLINICAL LECTURES ON THE TREATMENT OF RHEUMATISM, EPILEPSY, ASTHMA, FEVER: Rutherford Russell (T)
1865: HOMÖPATHISCHEN PHARMACOPOE AUFGENOMMENEN PFLANZEN: Dr. H. Goullon (PH)
1865: THE GEOMETRY OF VITAL FORCES: Federal Vandenburgh, MD (O)
1865: ON HIGH POTENCIES AND HOMŒOPATHICS: Bernhardt Fincke, MD (PR)
1865: ORGANON DER HEILKUNST: Samuel Hahnemann, MD (Lutze edition)
1866: A SYSTEMATIC TREATISE ON ABORTION: Edwin M. Hale, MD (T)
1866: TEXTBOOK OF MATERIA MEDICA: Adolph Lippe, MD (MM)
1867: A MANUAL OF PHARMACODYNAMICS: Richard Hughes, MD (MM)
1867: DR. H GROSS' COMPARATIVE MATERIA MEDICA: Edited by Constantine Hering, MD (MM)
1867: THE APPLICATION OF THE PRINCIPLES AND PRACTICE OF HOMŒOPATHY TO OBSTETRICS, AND DISORDERS PECULIAR TO WOMEN AND YOUNG CHILDREN: Henry N. Guernsey, MD (T)
1867: RINDPEST: A. B. Conger (V)
1867: DIE HOMÖOPATHISCHEN THIER ARZNEIMITTEL: Carl Ludwig Boehm (V)
1867: THE SCIENCE AND ART OF SURGERY: Edward C. Franklin, MD (AP)
1868: HINTS FOR THE PRACTICAL STUDY OF THE HOMŒOPATHIC METHOD, IN THE ABSENCE OF ORAL INSTRUCTION WITH CASES FOR CLINICAL COMMENT: Edward D. Chepmell, MD (O)
1868: HOMOEOPATHIC HOME AND SELF TREATMENT OF DISEASE. FOR THE USE OF FAMILY AND TRAVELLERS: Charles Woodhouse, MD (D)
1868: REPERTORY OF THE NEW REMEDIES: Temple Hoyne, MD (R)
1868: SPECIAL PATHOLOGY AND DIAGNOSTICS, WITH THERAPEUTIC HINTS: Charles G. Raue, MD (T)
1869: A MANUAL OF THERAPEUTICS: Richard Hughes, MD (T)
1869: A REPERTORY OF THE SYMPTOMS OF THE EYES AND HEAD: Edward W. Berridge, MD (R)
1869: CHARACTERISTIC MATERIA MEDICA: William Burt, MD (MM)
1869: EPITOME OF HOMEOPATHIC MEDICINES: William L. Breyfogle, MD (MM)
1869: HOMŒOPATHIC THERAPEUTICS OF DIARRHEA: James B. Bell, MD (T)
1869: THE HOMŒOPATHIC TREATMENT OF SYPHILIS, GONORRHOEA, SPERMATORRHOEA AND URINARY DISEASES: Dr. J. Ph. Berjeau (T)
1869: THE SCIENCE OF THERAPEUTICS ACCORDING TO THE PRINCIPLES OF HOMŒOPATHY: Bernard Baehr, MD (T)
1869: THERAPEUTIC GUIDE: G. H. G. Jahr (T)
1870: ANNUAL: RECORD OF HOMŒOPATHIC LITERATURE: Charles G. Raue, MD, editor (H)
1870: BRITISH HOMŒOPATHIC PHARMACOPŒIA (PH)
1870: VETERINARY HOMŒOPATHY: James S. Beach (V)
1870: HOMŒOPATHIC TREATMENT OF HOOPING COUGH: C. von Bönninghausen (T)
1870: MATERNITY: A POPULAR TREATISE FOR YOUNG WIVES AND MOTHERS: Tullio Verdi, MD (D)
1870: TEXTBOOK OF HOMŒOPATHY: Eduard von Grauvogl, MD (PR)
1871: APPLIED HOMŒOPATHY OR SPECIFIC RESTORATIVE MEDICINE: William Bayes, MD (T)
1871: ON INTERMITTENT FEVER AND OTHER MALARIOUS DISEASES: I. S. P. Lord, MD (T)
1871: THERAPEUTIC KEY; OR PRACTICAL GUIDE FOR THE TREATMENT OF ACUTE DISEASES: Isaac D. Johnson, MD (T)
1871: THE REJECTED ADDRESS. MAN'S TRUE RELATION TO NATURE; HIS ORIGIN, CHARACTER AND DESTINY: Thomas P. Wilson, MD (O)
1872: HUMPHREYS' HOMEOPATHIC MENTOR: Frederick Humphreys, MD (D)
1872: LEUCORRHOEA, ITS CONCOMITANT SYMPTOMS AND ITS HOMŒOPATHIC TREATMENT: Alvin Matthew Cushing, MD (T)
1872: PHARMACOPOEA HOMÖOPATHICA POLYGLOTTA: Dr. Willmar Schwabe (PH)
1872: REPERTORY OF LEUCORRHOEA: Alvin Matthew Cushing, MD (R)
1873: CLEAVE'S BIOGRAPHICAL CYCLOPEDIA: Egbert Cleave (B)
1873: COMPLETE REPERTORY TO THE HOMŒOPATHIC MATERIA MEDICA/ DISEASES OF THE EYES: Edward W. Berridge, MD (R)

1873: INSTRUCTIONS FOR THE USE OF N. F. COOKE'S FAMILY MEDICINES: N. F. Cooke (O)
1873: MATERIA MEDICA VOL. 1: Constantine Hering, MD (MM)
1873: OPHIDIANS; ZOOLOGICAL ARRANGEMENT OF THE DIFFERENT GENERA: S. B. Higgins (O)
1873: THE TREATMENT OF TYPHOID FEVERS, WITH A FEW ADDITIONS: Constantine Hering, MD (T)
1873: THERAPEUTICS OF INTERMITTENT FEVERS: C. von Bönninghausen (T)
1873: THE HOMEOPATHIC TREATMENT OF SURGICAL DISEASES: J. Grant Gilchrest, MD (T)
1874: THE SCIENCE OF HOMŒOPATHY: Charles Julius Hempel, MD (PR)
1874: A MANUAL OF HOMŒOPATHIC VETERINARY PRACTICE DESIGNED FOR HORSES, ALL KINDS OF DOMESTIC ANIMALS, AND FOWLS: Anonymous (V)
1874: ON THE UNIVERSALITY OF THE HOMŒOPATHIC LAW OF CURE: Charles Neidhard, MD (PR)
1874: SUPPLEMENT TO GROSS' COMPARATIVE MATERIA MEDICA: E. A. Farrington, MD (MM)
1874: THE ENCYCLOPEDIA OF PURE MATERIA MEDICA; A RECORD OF THE POSITIVE EFFECTS OF DRUGS UPON THE HEALTHY HUMAN ORGANISM: Timothy F. Allen, MD (10 volumes) (MM)
1875: ANALYTICAL THERAPEUTICS: Constantine Hering, MD (R)
1875: A RECORD OF THE SURGICAL CLINICS OF WILLIAM TOD HELMUTH, MD, HELD AT THE NEW YORK HOMŒOPATHIC MEDICAL COLLEGE DURING THE SESSION OF 1874-75: Philetus J. Stephens (AP)
1876: HOMŒOPATHY IN ITS RELATION TO THE DISEASES OF WOMEN: Thomas Skinner, MD (T)
1876: OPHTHALMIC THERAPEUTICS: George S. Norton, MD and T. F. Allen, MD (T)
1876: ORGANON OF THE ART OF HEALING: Samuel Hahnemann (Wesselhoeft Translation)
1876: REPERTORY OF NEW REMEDIES: Charles Porter Hart, MD (R)
1876: TRANSACTIONS OF THE WORLD'S HOMŒOPATHIC CONVENTION UNDER THE AUSPICES OF THE AMERICAN INSTITUTE OF HOMŒOPATHY. VOL. 2. HISTORY OF HOMŒOPATHY (H)
1876: UNITED STATES HOMŒOPATHIC PHARMACOPOEIA (PH)
1877: CONDENSED MATERIA MEDICA: Constantine Hering, MD (MM)
1877: THE SCIENCE OF THERAPEUTICS: Carroll Dunham, MD (PR)
1877: THE KABBALA; OR THE TRUE SCIENCE OF LIGHT: Seth Pancoast, MD (O)
1877: ON THE APPLICATION OF ELECTRICITY AS A THERAPEUTIC AGENT: Julius H. Rae (O)
1878: THREE LECTURES ON HOMŒOPATHIC PHARMACEUTICS: Francis E. Boericke, MD (PH)
1878: A TREATISE ON TYPHOID FEVER: Cav. Francesco Panelli (T)
1878: AN ELEMENTARY TEXTBOOK OF MATERIA MEDICA: A. C. Cowperthwaite, MD (MM)
1878: CLINICAL THERAPEUTICS: Temple Hoyne, MD (MM)
1878: HOMŒOPATHIC THERAPEUTICS: Samuel Lilienthal, MD (T)
1878: HOW TO BE PLUMP: Thomas Cation Duncan, MD (O)
1878: LECTURES ON MATERIA MEDICA: Carroll Dunham, MD (MM)
1878: ON STERILITY: Edwin M. Hale, MD (T)
1878: POCKET MANUAL OF HOMŒOPATHIC VETERINARY MEDICINE: E. Harris Ruddock (V)
1878: POULTRY PHYSICIAN: Fr. Schröter (V)
1878: NATRUM MUR AS A TEST OF THE DOCTRINE OF DRUG DYNAMIZATION: James Compton Burnett, MD (MM)
1878: TERATOLOGY, OR THE SCIENCE OF MONSTERS: Mahlon Walker, MD (O)
1879: GOLD AS A REMEDY IN DISEASE: James Compton Burnett, MD (MM)
1879: A REPERTORY OF HEADACHES: John C. King, MD (R)
1879: A REPERTORY OF MENSTRUATION: William Jefferson Guernsey, MD (R)
1879: A SYSTEM OF SURGERY: William Tod Helmuth, MD (AP)
1879: AN ILLUSTRATED REPERTORY OF PAINS IN CHEST, SIDES AND BACK: Rollin R. Gregg, MD (R)
1879: HEADACHES AND THEIR CONCOMITANT SYMPTOMS: John C. King, MD (T)
1879: ON THE TREATMENT, DIET, AND NURSING OF YELLOW FEVER: William H. Holcombe, MD (T)
1879: REPERTORY TO THE MORE CHARACTERISTIC SYMPTOMS OF THE MATERIA MEDICA: Constantine Lippe, MD (R)

1879: SCRATCHES OF A SURGEON: William Tod Helmuth, MD (O)
1879: THE GUIDING SYMPTOMS OF THE MATERIA MEDICA: Constantine Hering, MD
1879: THE INCOMPATIBLE REMEDIES: Charles Mohr, MD (MM)
1879: THERAPEUTICS OF INTERMITTENT FEVER: H. C. Allen, MD (T)
1879: SEXUAL NEUROSES: James Tyler Kent, MD
1879: UTERINE AND VAGINAL DISCHARGES: William Eggert, MD (R)
1879: TRAVELLER'S MEDICAL REPERTORY AND FAMILY ADVISOR FOR HOMŒOPATHIC TREATMENT OF ACUTE DISEASES: William Jefferson Guernsey, MD (D)
1879: A GUIDE TO HOMEOPATHIC PRACTICE: Isaac D. Johnson, MD (D)
1879: LIST OF MEDICINES MENTIONED IN HOMŒOPATHIC LITERATURE: Henry M. Smith (PH)
1879: HOMŒOPATHIC VETERINARY HANDBOOK: J. W. Johnson, VS (V)
1880: HOMŒOPATHY: WHAT IS IT?: A. B. Palmer, MD (CR)
1880: THE HOMŒOPATHIC TREATMENT OF DIPHTHERIA: DeForest Hunt, MD (T)
c. 1880: COMPANION TO BRITISH AND AMERICAN HOMŒOPATHIC PHARMACOPŒIAS, ARRANGED IN THE FORM OF A DICTIONARY: Lawrence T. Ashwell (PH)
1880: CURABILITY OF CATARACTS WITH MEDICINES: James Compton Burnett, MD (T)
1880: DIPHTHERIA; ITS CAUSES, NATURE, AND TREATMENT: Rollin Robinson Gregg, MD (T)
1880: ELECTRICITY: ITS NATURE AND FORMS, WITH A STUDY ON ELECTRO-THERAPEUTICS: Captain William Boyce, MD (O)
1880: ON THE PREVENTION OF HARE-LIP, CLEFT PALATE, AND OTHER CONGENITAL DEFECTS: James Compton Burnett, MD (T)
1880: REPERTORY TO THE MODALITIES: Samuel Worcester, MD (R)
1880: SAFETY IN CHOLERA TIMES: Boericke and Tafel (T)
1880: THE GROUNDS OF A HOMŒOPATH'S FAITH: Samuel A. Jones, MD (PR)
1880: THE SYMPTOM REGISTER: Timothy F. Allen, MD (R)
1881: A TREATISE ON DIPHTHERIA: A. McNeil, MD (T)
1881: BILIARY CALCULI: C. H. Von Tagen, MD (AP)
1881: ECCE MEDICUS, OR HAHNEMANN AS A MAN AND AS A PHYSICIAN, AND THE LESSONS OF HIS LIFE: James Compton Burnett, MD (B)
1881: THE MEDICINAL TREATMENT OF DISEASES OF THE VEINS: James Compton Burnett, MD (T)
1882: A REPERTORY OF HAEMORRHOIDS: William Jefferson Guernsey, MD (R)
1882: AMERICAN HOMŒOPATHIC PHARMACOPŒIA (PH)
1882: ELECTRICITY IN SURGERY: John Butler, MD (O)
1882: MATERIA MEDICA MEMORIZER: Andrew Leight Monroe, MD (MM)
1882: PHTHISIS PULMONALIS; OR, TUBERCULAR CONSUMPTION: Gershom Nelson Brigham, MD (T)
1882: PLAIN TALKS ON AVOIDED SUBJECTS: Henry Newell Guernsey, MD (O)
1882: SUPRAPUBIC LITHOTOMY: William Tod Helmuth, MD (AP)
1883: A REPERTORY OF DESIRES AND AVERSIONS: William Jefferson Guernsey, MD (R)
1883: DISEASES AND INJURIES OF THE EYE: J. E. Buffam, MD (AP)
1883: KEY NOTES OF MEDICAL PRACTICE: Charles Gatchell, MD (AP)
1883: MEDIZINAL PFLANZEN: Hermann A. Köhler (PH)
1883: REPERTORY TO THE SYMPTOMS OF INTERMITTENT FEVER: William A. Allen, MD (R)
1883: THERAPEUTICS OF CHOLERA: Dr. P. C. Majumdar (T)
1883: UTERINE THERAPEUTICS: Henry Minton, MD (T)
1883: VENEREAL AND URINARY DISEASES: Temple S. Hoyne, MD (AP)
1884: A MEMORIAL TO CONSTANTINE HERING: Charles G. Raue, MD (B)
1884: AMERICAN HOMŒOPATHIC DISPENSATORY: Theo D. Williams, MD (PH)
1884: AMERICAN MEDICINAL PLANTS: Charles F. Millspaugh, MD (PH)
1884: COUGH AND EXPECTORATION: Edmund Jennings Lee, MD, and George Henry Clark, MD (R)
1884: REJECTED: An Address Delivered Before the Massachusetts Homœopathic Medical Society and Rejected by the Publication Committee: A. M. Cushing, MD (H)
1884: THE CAT AND ITS DISEASES: Edwin M. Hale, MD (V)
1885: A CARD REPERTORY FOR DIPHTHERIA: William Jefferson Guernsey, MD (R)

1885: A CYCLOPEDIA OF DRUG PATHOGENESY (4 volumes): Richard Hughes, MD and Jabez P. Dake, MD, editors (MM)
1885: A SYSTEM OF MEDICINE BASED UPON THE LAW OF HOMŒOPATHY: H. R. Arndt, MD (AP)
1885: DOMESTIC GUIDE TO HOMOEOPATHIC TREATMENT, ALSO THE HYGIENIC MEASURES REQUIRED IN THE MANAGEMENT OF EPIDEMIC CHOLERA: Joseph A. Biegler, MD (D)
1885: HISTORY OF HOMŒOPATHY: IT'S ORIGINS; IT'S CONFLICTS: Wilhelm Ameke (H)
1885: HUMPHREYS' VETERINARY GUIDE: Frederick Humphreys (V)
1885: LECTURES ON CLINICAL OTOLOGY: Henry M. Houghton, MD (T)
1885: REPERTORY OF ECZEMA: Charles F. Millspaugh, MD (R)
1885: THE PRESCRIBER; A DICTIONARY OF THE NEW THERAPEUTICS: John Henry Clarke, MD (T)
1885: VALVULAR DISEASE OF THE HEART FROM A NEW STANDPOINT: James Compton Burnett, MD (T)
1886: DISEASES OF THE SKIN FROM THE ORGANISMIC STANDPOINT: James Compton Burnett, MD (T)
1886: REPERTORY OF THE MOST CHARACTERISTIC SYMPTOMS: George W. Winterburn, MD (R)
1886: SEXUAL ILLS AND DISEASES; A POPULAR MANUAL: anonymous (D)
1886: DOGS IN HEALTH AND DISEASE AS TYPIFIED BY THE GREYHOUND: John Sutcliffe Hurndall (V)
1886: THERAPEUTIC METHODS; AN OUTLINE OF PRINCIPLES OBSERVED IN THE ART OF HEALING: Jabez Dake, MD (T)
1887: REPERTORY TO HAEMORRHAGES OF THE BOWELS: J. V. Allen, MD (R)
1887: A CLINICAL MATERIA MEDICA: Ernest A. Farrington, MD (MM)
1887: A COUGH TIME TABLE: J. E. Winans, MD (R)
1887: DISEASES OF THE SPLEEN: James Compton Burnett, MD (T)
1887: KEYNOTES TO THE MATERIA MEDICA: Henry N. Guernsey, MD (MM)
1887: PRACTICAL GUIDE TO HOMEOPATHY: A. Worthington, MD (D)
1887: THE ELEMENTS OF MODERN DOMESTIC MEDICINE: Henry G. Hanchett, MD (D)
1887: THE MEDICAL GENIUS: A GUIDE TO THE CURE: Stacy Jones, MD (T)
1887: THE PAST, PRESENT, AND FUTURE TREATMENT OF HOMŒOPATHY, ECCLECTICISM, AND KINDRED DELUSIONS: Henry I. Bowditch, MD (CR)
1888: A MATERIA MEDICA CONTAINING PROVINGS AND CLINICAL VERIFICATIONS OF NOSODES AND MORBIFIC PRODUCTS: Samuel Swan, MD (MM)
1888: CATALOGUE OF MORBIFIC PRODUCTS, NOSODES, AND OTHER REMEDIES, IN HIGH POTENCIES: Samuel Swan, MD (O)
1888: A REPERTORY OF GONORRHEA: Samuel A. Kimball, MD (R)
1888: FEVERS AND BLOOD POISONING, AND THEIR TREATMENT WITH SPECIAL REFERENCE TO THE USE OF PYROGENIUM: James Compton Burnett, MD (T)
1888: FIFTY REASONS FOR BEING A HOMŒOPATH: James Compton Burnett, MD (PR)
1888: ODIUM MEDICUM AND HOMŒOPATHY: THE "TIMES" CORRESPONDENCE: edited by John Henry Clarke, MD (H)
1888: PATHOGENIC AND CLINICAL REPERTORY OF THE MOST PROMINENT SYMPTOMS OF THE HEAD, WITH THEIR CONCOMITANTS AND CONDITIONS: Charles Neidhard, MD (R)
1888: REPERTORY OF HEART SYMPTOMS: Edwin Snader, MD (R)
1888: SALIENT MATERIA MEDICA AND THERAPEUTICS: Charles Luther Cleveland, MD (MM)
1888: SEMI-CENTENNIAL CELEBRATION OF THE INTRODUCTION OF HOMŒOPATHY WEST OF THE ALLEGHENY MOUNTAINS: J. C. Burgher, MD (H)
1888: SIMILIA SIMILIBUS CURANTUR? ADDRESSED TO THE MEDICAL PROFESSION: Charles S. Mack, MD (PR)
1888: THE HOMŒOPATHIC TREATMENT OF RHEUMATISM: Daniel C. Perkins, MD (T)
1888: THE TWELVE TISSUE REMEDIES: William A. Boericke, MD and Willis A. Dewey, MD (MM)
1888: TUMOURS OF THE BREAST AND THEIR CURE: James Compton Burnett, MD (T)
1888: REPERTORY OF THE URINARY SYMPTOMS: Theodore J. Gramm, MD (R)
1889: REPERTORY TO LABOR AND AFTER PAINS: J. V. Allen, MD (R)
1889: REPERTORY TO MASTITIS: William Jefferson Guernsey, MD (R)

1889: CATARACT ITS NATURE AND CURE: James Compton Burnett, MD (T)
1889: GUERNSEY'S BÖNNINGHAUSEN: assembled by William Jefferson Guernsey, MD (R)
1889: HANDBOOK OF MATERIA MEDICA AND HOMEOPATHIC THERAPEUTICS: Timothy Field Allen, MD (MM)
1889: ON FISTULA AND ITS RADICAL CURE BY MEDICINES: James Compton Burnett, MD (T)
1889: ON NEURALGIA: ITS CAUSES AND REMEDIES: James Compton Burnett, MD (T)
1889: REPERTORY OF THE CHARACTERISTIC SYMPTOMS OF THE HOMŒOPATHIC MATERIA MEDICA: Edmund Jennings Lee, MD (R)
1889: REPERTORY TO HERING'S CONDENSED MATERIA MEDICA: J. C. Guernsey (R)
1889: THE ORGANON: Samuel Hahnemann (Fincke Translation)
1890: CONSUMPTION AND ITS CURE BY ITS OWN VIRUS: James Compton Burnett, MD (T)
1890: DICTIONARY OF DOMESTIC MEDICINE: John Henry Clarke, MD (D)
1890: GENTRY'S CONCORDANCE REPERTORY OF THE MATERIA MEDICA: William D. Gentry, MD (R)
1890: REPERTORY OF CONVULSIONS: Ellis M. Santee, MD (R)
1890: THE HOMŒOPATHC CURE OF DOMESTIC ANIMALS: M. A. A. Wolff (V)
1890: THE HOMŒOPATHIC TREATMENT OF ALCOHOLISM: Jean Pierre Gallivardin, MD (T)
1890: THE HOMŒOPATHIC VETERINARY DOCTOR: George Hammerton (V)
1890: THE RUBRICAL AND REGIONAL TEXTBOOK OF THE HOMEOPATHIC MATERIA MEDICA, WITH SECTIONS ON URINE AND THE URINARY ORGANS: William Gentry, MD (MM)
c. 1890: PSYCHISME ET HOMOEOPATHIE: Jean-Pierre Gallavardin, MD (R)
1891: THE GREATER DISEASES OF THE LIVER: James Compton Burnett, MD (T)
1891: THE POCKET MEDICAL DICTIONARY: Charles Gatchell, MD (O)
1891: THE POULTRY DOCTOR: P. H. Jacobs (V)
1891: THE TEXT BOOK FOR DOMESTIC PRACTICE: Samuel Morgan, MD (D)
1892: A PRIMER OF MATERIA MEDICA: T. F. Allen, MD (MM)
1892: A REPERTORY FOR DIPHTHERIA: William Jefferson Guernsey, MD (R)
1892: COMPENDIUM OF MATERIA MEDICA, THERAPEUTICS, AND REPERTORY OF THE DIGESTIVE SYSTEM: Arkell McMichael, MD (MM)
1892: HOMŒOPATHIC BIBLIOGRAPHY: Thomas Lindsley Bradford, MD (H)
1892: "INCURABLE" DISEASES OF BEAST AND FOWL: James Moore (V)
1892: OPHTHALMIC DISEASES AND THERAPEUTICS: Arthur B. Norton, MD (T)
1892: RINGWORM: ITS CONSTITUTIONAL NATURE AND CURE: James Compton Burnett, MD (T)
1892: THE HOMŒOPATHIC THERAPEUTICS OF HAEMORRHOIDS: William Jefferson Guernsey, MD (T)
1892: WITH THE "POUSSE CAFÉ;" BEING A COLLECTION OF POST-PRANDIAL VERSES: William Tod Helmuth, MD (O)
1892: NOTES ON SCIATICA: B. Simmons, MD (R)
1893: COMPLETE REPERTORY TO THE TISSUE REMEDIES OF SCHÜSSLER: S. F. Shannon (R)
1893: CURABILITY OF TUMOURS: James Compton Burnett, MD (T)
1893: DIE PFLANZEN DES HOMÖOPATHICHEN ARZNEISCHATZES. Dr. A. von Villers and F. von Thümen (PH)
1893: DISEASES OF THE NOSE AND THROAT: Horace F. Ivins, MD (AP)
1893: REPERTORY OF SYMPTOMS OF THE OVARIES: Cyrus M. Boger, MD (R)
1893: SPECIAL DIAGNOSIS AND HOMŒOPATHIC TRATMENT OF DISEASE FOR POPULAR USE: Tullio S. Verdi, MD (D)
1894: A TEXTBOOK OF GYNECOLOGY: James Craven Wood, MD (AP)
1894: BEE-LINE REPERTORY: Stacy Jones, MD (R)
1894: ESSENTIALS OF MATERIA MEDICA: Willis A. Dewey, MD (MM)
1894: POCKET CHARACTERISTICS: T. F. Allen, MD (MM)
1894: PROVINGS AND CLINICAL OBSERVATIONS WITH HIGH POTENCIES: Malcolm Macfarlan, MD (MM)
1894: REPERTORY OF FOOT SWEATS: Olin M. Drake, MD (R)
1894: SEMI CENTENNIAL SECTION ON MATERIA MEDICA AND THERAPEUTICS (PR)

1894: SENSATIONS AS IF: A. W. Holcomb, MD (R)
1894: THE PRACTICE OF MEDICINE: William C. Goodno, MD (AP)
1894: THE TRUTH ABOUT HOMŒOPATHY: William H. Holcombe, MD (PR)
1895: A MANUAL OF GENITO-URINARY AND VENEREAL DISEASES: Bukk Carleton, MD (AP)
1895: A HANDBOOK ON THE DISEASES OF CHILDREN AND THEIR HOMŒOPATHIC TREATMENT: Charles E. Fischer, MD (T)
1895: A HOMŒOPATHIC TEXTBOOK OF SURGERY: C. E. Fischer and T. L. MacDonald, editors (AP)
1895: ACCOUCHEUR'S EMERGENCY MANUAL: William A. Yingling, MD (T)
1895: COMPARATIVE MATERIA MEDICA: John Malcom, MD and Oscar Moss, MD (MM)
1895: COUGH BY LYING: Willard Ide Pierce, MD (R)
1895: DELICATE, BACKWARD, PUNY AND STUNTED CHILDREN: James Compton Burnett, MD (T)
1895: GOUT AND ITS CURE: James Compton Burnett, MD (T)
1895: HOMŒOPATHY IN VETERINARY PRACTICE: John Sutcliff Hurndall, MRCVS (V)
1895: PATHOGENIC MATERIA MEDICA: Medical Investigation Club of Baltimore, MD (MM)
1895: PRESCRIPTION CARD: Stacy Jones, MD (O)
1895: REPERTORY OF APPENDICITIS: William A. Yingling, MD (R)
1895: REPERTORY OF SCARLET FEVER: Edward Rushmore, MD (R)
1895: REPERTORY OF SPASMS AND CONVULSIONS: A. W. Holcomb, MD (R)
1895: THE LIFE AND LETTERS OF DR. SAMUEL HAHNEMANN: Thomas Lindsley Bradford, MD (B)
1896: A REPERTORY OF THE GUIDING SYMPTOMS: Calvin Knerr, MD (R)
1896: A REPERTORY OF TONGUE SYMPTOMS: M. E. Douglas, MD (R)
1896: DEFENSE OF THE ORGANON: Samuel Hahnemann, MD (PR)
1896: HEART REPERTORY: John Henry Clarke, MD (R)
1896: MANUAL OF THE ESSENTIAL DISEASES OF THE EYE AND EAR: Joseph H. Buffam, MD (AP)
1896: ORGAN DISEASES OF WOMEN: James Compton Burnett, MD (T)
1896: VETERINARY HOMŒOPATHY IN ITS APPLICATION TO THE HORSE: J. S. Hurndall (V)
1896: THE PRACTICE OF MEDICINE; A CONDENSED MANUAL FOR THE BUSY PRACTITIONER: Marvin A. Custis, MD (T)
1896: A COMPEND OF THE PRINCIPLES OF HOMEOPATHY: William Boericke, MD (PR)
1897: LECTURES ON NERVOUS AND MENTAL DISEASES: Charles S. Elliott, MD (AP)
1897-1899: REPERTORY OF THE BACK: E. H. Wilsey, MD (R)
1897: A PRACTICAL WORKING HANDBOOK IN THE DIAGNOSIS AND TREATMENT OF THE DISEASES OF THE GENITO-URINARY SYSTEM AND SYPHILIS: George Parker Holden, MD (AP)
1897: A REPERTORY OF HOMŒOPATHIC MATERIA MEDICA: James Tyler Kent, MD (R)
1897: NOTES ON MATERIA MEDICA LECTURES: W. W. Winans, MD (MM)
1897: REPERTORY OF THERAPEUTICS OF THE EYE: C. C. Boyle, MD (R)
1897: REPERTORY OF WARTS AND CONDYLOMATA: Olin M. Drake, MD (R)
1897: THE BED FEELS HARD: H. C. Morrow, MD (R)
1897: THE PHARMACOPŒIA OF THE AMERICAN INSTITUTE OF HOMEOPATHY: The Committee on Pharmacopœia of the American Institute of Homœopathy (PH)
1897: THE PIONEERS OF HOMŒOPATHY: Thomas Lindsley Bradford, MD (B)
1897: THE SCIENTIFIC BASIS OF MEDICINE: Isaac W. Heysinger, MD (PR)
1897: VACCINOSIS AND ITS CURE BY THUJA: James Compton Burnett, MD (T)
1898: REPERTORY OF RHEUMATISM, SCIATICA, AND ETC.: Alfred Pulford, MD (R)
1898: A HANDBOOK OF THE DISEASES OF THE HEART AND THEIR HOMŒOPATHIC TREATMENT: T. C. Duncan, MD (T)
1898: THE HOMŒOPATHIC THERAPEUTICS OF DIPHTHERIA: Cyrus M. Boger, MD (T)
1898: A PRACTICAL TREATISE ON THE SEXUAL DISORDERS OF MEN: Bukk Carleton, MD (AP)
1898: CHANGE OF LIFE IN WOMEN: James Compton Burnett, MD (T)
1898: ESSENTIALS OF HOMŒOPATHIC THERAPEUTICS: Willis A. Dewey, MD (T)
1898: HISTORY OF THE HOMŒOPATHIC MEDICAL COLLEGE OF PENNSYLVANIA: Thomas Lindsley Bradford, MD (H)
1898: KEYNOTES TO THE MATERIA MEDICA: Henry C. Allen, MD (MM)
1898: MEDICAL AND SURGICAL DISEASES OF THE KIDNEYS AND URETERS: Bukk Carleton, MD (AP)

1898: NERVOUS DISEASES WITH HOMŒOPATHIC TREATMENT: Joseph O'Connor, MD (T)
1898: PHARMACOPÉE HOMŒOPATHIQUE FRANÇAISE: Edited by Drs. Marc Jousset and Vincent Leon-Simon (PH)
1898: RENAL THERAPEUTICS: Clifford Mitchell, MD (AP)
1898: REPERTORY FACIAL AND SCIATIC NEURALGIAS: F. H. Lutze, MD (R)
1898: SAW PALMETTO: Edwin B. Hale, MD (MM)
1898: THE PORCELAIN PAINTER'S SON: A FANTASY: Samuel A. Jones, MD (B)
1898: THERAPEUTICS OF FACIAL AND SCIATIC NEURALGIA WITH CLINICAL CASES AND REPERTORIES: F. H. Lutze, MD (T)
1899: CATARRH, COLDS, AND GRIPPE: John Henry Clarke, MD (T)
1899: HOMŒOPATHIC PAMPHLET SERIES: F. M. Adams, MD (P)
1899: LEADERS IN THERAPEUTICS: E. B. Nash, MD (MM)
1899: POCKET BOOK OF MEDICAL PRACTICE: Charles Gatchell, MD (T)
1899: REPERTORY OF THE URINARY ORGANS: Alonzo Richard Morgan, MD (R)
1900: A DICTIONARY OF PRACTICAL MATERIA MEDICA: John Henry Clarke, MD (MM)
1900: A SYSTEMATIC, ALPHABETIC REPERTORY OF HOMŒOPATHIC REMEDIES: C. von Bönninghausen, edited by Cyrus M. Boger, MD (R)
1900: AN HISTORIC SKETCH OF THE MONUMENT ERECTED IN WASHINGTON CITY (The History of the Hahnemann Monument): Rev. B. F. Bittinger (H)
1900: LEADERS IN TYPHOID: E. B. Nash, MD (T)
1900: LECTURES ON HOMŒOPATHIC PHILOSOPHY: James Tyler Kent, MD (PR)
1900: NEW, OLD, AND FORGOTTEN REMEDIES: Edward Pollock Anschutz (MM)
1900: REPERTORY OF THE CYCLOPEDIA OF DRUG PATHOGENESY: Richard Hughes, MD (R)
1900: THE LOGIC OF FIGURES OR COMPARATIVE RESULTS OF HOMŒOPATHIC AND OTHER TREATMENTS: Thomas Lindsley Bradford, MD (H)
1901: ABC MANUAL OF MATERIA MEDICA: George Hardy Clark, MD (MM)
1901: CHARACTERISTICS OF MATERIA MEDICA: M. E. Douglas, MD (MM)
1901: DEUTSCHES HOMÖOPATHISCHES ARZNEIBUCH (PH)
1901: ENLARGED TONSILS CURED BY MEDICINE: James Compton Burnett, MD (T)
1901: INDEX TO PROVINGS: Thomas Lindsley Bradford, MD (O)
1901: MATERIA MEDICA: William Boericke, MD (MM)
1901: MENTAL DISEASES AND THEIR MODERN TREATMENT: Selden H. Talcott, MD (T)
1901: PRACTICAL HOMŒOTHERAPEUTICS: Willis A. Dewey, MD (T)
1901: PRACTICAL MEDICINE: Frederic Mortimer Lawrence, MD (AP)
1901: PRACTICE OF MEDICINE CONTAINING THE HOMŒOPATHIC TREATMENT OF DISEASES: Dr. Pierre Jousset (AP)
1901: REGIONAL LEADERS: E. B. Nash, MD (MM)
1901: A MANUAL OF HOMŒOPATHIC MATERIA MEDICA: J. C. Fahnestock, MD (MM)
1902: CATS. HOW TO CARE FOR THEM: Edith K. Neel, MD (V)
1902: DISEASES AND THERAPEUTICS OF THE SKIN: James Henry Allen, MD (T)
1902: DISEASES OF THE LUNGS: A. L. Blackwood, MD (AP)
1902: THERAPEUTICS OF FEVERS: Henry C. Allen, MD (T)
1903: DISEASES OF THE SKIN: Henry M. Dearborn, MD (AP)
1903: HAY FEVER: ITS PREVENTION AND CURE: Perry Dickie, MD (T)
1903: STEPPING STONES TO NEUROLOGY A MANUAL FOR THE STUDENT AND GENERAL PRACTITIONER: E. R. McIntyer, MD (AP)
1903: A CLASSIFIED INDEX OF THE HOMŒOPATHIC MATERIA MEDICA FOR UROGENITAL DISEASES: Bukk G. Carleton, MD and Howard Coles, MD (T)
1903: DOGS. HOW TO CARE FOR THEM IN HEALTH AND TREAT THEM WHEN ILL: Edward Pollock Anshutz (V)
1904: A PHILOSOPHY OF THERAPEUTICS: Eldridge C. Price, MD (PR)
1904: ARE WE TO HAVE A UNITED MEDICAL PROFESSION: Charles S. Mack, MD (H)
1904: CLINICAL REPERTORY OF MATERIA MEDICA: John Henry Clarke, MD (R)
1904: LIFE AND WORK OF JAMES COMPTON BURNETT: John Henry Clarke, MD (B)

1904: MEDICAL UNION NUMBER SIX: William Harvey King, MD (O)
1904: THE MNEMONIC SIMILIAD: Stacy Jones, MD (MM)
1904: THOMAS SKINNER, MD: John Henry Clarke, MD (B)
1905: A TREATISE ON UROLOGICAL AND VENEREAL DISEASES: Bukk G. Carleton, MD (AP)
1905: CHARACTERISTIC AND REPERTORY OF BÖNNINGHAUSEN: Cyrus M. Boger, MD (R)
1905: HISTORY OF HOMŒOPATHY AND IT'S INSTITUTIONS IN AMERICA: William Harvey King, MD (B) (H)
1905: HOMŒOPATHY EXPLAINED: John H. Clarke, MD (P)
1905: LECTURES ON MATERIA MEDICA: James Tyler Kent, MD (MM)
1906: BEFORE AND AFTER SURGICAL OPERATIONS: Dean T. Smith, MD (T)
1906: HOMŒOPATHIC MATERIA MEDICA WITH REPERTORY: Oscar Boericke, MD (R)
1906: MANUAL OF MATERIA MEDICA, THERAPEUTICS, AND PHARMACOLOGY: A. L. Blackwood, MD (MM)
1906: TEST DRUG PROVING: The O.O. & L. Society (MM)
1906: WHAT TO DO FOR THE HEAD: George E. Dienst, MD (T)
1907: WHAT TO DO FOR THE STOMACH: George E. Dienst, MD (T)
1907: THE ELEMENTS OF HOMŒOPATHIC THEORY, MATERIA MEDICA, PRACTICE, AND PHARMACY: Felix A. Boericke and Edward Pollock Anshutz (O)
1907: THE LIBRARY OF HOMŒOPATHIC CLASSICS, Volume I: P. W. Shedd, editor (MM)
1907: HOW TO TAKE THE CASE AND FIND THE SIMILLIMUM: E. B. Nash, MD (O)
1907: COUGH BETTER AND WORSE: Willard Ide Pierce, MD (R)
1907: SULPHUR AND COMPARISONS: E. B. Nash, MD (MM)
1908: A NURSERY MANUAL: Ruel Benson, MD (D)
1908: BÖNNINGHAUSEN'S LESSER WRITINGS: C. von Bönninghausen (PR)
1908: CLINICAL REPERTORY: P. W. Shedd, MD (R)
1908: THE CURE OF TUMOURS BY MEDICINES: John Henry Clarke, MD (T)
1908: THE CHRONIC MIASMS: PSORA AND PSEUDO PSORA: James Henry Allen, MD (PR)
1908: THE CHRONIC MIASMS: SYCOSIS: James Henry Allen, MD (PR)
1909: HYDROTHERAPY: William Diffenbach, MD (O)
1909: DISEASES OF THE PERSONALITY: Th. Ribot (AP)
1909: LEADERS IN RESPIRATORY ORGANS: E. B. Nash, MD (T)
1909: POCKET BOOK OF VETERINARY MEDICAL PRACTICE: A. Von Rosenberg (V)
1909: THE SCIENTIFIC REASONABLENESS OF HOMŒOPATHY: Royal S. Copeland, MD (PR)
1910: DISEASES OF THE DIGESTIVE SYSTEM: E. O. Adams (AP)
1910: MEDICAL EDUCATION IN THE UNITED STATES AND CANADA: A REPORT TO THE CARNEGIE FOUNDATION FOR THE ADVANCEMENT OF TEACHING: Abraham Flexner (H)
1910: THE AGNOSTIC IN MEDICINE: James William Ward, MD (PR)
1910: THE MATERIA MEDICA OF THE NOSODES: Henry C. Allen, MD (MM)
1910: TIMES OF THE REMEDIES: Cyrus M. Boger, MD (R)
1911: PATHOGENIC MATERIA MEDICA: Elizabeth Enz, MD (MM)
1911: PLAIN TALKS ON MATERIA MEDICA: Willard Ide Pierce, MD (MM)
1911: POULTRY SENSE: A TREATISE ON THE MANAGEMENT AND CARE OF CHICKENS: James P. Pursell (V)
1911: MENTAL DISEASES AND THEIR HOMŒOPATHIC TREATMENT: William Morris Butler, MD (T)
1911: THE TESTIMONY OF THE CLINIC: E. B. Nash, MD (T)
1912: A CARD REPERTORY: Margaret M. Tyler, MD (R)
1913: EDUCATIONAL REPORT OF THE COUNCIL ON MEDICAL EDUCATION: AIH
1913: HOMŒOPATHY IN MEDICINE AND SURGERY: Edmund Carleton, MD (T)
1913: THE ORGANON OF RATIONAL HEALING: Samuel Hahnemann, MD (Wheeler translation)
1914: THE HOMŒOPATHIC PHARMACOPŒIA OF THE UNITED STATES: The Committee on Pharmacopœia of the American Institute of Homœopathy (PH)
1914: THE CASE FOR HOMŒOPATHY: Charles E. Wheeler, MD (PR)
1915: CATALOGUE OF THE HOMŒOPATHIC BOOKS OF BOERICKE AND TAFEL (O)
1915: CONSTANTINE HERING, MD: A BIOGRAPHICAL SKETCH: Herman Faber (B)

1915: GUNPOWDER AS A WAR REMEDY: John Henry Clarke, MD (MM)
1915: HOW TO USE THE REPERTORY: Glenn Bidwell, MD (O)
1915: PRACTICE OF MEDICINE: Walter Sands Mills, MD (AP)
1915: THE SYNOPTIC KEY: Cyrus M. Boger, MD (MM)
1916: A STUDY ON MATERIA MEDICA: Dr. N. M. Choudhuri (MM)
1916: DISEASES OF THE NERVOUS SYSTEM: John Eastman Wilson, MD (AP)
1916: DISEASES OF THE RESPIRATORY ORGANS: F. H. Lutze, MD (R)
1916: HOSPITALS AND SANITARIUMS OF THE HOMŒOPATHIC SCHOOL OF MEDICINES (H)
1916: SOME CLINICAL EXPERIENCES: Erastus E. Case, MD (T)
1916: THERAPEUTICS OF THE RESPIRATORY SYSTEM: M. W. VanDenburg, MD (T)
1917: CLINICAL GYNECOLOGY: James Craven Wood, MD (AP)
1917: MATERIA MEDICA FOR NURSES: Benjamin Woodbury, MD (T)
1917: REMINICINCES OF CONSTANTINE HERING: Arthur M. Eastman, MD (B)
1918: CHRONOLOGY OF EVENTS IN THE LIFE OF CONSTANTINE HERING, MD: Carl Hering (B)
1919: CONSTANTINE HERING— AN APPRECIATION: Rudolph Hering (B)
1919: AN INTRODUCTION TO THE PRINCIPLES AND PRACTICE OF HOMŒOPATHY:
  Charles E. Wheeler, MD (MM)
1919: THERAPEUTICS OF THE RESPIRATORY ORGANS: Francois Carter, MD (T)
1920: CARD REPERTORY: Enrique Jiminez-Nuñez (R)
1920: TEXTBOOK OF HOMEOPATHIC MATERIA MEDICA: George Royal, MD (MM)
1921: ORGANON DER HEILKUNST: Samuel Hahnemann, MD (sixth German)
1922: SAMUEL HAHNEMANN, HIS LIFE AND WORK: Richard Haehl, MD (B)
1922: SYMPTOM REGISTER: Richard Field, MD (R)
1922: THE ORGANON OF MEDICINE: Samuel Hahnemann, MD (sixth English/Boericke)
1923: A TREATISE ON THE PRACTICE OF MEDICINE: Clarence Bartlett, MD (AP)
1923: AMERICAN HOMŒOPATHY IN THE WORLD WAR: Frederick M. Dearborn, MD (H)
1923: THE TREND OF MODERN MEDICINE: John Weir, MD (PR)
1924: 700 RED-LINE SYMPTOMS: J. W. Hutchinson, MD (MM)
1924: THE GENIUS OF HOMŒOPATHY: Stuart N. Close, MD (PR)
1924: THE VALUE AND LIMITATIONS OF HOMŒOPATHY: James C. Wood, MD (PR)
1925: HAHNEMANN'S ORGANON OF THE ART OF HEALING RESTATED: C. A. Baldwin, MD
1925: HOMŒOPATHY: A PAMPHLET FOR THE PEOPLE: AFH (P)
1925: THE PRINCIPLES AND SCOPE OF HOMŒOPATHY: James William Ward, MD (PR)
1925: WHAT SHALL BE OUR ATTITUDE TOWARD HOMŒOPATHY?: Dr. August Bier (PR)
1926: FORTY-ONE YEARS OF HOMEOPATHY: Alfred Pulford, MD (B)
1926: NEW REMEDIES; CLINICAL CASES, LESSER WRITINGS, APHORISMS, AND PRECEPTS:
  James Tyler Kent, MD (PR)
1926: THE GENERAL ANALYSIS: Cyrus Maxwell Boger, MD (R)
1927: CONSTITUTIONAL MEDICINE WITH ESPECIAL REFERENCE TO THE THREE
  CONSTITUTIONS OF VON GRAUVOGL: John Henry Clarke, MD (PR)
1927: MANUAL OF HOMŒOTHERAPEUTICS: Edwin A. Neatby, MD and
  Thomas George Stonham, MD (MM)
1927: THE CANCER PROBLEM: SOME DEDUCTIONS BASED ON CLINICAL EXPERIENCE:
  R. Le Hunte Cooper (T)
1927: THE PRESENT-DAY ATTITUDE OF THE MEDICAL PROFESSION TOWARDS
  HOMŒOPATHY: John Weir, MD (H)
1928: HOMŒOPATHIC THERAPY OF THE DISEASES OF THE BRAIN AND NERVES:
  George Royal, MD (T)
1928: LEADERS IN PNEUMONIA: Alfred Pulford, MD and Dayton Pulford, MD (T)
1928: RADIUM: William H. Diffenbach, MD (MM)
1928: TEN REMEDIES IN THE TREATMENT OF SCARLET FEVER: Elizabeth Wright, MD (T)
1929: A COMPEND OF THE PRINCIPLES OF HOMŒOPATHY FOR STUDENTS OF MEDICINE:
  Garth Boericke, MD (PR)
1929: CORRECTIONS TO KENT'S REPERTORY: J. S. Pugh, MD (R)

1929: THE PRACTITIONER OTOLOGY: Gilbert Palen, MD and Joseph Clay, MD (AP)
1929: TREATMENT OF CANINE DISTEMPER WITH THE POTENTIZED VIRUS:
   Dr. Horace B. Jervis (V)
1930: A HANDY BOOK OF REFERENCE: George Royal, MD (T)
1930: MATERIA MEDICA IN VERSE: V. M. Kulkarni (MM)
1931: MIRACLES OF HEALING AND HOW THEY ARE DONE: A NEW PATH TO HEALTH:
   J. Ellis Barker (P)
1931: PHYSICS OF HIGH DILUTIONS: Guy Beckley Stearns, MD (PR)
1932: THE HOMEOPATHIC PRINCIPLE IN THERAPEUTICS: Thomas Hodge McGavack, MD (PR)
1932: ADDITIONS TO KENT'S REPERTORY: Cyrus M. Boger, MD (R)
1932: DISEASES OF THE NOSE AND THROAT: Joseph Clay, MD (AP)
1932: FADS AND QUACKERY IN HEALING: Morris Fishbein, MD (CR)
1933: LIFE OF CHRISTIAN SAMUEL HAHNEMANN, FOUNDER OF HOMŒOPATHY:
   Rosa Waugh Hobhouse (B)
1934: NEW LIVES FOR OLD: HOW TO CURE THE INCURABLE: J. Ellis Barker (P)
1935: LIFE OF MAHENDRA LAL SIRCAR: Dr. Sarat Chandra Ghose (B)
1935: SPEEDY DOG CURES: F. J. Bennett (V)
1935: TEXTBOOK OF MATERIA MEDICA: Otto Leeser, MD (MM)
1935: THE PRINCIPLES AND PRACTICALITY OF BÖNNINGHAUSEN'S THERAPEUTIC POCKET
   BOOK: H. A. Roberts, MD and Annie C. Wilson (R)
1936: A STUDY OF THE SIMILE IN MEDICINE: Linn J. Boyd, MD (PR)
1936: CONCISE PICTURES OF DRUGS PERSONALLY PROVEN: Donald Macfarlan, MD (MM)
1936: KEYS TO HOMEOPATHIC MATERIA MEDICA: Alfred Pulford, MD & Dayton Pulford, MD (MM)
1936: THE PRINCIPLES AND ART OF CURE BY HOMŒOPATHY: Herbert A. Roberts, MD (PR)
1937: SENSATIONS AS IF: Herbert A. Roberts, MD (R)
1937: THE METROPOLITAN HOSPITAL: Frederick M. Dearborn, MD (H)
1938: CARROLL DUNHAM HIS LIFE AND WORKS: E. Wallace MacAdam, MD (B)
1939: A REPERTORY OF LEUCORRHOEA: Alfred Pulford, MD (R)
1939: CHILDREN'S TYPES: Dr. Douglas Borland (T)
1939: INFULENZAS: Dr. Douglas Borland (T)
1939: MATERIA MEDICA CARDS: Garth Boericke, MD (MM)
1939: MY TESTAMENT OF HEALING: J. Ellis Barker (P)
1939: PNEUMONIAS: Dr. Douglas Borland, MD (T)
1939: THE RHEUMATIC REMEDIES: Herbert A. Roberts, MD (T)
1939: GESCHICHTE DER HOMÖOPATHIE: R. Tischner (H) (B)
1939: THE UNABRIDGED DICTIONARY OF SENSATIONS AS IF: James A. Ward, MD (R)
c. 1939: POINTERS TO THE COMMON REMEDIES: Margaret L. Tyler, MD (T)
1940: LIFE OF HERING: Calvin B. Knerr, MD (B)
1940: THE LITTLE HOMEOPATHIC PHYSICIAN: William Gutman, MD (D)
1941: THE STUDY OF REMEDIES BY COMPARISON: Herbert A. Roberts, MD (MM)
1942: A NEW SYNTHESIS: Guy Beckley Stearns, MD and Edgar D. Evia (PR)
1942: AN OLD DOCTOR OF THE NEW SCHOOL: James Craven Wood, MD (B)
1942: HOMEOPATHIC DRUG PICTURES: Margaret L. Tyler, MD (MM)
1944: DRUGS OF HINDOOSTAN: Sarat Chandra Ghose, MD (MM)
1944: MATERIA MEDICA OF GRAPHIC DRUG PICTURES: Alfred Pulford, MD and
   Dayton Pulford, MD (MM)
1944: THE HOMEOPATHIC MATERIA MEDICA AND HOW IT SHOULD BE STUDIED:
   Noel Puddephatt (MM)
c.1944: DIGESTIVE DRUGS: Dr. Douglas Borland (MM)
1945: HAHNEMANN; THE ADVENTUROUS CAREER OF A MEDICAL REBEL: Martin Gumpert (B)
1945: HOMEOPATHY FOR THE FIRST AIDER: Dorothy Shepherd, MD (D)
c. 1945: THE MIRACLE OF HOMŒOPATHY: A Live Explanation of What Homœopathy is and What it
   Means to Your Health: C. Frazer McKenzie (P)
c. 1945: WHY I BECAME A HOMŒOPATH: Assorted authors (B)

1946: A QUALIFYING COURSE FOR LAYMEN: AFH (P)
1946: MAGIC OF THE MINIMUM DOSE: Dorothy Shepherd, MD (P)
1947: MASTER KEY TO HOMŒOPATHIC MATERIA MEDICA: K. C. Bhanja, MD (MM)
1948: PRACTICAL HOMEOPATHIC REPERTORY IN COLORED AND PERFORATED CARDS: Marcos Jimenez, MD (R)
1949: A PHILOSOPHY OF HEALING AND A PRACTICAL PRESENTATION OF HOMŒOPATHIC PRINCIPLES: Frank Watt (P)
1949: ROYAL LONDON HOMŒOPATHIC HOSPITAL CENTENARY (H)
1949: SONG OF SYMPTOMS: Patersimilias (MM)
1950: ESSENTIALS OF HOMEOPATHIC TREATMENT: H. Fergie Woods, MD (D)
1950: HOMEOPATHY FOR MOTHER AND INFANT: Dr. Douglas Borland (D)
1950: HOMEOPATHY: Garth Boericke, MD (D)
1950: HOMŒOPATHY FOR MOTHER AND INFANT: Dr. Douglas Borland (T)
1950: PUNCH CARD SPINDLE REPERTORY: Robert H. Farley, MD (R)
c. 1950: CHILDREN'S TYPES: Dr. Douglas Borland (D)
1951: A PHYSICIAN'S POSY: Dorothy Shepherd, MD (MM)
1952: THE PLACE OF HOMŒOPATHY IN MODERN MEDICINE: Elinore Peebles (P)
1955: HOMŒOPATHY: A RATIONAL AND SCIENTIFIC METHOD: A. Dwight Smith, MD (P)
1955: HOMEOPATHY AND HOMEOPATHIC PRESCRIBING: Harvey Farrington, MD (O)
1955: MARASMUS AND RICKETS: Dr. P. S. Kamthan (T)
c. 1955: HOMŒOPATHY: HUMAN MEDICINE: Dr. Leon Vannier (PR)
1958: THE CARCINOSIN DRUG PICTURE: Donald Foubister, MD (MM)
1958: WHO IS YOUR DOCTOR AND WHY?: Alonzo Shadman, MD (P)
1959: CARD REPERTORY: Dr. Jugal Kishore (R)
1960: THE HOME PRESCRIBER: A. Dwight Smith, MD (D)
1960: TREATMENT OF CATS BY HOMEOPATHY: K. Sheppard (V)
c. 1960: HOMEOPATHIC TREATMENT IN THE NURSERY: H. Fergie Woods, MD (D)
1963: HAHNEMANNIAN PROVINGS: James H. Stephenson, MD (MM)
1963: THE CONCISE REPERTORY: Dr. S. R. Phatak (R)
1963: TREATMENT OF DOGS BY HOMEOPATHY: K. Sheppard (V)
1964: THE HOMŒOPATHIC PHARMACOPŒIA OF THE UNITED STATES: The Committee on Pharmacopœia of the American Institute of Homœopathy (PH)
1965: THE GIFT THAT GREW. THE HISTORY OF THE GENESEE HOSPITAL: Anonymous (H)
1965: CARD REPERTORY: Dr. P. Sankaran (R)
1965: DRAINAGE IN HOMŒOPATHY (DETOXIFICATION): E. A. Maury, MD (T)
1967: HOMŒOPATHY IN EPIDEMIC DISEASES: Dorothy Shepherd, MD (T)
1967: ONE HUNDRED YEARS OF MEDICAL PROGRESS: A HISTORY OF NY MEDICAL COLLEGE AND FLOWER HOSPITAL: Leonard Paul Wershub (H)
1967: PRINCIPLES AND PRACTICE OF HOMŒOPATHY VOLUME 1: M. L. Dhawale (PR)
1968: ESSAYS ON HOMEOPATHY: B. K. Sarkar (O)
1969: CARD REPERTORY: George Broussalian (R)
1970: QUICK BEDSIDE PRESCRIBER: Dr. J. N. Shinghal (T)
1970: THE ORGANON OF MEDICINE: Samuel Hahnemann, MD (5th and 6th combined)
c. 1970: FIRST AID HOMEOPATHY IN ACCIDENTS AND AILMENTS: Dr. Douglas M. Gibson (D)
1971: HOMEOPATHY IN AMERICA: THE RISE AND FALL OF A MEDICAL HERESY: Martin Kaufman, PhD (H)
1971: HOMEOPATHY: MEDICINE OF THE NEW MAN: George Vithoulkas (P)
1971: MATERIA MEDICA OF NEW REMEDIES: O. A. Julian, MD (MM)
1972: HOMŒOPATHIC MEDICINE: Harris L. Coulter , PhD (P)
1972: SYSTEMATIC MATERIA MEDICA: Dr. Kailash Narain Mathur (MM)
1973: DIVIDED LEGACY: A HISTORY OF THE SCHISM IN MEDICAL THOUGHT. SCIENCE AND ETHICS IN AMERICAN MEDICINE, 1800-1914: Harris L. Coulter, PhD (H)
1973: HOMŒOPATHIC INFLUENCES: IN 19TH CENTURY ALLOPATHIC MEDICINE: Harris L. Coulter, PhD (H)

1973: THE SYNTHETIC REPERTORY: ed. Horst Barthel, MD and Will Klunker, MD (R)
1974: ADDITIONS TO KENT'S REPERTORY: George Vithoulkas (R)
1974: COMPENDIUM OF HOMEOTHERAPEUTICS: Wyrth Post Baker, MD, editor (PH)
1974: INTRODUCTION TO HOMEOTHERAPEUTICS: Wyrth Post Baker, MD, William W. Young, MD, Alan Neiswander, MD (MM)
1974: THE PEOPLE OF THE MATERIA MEDICA WORLD: Frederica E. Gladwin, MD (MM)
1974: WINE IS THE BEST MEDICINE: E. A. Maury, MD (O)
1975: CARD REPERTORY: Hans Lees (R)
1975: DIVIDED LEGACY: A HISTORY OF THE SCHISM IN MEDICAL THOUGHT. THE PATTERNS EMERGE: HIPPOCRATES TO PARACELSUS: Harris L. Coulter, PhD (H)
1975: HOMEOPATHY IN VETERINARY PRACTICE: K. J. Biddis, MRCVS (V)
1975: HOMŒOPATHY; THE FIRST AUTHORITATIVE STUDY OF ITS PLACE IN MEDICINE TODAY: Dr. G. Ruthven Mitchel (H)
1975: WHAT IS HOMŒOPATHY?: Kay Vargo (P)
1976: A DOCTORS' GUIDE TO HELPING YOURSELF WITH HOMEOPATHIC REMEDIES: James Stephenson, MD (D)
1976: BEFORE THE DOCTOR COMES: Donovan Cox and T. W. Hyne Jones (D)
1976: HOMEOPATHIC TREATMENT FOR BIRDS: Beryl Chapman (V)
1976: SIGNPOSTS TO THE HOMEOPATHIC REMEDIES: Noel Puddephatt and Marjorie Kincaid Smith (MM)
1976: THE PATIENT NOT THE CURE: THE CHALLENGE OF HOMŒOPATHY: Margery Blackie, MD (P)
1977: A BRIEF STUDY COURSE IN HOMEOPATHY: Elizabeth Wright Hubbard, MD (PR)
1977: DIVIDED LEGACY: A HISTORY OF THE SCHISM IN MEDICAL THOUGHT; PROGRESS AND REGRESS: J. B. VAN HELMONT TO CLAUDE BERNARD: Harris L. Coulter, PhD (H)
1977: EMERGENCY HOMEOPATHY AND FIRST AID: Paul Chavanon, MD & René Levannier, MD (T)
1977: MATERIA MEDICA OF HOMEOPATHIC REMEDIES: Dr. S. R. Phatak (MM)
1977: THE AMAZING HEALER ARNICA, AND A DOZEN OTHER HOMEOPATHIC REMEDIES: Dr. A. C. Gordon Ross (D)
1977: TREATISE ON DYNAMIZED IMMUNOLOGY: O. A. Julian, MD (T)
1977: TREATMENT OF HORSES BY HOMEOPATHY: George MacLeod, MRCVS (V)
1978: AUTOVISUAL REPERTORY: Dr. Ramanlal Patel (R)
1978: HOMEOPATHIC REMEDIES FOR PHYSICIANS, LAYMEN, AND THERAPISTS: David Anderson, MD, Dennis Chernin, MD, Dale Buegel, MD (D)
1978: THE SCIENCE OF HOMŒOPATHY: George Vithoulkas (PR)
1979: HOMOEOPATHIC PRESCRIBING; REMEDIES FOR THE HOME AND SURGERY: Dr. Adolph Voegeli (D)
1979: THE HEALING ART OF HOMOEOPATHY; THE ORGANON OF SAMUEL HAHNEMANN: Edward Hamlyn
1979: THE HOMŒOPATHIC PHARMACOPŒIA OF THE UNITED STATES: The Committee on Pharmacopœia of the American Institute of Homœopathy (PH)
1979: THE ORGANON OF MEDICINE: Samuel Hahnemann, MD (Kurt Hochstetter)
1980: A SCIENTIFIC APPROACH TO HOMEOPATHY: George Russell Henshaw, MD (O)
1980: ESSENTIALS OF HOMEOPATHIC MATERIA MEDICA: Jacques Jouanny, MD (MM)
1980: NOTES ON THE MIASMS OR HAHNEMANN'S CHRONIC DISEASES: Dr. Proceso Sanchez Ortega (PR)
1980: HOMEOPATHIC MEDICINE AT HOME: Maesimund B. Panos, MD and Jane Heimlich (D)
1980: HOMEOPATHIC PRESCRIBING: Noel Pratt (T)
1980: HOMŒOPATHY: QUESTIONS AND ANSWERS: Karl Robinson, MD (P)
1980: HOMŒOPATHIC REASONING: Richard Moskowitz, MD (P)
1980: PSYCHE AND SUBSTANCE: Edward Whitmont, MD (PR)
1980: REPERTORY OF DESIRES AND AVERSIONS: Dr. V. R. Agrawal (R)
1980: THE ESSENTIALS OF THERAPEUTICS: Jacques Jouanny, MD (T)
1980: THE FINAL GENERAL REPERTORY: Diwan Harish Chand, MD and Pierre Schmidt, MD (R)
1981: DICTIONARY OF MATERIA MEDICA: O. A. Julian, MD (MM)

1981: HOMEOPATHY FOR PETS: George MacLeod, MRCVS (V)
1981: HOMEOPATHY IN PRACTICE: Dr. Douglas Borland, edited by Dr. Kathleen Priestman (T)
1981: SAMUEL HAHNEMANN: THE FOUNDER OF HOMEOPATHIC MEDICINE: Trevor Cook (B)
1981: SEQUELAE: Dr. G. S. R. Sastry (R)
1981: TREATMENT OF CATTLE BY HOMEOPATHY: George MacLeod, MRCVS (V)
1982: INTRODUCTION TO HOMŒOPATHIC PRESCRIBING: S. W. Gunavante (PR)
1982: DR. PITCAIRN'S COMPLETE GUIDE TO NATURAL HEALTH FOR DOGS AND CATS: Richard H. Pitcairn, DVM, PhD and Susan Hubble Pitcairn (V)
1982: HOMOEOPATHIC MEDICINE: A DOCTORS GUIDE TO REMEDIES FOR COMMON AILMENTS: Dr. Trevor Smith (D)
1982: HPUS SUPPLEMENT A (PH)
1982: THE COMPLETE BOOK OF HOMEOPATHY: Michael Weiner, PhD and Kathleen Goss (P)
1982: THE ORGANON OF MEDICINE: Samuel Hahnemann, MD (Naudé, Kunzli, Pendelton translation)
1983: ESSENTIAL THEORY GUIDE TO MATERIA MEDICA: Subatra Kumar Banerjea, BMS (MM)
1983: HOMEOPATHIC REMEDIES FOR CHILDREN: Phyllis Speight (D)
1983: HOMEOPATHIC TREATMENT OF DOGS: George MacLeod, MRCVS (V)
1983: SOME NOTES AND OBSERVATIONS: Julian Winston (H)
1983: THE DENTAL PRESCRIBER: Dr. Colin Lessell (T)
1983: THE ENCYCLOPEDIA OF HOMŒOPATHY: Trevor Smith, MFHom, BChir. (O)
1983: VETERINARY MATERIA MEDICA WITH REPERTORY: George MacLeod, MRCVS (V)
1984: BIBLIOTHECA HOMŒOPATHICA: Jacques Baur, Klaus-Henning Gypser, Georg von Keller, Philip W. Thomas (O)
1984: A WOMAN'S GUIDE TO HOMOEOPATHIC MEDICINE: : Trevor Smith, MD (D)
1984: EVERYBODY'S GUIDE TO HOMEOPATHIC MEDICINES: Dana Ullman, MPH and Stephen Cummings, MD (D)
1984: HOMEOPATHIC FIRST AID TREATMENT FOR PETS: Francis Hunter, MRCVS (V)
1984: HOMEOPATHIC TREATMENT OF SMALL ANIMALS: Christopher Day, MRCVS (V)
1984: MEDICINE FOR BEGINNERS: Tony Pinchuck and Richard Clark (O)
1984: SYNOPTIC MEMORIZER: Subatra Kumar Banerjea, BMS (MM)
1984: THE HOMOEOPATHIC TREATMENT OF EMOTIONAL ILLNESS: Trevor Smith, MD (D)
1984: THE TWO FACES OF HOMŒOPATHY: Dr. Anthony Campbell (H)
1985: ANIMAL EMERGENCY HANDBOOK: Gloria Dodd (V)
1985: BRASS TACKS: THE ORAL BIOGRAPHY OF A 20TH CENTURY PHYSICIAN: Adelaide Suits (B)
1985: HOMEOPATHY FOR WOMEN'S AILMENTS: Phyllis Speight (D)
1985: HOMEOPATHY: H. J. Bopp (CR)
1985: THE BIBLE AND HOMEOPATHY: A DEFENCE OF PURIST HOMEOPATHIC MEDICINE: Ronald Male (O)
1985: THE MATERIA MEDICA OF THE HUMAN MIND: Dr. M. L. Agrawal (MM)
1986: CHAMPION OF HOMŒOPATHY; THE LIFE OF MARGERY BLACKIE: Constance Babington Smith (B)
1986: CHARACTERISTICS OF THE HOMEOPATHIC MATERIA MEDICA: Horst Barthels, MD (MM)
1986: CLASSICAL HOMEOPATHY: Margery Blackie, MD (O)
1986: HOMEOPATHIC PRACTICE IN CHILDHOOD DISORDERS: Denis Demarque, MD, et. al. (T)
1986: MANAGEMENT OF OTITS MEDIA WITH EFFUSION IN HOMEOPATHIC PRACTICE: Randall Neustaedter, OMD (T)
1986: PORTRAITS OF HOMEOPATHIC MEDICINES VOL. I: Catherine R. Coulter (MM)
1986: SCORPION: Jeremy Sherr, FSHom (MM)
1986: THE FAMILY GUIDE TO HOMEOPATHY: Alain Horvilleur, MD (D)
1986: THE HANDBOOK OF HOMEOPATHY; ITS PRINCIPLES AND PRACTICE: Gerhard Koehler, MD (PR)
1986: TUTORIALS ON HOMŒOPATHY: Donald Foubister, MD (O)
1986: HOMEOPATHIC GUIDE FOR THE FAMILY: Allan Neiswander, MD (D)
1987: CATCHING GOOD HEALTH WITH HOMEOPATHIC MEDICINE: Ray Garrett (P)
1987: CURING COLIC AND LACTOSE INTOLERANCE: Jana Shiloh (D)

1987: EVERYDAY HOMOEOPATHY: A SAFE GUIDE FOR SELF-TREATMENT: Dr. David Gemmell (D)
1987: HOMŒOPATHY FOR EVERYONE: WHAT IT IS, HOW IT DEVELOPED, HOW IT CAN HELP YOU, WHERE YOU CAN FIND TREATMENT: Drs. Robin and Shelia Gibson (P)
1987: KENT'S MINOR WRITINGS ON HOMŒOPATHY: Klaus-Henning Gypser, MD, editor (PR)
1987: REPERTORIUM GENERALE: Jost Künzli, MD (R)
1987: STUDIES OF HOMEOPATHIC REMEDIES: Douglas Gibson, MD (MM)
1988: ESSENCES OF MATERIA MEDICA: George Vithoulkas (MM)
1988: HOMEOPATHY IN PEDIATRIC PRACTICE: Hedwig Imhäuser, MD (T)
1988: HOMEOPATHY: MEDICINE FOR THE 21ST CENTURY: Dana Ullman, MPH (P)
1988: HOMŒOPATHY AND THE MEDICAL PROFESSION: Philip A. Nicholls, PhD (H)
1988: KENT'S COMPARATIVE REPERTORY OF THE HOMŒOPATHIC MATERIA MEDICA: Rene Dockx, MD and Guy Kokelenberg, MD (T)
1988: OTHER HEALERS: UNORTHODOX MEDICINE IN AMERICA: Norman Gevitz, Editor (H)
1988: PORTRAITS OF HOMEOPATHIC MEDICINES VOL. II: Catherine R. Coulter (MM)
1989: THE HOMEOPATHIC RECORDER AND PROCEEDINGS OF THE INTERNATIONAL HAHNEMANNIAN ASSOCIATION, CUMULATIVE INDICES 1881-1958: Maesimund B. Panos, MD, and Della P. Desrosiers (O)
1989: COMPARATIVE MATERIA MEDICA: Eugenio Candegabe, MD (MM)
1989: ENCYCLOPEDIA OF REPERTORIES: Dr. J. Benedict D'Castro (O)
1989: HER PREFERENCE WAS TO HEAL: WOMEN'S CHOICE OF HOMEOPATHIC MEDICINE IN THE NINETEENTH CENTURY UNITED STATES: Kristen M. Mitchel (H)
1989: PORTRAITS OF INDIFFERENCE: Catherine R. Coulter (MM)
1989: REPERTORY OF PREGNANCY, PARTURITION, AND PUERPERIUM: Alberto Soler-Medina, MD (R)
1989: THE FAMILY GUIDE TO HOMEOPATHY: THE SAFE FORM OF MEDICINE FOR THE FUTURE: Dr. Andrew Lockie (D)
1990: A DICTIONARY OF HOMEOPATHIC MEDICAL TERMINOLOGY: Jay Yasgur (O)
1990: A FIELD GUIDE TO MEDICINAL PLANTS: Steven Foster and James A. Duke (PH)
1990: A HOMEOPATHIC LOVE STORY: Rima Handley (B)
1990: A MODERN GUIDE AND INDEX TO THE MENTAL RUBRICS IN KENT'S REPERTORY: David Sault (O)
1990: CATS: HOMEOPATHIC REMEDIES: George MacLeod, MRCVS (V)
1990: INSIGHTS INTO HOMEOPATHY: Frank Bodman, MD (O)
1990: SYNTHETIC MATERIA MEDICA OF THE MIND: Dr. Hari Singh (MM)
1990: THE APPLIED REPERTORY: Dr. Devika Aggarwal (R)
1990: THE COMPLETE HOMEOPATHY HANDBOOK: Miranda Castro, FSHom (D)
1990: THE MAGICAL STAFF; THE VITALIST TRADITION IN WESTERN MEDICINE: Matthew Wood (H)
1991: KRANKENJOURNAL: Samuel Hahnemann, MD (O)
1991: A GUIDE TO THE METHODOLOGIES OF HOMEOPATHY: Ian Watson (PR)
1991: A NEW MODEL OF HEALTH AND DISEASE: George Vithoulkas (PR)
1991: EVERYDAY MIRACLES: HOMEOPATHY IN ACTION: Linda Johnston, MD (P)
1991: HOMEOPATHIC PEDIATRICS ASSESSMENT AND CASE MANAGEMENT: Randall Neustaedter, OMD (AP)
1991: HOMŒOPATHY IN THE UNITED STATES: A BIBLIOGRAPHY OF HOMŒOPATHIC MEDICAL IMPRINTS, 1825-1925: Francisco Cordasco (O)
1991: HOW TO USE HOMOEOPATHY: Dr. Christopher Hammond (D)
1991: IKONOGRAPHIE SAMMLUNG, DOKUMENTATION, HISTORIE, UND LEGENDEN DER BILDER DES HOFRATES, DR. MED. HABIL. C. F. S. HAHNEMANN: Wolfgang Schweitzer (B)
1991: LACHESIS; METAPHOR AS MEDICINE: Greg Bedayn, RSHom.(NA) (MM)
1991: SPORTS AND EXERCISE INJURIES: Stephen Subotnick, DPM (D)
1991: THE HOMEOPATHIC TREATMENT OF CHILDREN: Paul Herscu, ND (MM)
1991: THE HOMŒOPATHIC PHARMACOPŒIA OF THE UNITED STATES, REVISION SERVICE: HPCUS (PH)

1991: THE SPIRIT OF HOMEOPATHY: Rajan Sankaran (PR)
1991: THORSONS ENCYCLOPAEDIC DICTIONARY OF HOMEOPATHY: Harald Gaier, DHomM (O)
1991: TREATISE ON HOMEOPATHIC MEDICINE: Francisco Eizayaga, MD (PR)
1991: TREATMENT OF GOATS BY HOMEOPATHY: George MacLeod, MRCVS (V)
1991: YOUR HEALTHY CAT: HOMEOPATHIC MEDICINES FOR COMMON FELINE AILMENTS: Hans Gunther Wolff, DVM (V)
1992: A CONSUMER'S GUIDE TO ALTERNATIVE MEDICINE: Kurt Butler (CR)
1992: HOMEOPATHIC EMERGENCY GUIDE: Thomas Kruzel, ND (T)
1992: HOMEOPATHIC MEDICINE FOR CHILDREN AND INFANTS: Dana Ullman, MPH (D)
1992: HOMEOPATHIC MEDICINES FOR PREGNANCY AND CHILDBIRTH: Richard Moskowitz, MD (T)
1992: MATERIA MEDICA VIVA VOLUME 1: George Vithoulkas (MM)
1992: ORGANON DER HEILKUNST: Samuel Hahnemann, MD (full 6th in German)
1992: PROVING OF HYDROGEN: Jeremy Sherr, FSHom (MM)
1992: THE COMPLETE REPERTORY: Roger van Zandvoort. (R)
1992: THE CONTROLLED CLINICAL TRIAL: AN ANALYSIS: Harris L. Coulter, PhD (O)
1992: THE SYNOPTIC MATERIA MEDICA: Frans Vermeulen (MM)
1992: TYPOLOGY IN HOMŒOPATHY: Dr. Leon Vannier (PR)
1993: 24 CHAPTERS ON HOMEOPATHY: Joseph Reves (PR)
1993: CHRISTIAN COMMON SENSE AND MEDICAL CONTROVERSY: Richard Culp, DO (O)
1993: DIRECTORY OF DECEASED AMERICAN PHYSICIANS 1804-1929: Arthur W. Hafner, PhD (B)
1993: HOMEOPATHY AND MINERALS: Jan Scholten (MM)
1993: HOMEOPATHY FOR COMMON AILMENTS: Robin Hayfield, RSHom (D)
1993: HOMEOPATHY FOR PREGNANCY, BIRTH, AND YOUR BABY'S FIRST YEAR: Miranda Castro, FSHom (D)
1993: HOMEOPATHY: AN INTRODUCTION FOR SKEPTICS AND BEGINNERS: Richard Grossinger (P)
1993: METAPHORIC NATURALISM: Greg Bedayn, RSHom.(NA) (MM)
1993: THE ALCHEMY OF HEALING: Edward Whitmont, MD (PR)
1993: THE DESKTOP GUIDE: Roger Morrison, MD (MM)
1993: THE HOMEOPATHIC MEDICAL REPERTORY: Robin Murphy, ND (R)
1993: THE PROVING OF CHOCOLATE: Jeremy Sherr, FSHom (MM)
1993: THE SYNTHESIS REPERTORY: Frederik Schroyens, MD (R)
1994: A TUTORIAL AND WORKBOOK FOR THE HOMEOPATHIC REPERTORY: Karen B. Allen (O)
1994: COMPREHENSIVE HOMEOPATHIC MATERIA MEDICA OF THE MIND: Dr. H. L. Chitkara (MM)
1994: CONCORDANT MATERIA MEDICA: Frans Vermeulen (MM)
1994: CORE ELEMENTS OF THE MATERIA MEDICA OF THE MIND: Ananda Zaren (MM)
1994: DIVIDED LEGACY: TWENTIETH CENTURY MEDICINE: THE BACTERIOLOGICAL ERA: Harris L. Coulter, PhD (H)
1994: HOMEOPATHY UNVEILED: AN EXPLANATION OF HOW IT REALLY WORKS: Giri Westcott (P)
1994: HPUS ABSTRACTS 1994: HPCUS (PH)
1994: PIGS: A HOMEOPATHIC APPROACH TO THE TREATMENT AND PREVENTION OF DISEASES: George MacLeod, MRCVS (V)
1994: THE COLLECTED WRITINGS OF C. M. BOGER: edited by Robert Bannan (O)
1994: THE DYNAMICS AND METHODOLOGY OF HOMOEOPATHIC PROVINGS: Jeremy Sherr (O)
1994: THE MAD HATTER'S TEA PARTY: Melissa Assilem (MM)
1994: THE ORGANON OF MEDICINE: Samuel Hahnemann, MD; with explanation by Joseph Reves
1994: THE PROVING OF LAC HUMANUM: Jacquelyn Houghton and Elisabeth Halahan (MM)
1994: THE SUBSTANCE OF HOMEOPATHY: Rajan Sankaran (PR)
1994: THE VITAMIN PUSHERS: Stephen Barrett, MD and Victor Herbert, MD (CR)
1994: WHAT THE HELL IS HOMEOPATHY: Jacob Mirman, MD (P)
1995: 1001 SMALL REMEDIES: Frederik Schroyens, MD (MM)
1995: CONSUMER'S GUIDE TO HOMEOPATHY: Dana Ullman (D)
1995: ENCYCLOPEDIA OF HOMEOPATHIC PHARMACOPOEIA: P. N. Verna (PH)
1995: HOMEOPATHIC PSYCHOLOGY: Philip Bailey, MD (MM)

1995: A TEXTBOOK OF DENTAL HOMOEOPATHY: Dr. Colin Lessell (T)
1995: HOMEOPATHIC TREATMENT OF BEEF AND DAIRY CATTLE: Christopher Day, MRCVS (V)
1995: HOMEOPATHY RENEWED: Rudolph Verspoor and Patricia Smith (PR)
1995: HOMEOPATHY: A FRONTIER IN MEDICAL SCIENCE: Paolo Bellavite, MD and Andrea Signorini, MD (O)
1995: HOMEOPATHY: BEYOND FLAT EARTH MEDICINE: Timothy Dooley, MD, ND (P)
1995: HOMŒOPATHY IN THE IRISH POTATO FAMINE: Francis Treuherz, FSHom (H)
1995: HOMŒOPATHY: SOME THINGS ARE NOT WHAT THEY THEY SEEM: Branson Hopkins (CR)
1995: LOTUS MATERIA MEDICA: Robin Murphy, ND (MM)
1995: PATIENTS GUIDE TO HOMEOPATHIC MEDICINE: Judyth Reichenberg-Ullman, ND and Robert Ullman, ND (P)
1995: THE COMPLETE GUIDE TO HOMEOPATHY: Andrew Lockie, MD and Nicola Geddes, MD (P)
1995: THE COMPLETE MATERIA MEDICA OF THE MIND: Heli O. Retzek, MD (MM)
1995: THE COMPLETE REPERTORY: Roger van Zandvoort (R)
1995: THE UNFOLDED ORGANON: A PRÉCIS OF HAHNEMANN'S SIXTH EDITION: Peter Crockett
1996: A CHRISTIAN'S GUIDE TO HOMŒOPATHY: Alan Crook, MA, RSHom (O)
1996: THE COLLECTED WORKS OF ARTHUR HILL GRIMMER: Arthur H. Grimmer, MD (O)
1996: GUIDE TO KENT'S REPERTORY: Ahmed N. Currim, PhD, MD (O)
1996: AMBRA GRISEA: ROAD TO HOMEOPATHIC PRACTICE, VOL. I: Michael Thompson, FSHom. (MM)
1996: HEALING WITH HOMEOPATHY: THE NATURAL WAY TO PROMOTE RECOVERY AND RESTORE HEALTH: Wayne Jonas, MD and Jennifer Jacobs, MD (D)
1996: HOMEOPATHIC FIRST AID FOR ANIMALS: Kaetheryn Walker (V)
1996: HOMEOPATHY AND THE ELEMENTS: Jan Scholten (MM)
1996: HOMEOPATHY CHILDBIRTH MANUAL: Betty Idarius, LM, CHom (D)
1996: STRAMONIUM: Paul Herscu, ND (MM)
1996: THE ELEMENTS OF HOMEOPATHY: Dr. P. Sankaran (MM) (O)
1996: THE ORGANON OF THE MEDICAL ART: Samuel Hahnemann, MD (Decker/O'Reilly translation)
1996: RITALIN FREE KIDS: Judyth Reichenberg-Ullman, ND, and Robert Ullman, ND (P)
1996: THE SYNOPTIC MATERIA MEDICA, VOL. II: Frans Vermeulen (MM)
1996: THE VACCINE GUIDE: MAKING AN INFORMED CHOICE: Randall Neustaedter, OMD (O)
1996: WELTGESCHICHTE DER HOMÖOPATHIE: LÄNDER—SCHULEN—HEILKUNDIGE: Martin Dinges (H)
1996: CUMULATIVE INDEX TO THE HOMŒOPATHIC PHYSICIAN: Jay Yasgur (O)
1996: QUICK REMEDY INDEX TO THE HOMEOPATHIC MATERIA MEDICA: Bart Hiusmans. Edited by Rene Otter (O)
1997: DYNAMIC PROVINGS: Jeremy Sherr, FSHom (MM)
1997: HOMEOPATHIC HANDBOOK FOR POISON IVY AND POISON OAK: Joel Kreisberg, DC (T)
1997: HOMEOPATHIC PHARMACY: AN INTRODUCTION AND HANDBOOK: Stephen Kayne, MRPharmS (PH)
1997: HOMEOPATHIC SELF CARE: THE QUICK AND EASY GUIDE FOR THE WHOLE FAMILY: Judyth Reichenberg-Ullman, ND and Robert Ullman, ND (D)
1997: HOMŒOPATHIC HANDBOOK FOR DAIRY FARMING: Tineke Verkade (V)
1997: CRIES OF THE WILD; A WILDLIFE REHABILITATOR'S JOURNAL: Jeff Lederman (V)
1997: HOMEOPATHY FOR THE MODERN PREGNANT WOMAN AND HER INFANT: Sandra Perko, PhD (T)
1997: HOMEOPATHY IN PRIMARY CARE: Bob Leckridge, BSc, MB, MFHom (T)
1997: IN SEARCH OF THE LATER HAHNEMANN: Rima Handley (B)
1997: LET LIKE CURE LIKE: Vinton McCabe (P)
1997: NATURAL RELATIONSHIP OF REMEDIES: Jorg Wichmann and Anglica Bolte (O)
1997: PHARMACOLOGY AND HOMEOPATHIC MATERIA MEDICA: Jacques Jouanny, et. al. (MM)
1997: PROVING OF BAMBOO: Bernd Schuster (MM)
1997: PROVING OF GRANITE, MARBLE, LIMESTONE: Nuala Eising (MM)
1997: PROVING OF OZONE: Anne Schadde (MM)

1997: PROVING OF TUNGSTEN: Annette Bond (MM)
1997: REMEDY RELATIONSHIPS: Abdur Rehman (O)
1997: SIGNALS AND IMAGES: Madeleine Bastide, MD (O)
1997: THE SOUL OF REMEDIES: Rajan Sankaran (MM)
1998: AN ALTERNATIVE PATH: THE MAKING AND RE-MAKING OF HAHNEMANN MEDICAL COLLEGE AND HOSPITAL OF PHILADELPHIA: Naomi Rogers, PhD (H)
1998: ANIMAL MINDS, HUMAN VOICES: Nancy Herrick, PA (MM)
1998: CROSSROADS TO CURE: THE HOMEOPATH'S GUIDE TO THE SECOND PRESCRIPTION: Nicola Henriques (PR)
1998: CULTURE, KNOWLEDGE, AND HEALING: HISTORICAL PERSPECTIVES OF HOMEOPATHIC MEDICINE IN EUROPE AND NORTH AMERICA: Robert Jütte, editor (H)
1998: FUNDAMENTAL RESEARCH ON ULTRA HIGH DILUTIONS: assorted authors (O)
1998: HELP! AND HOMEOPATHY: WHAT TO DO IN AN EMERGENCY BEFORE 911 ARRIVES: Eileen Nauman, DIHom (D)
1998: MATERIA POETICA: Sylvia Seroussi Chatroux, MD (MM)
1998: MENOPAUSE AND HOMEOPATHY: A GUIDE FOR WOMEN IN MID-LIFE: Ifeoma Ikenze, MD (D)
1998: PORTRAITS OF HOMEOPATHIC MEDICINES VOL. III: Catherine R. Coulter (MM)
1998: PROVINGS: Rajan Sankaran (MM)
1998: THE DESKTOP COMPANION TO PHYSICAL PATHOLOGY: Roger Morrison, MD (T)
1998: THE HOMEOPATHIC TREATMENT OF ECZEMA: Robin Logan, FSHom (T)
1998: THE SPIRIT OF HOMEOPATHIC MEDICINES: Didier Grandgeorge, MD (MM)
1998: THEMATIC REPERTORY AND MATERIA MEDICA OF THE MIND SYMPTOMS: José Antonio Mirilli, MD (T)
1998: HERINGS MEDIZINISCHE SCHRIFTEN: Klaus-Henning Gypser, MD, editor (O)
1998: COMPLEMENTARY AND ALTERNATIVE VETERINARY MEDICINE: PRINCIPLES AND PRACTICE: Allen M. Schoen, DVM, and Susan G. Wynn, DVM, PhD, editors (V)
1999: *THE HERSCU LETTER*: Paul Herscu ND (PR)
1999: A VITAL FORCE: WOMEN PHYSICIANS AND PATIENTS IN AMERICAN HOMEOPATHY: 1850-1930: Anne Kirschmann (H)
1999: HAHNEMANN REVISITED: A TEXTBOOK OF CLASSICAL HOMEOPATHY FOR THE PROFESSIONAL: Luc De Schepper, MD (PR)
1999: PROZAC FREE: Judyth Reichenberg-Ullman, ND, and Robert Ullman, ND (P)
1999: HOMEOPATHIC CARE FOR CATS AND DOGS: A COMPREHENSIVE GUIDE: Donald Hamilton, DVM (V)
1999: HOMEOPATHY RE-EXAMINED: BEYOND THE CLASSICAL PARADIGM: Rudolph Verspoor and Stephen Decker (PR)
1999: HOMŒOPATHY BEFORE HAHNEMANN: THE FORGOTTEN MEN: Ian Oliver (H)
1999: HOMOEOPATHY: WHAT ARE WE SWALLOWING?: Steven Ransom (CR)
1999: PROVING OF COLA NITIDA: Bernd Schuster (MM)
1999: RHYMING REMEDIES: Sally Yamini (MM)
1999: THE FACES OF HOMŒOPATHY: AN ILLUSTRATED HISTORY OF THE FIRST 200 YEARS: Julian Winston (B) (H)
1999: THE HOMEOPATHIC TREATMENT OF INFLUENZA: Sandra Perko, PhD (T)
1999: THE PHOENIX REPERTORY: Dr. J. P. S. Bakshi (R)
2000: BÖNNINGHAUSENS THERAPEUTISCHES TASCHENBUCH: (German) edited by Klaus-Henning Gypser, MD (R)
2000: THE BÖNNINGHAUSEN REPERTORY; THERAPEUTIC POCKET BOOK METHOD: (English) edited by George Dimitriadis (R)
2000: INTERNATIONAL HOMEOPATHIC DICTIONARY: Jeremy Swayne, editor. (O)
2000: NATURE AND HUMAN PERSONALITY: Catherine R. Coulter (MM)
2000: PRACTICAL HOMEOPATHY: Vinton McCabe (D)
2000: THE SYSTEM OF HOMEOPATHY: Rajan Sankaran (PR)

The Heritage of Homœopathic Literature

The Book by Author

Key:
Materia Medica (MM); Repertory (R); Therapeutics (T); Anatomy and Physiology (AP); Domestic (D); Popular (P); Veterinary (V); Pharmacy (PH); Principles (PR); History (H); Biography (B); Other (O); Critical (CR).

A. Z. **1859:** THE HOMŒOPATHIC SURGICAL ADVISOR AND TRAVELLER'S COMPANION (D)
Adams, E. O. **1910:** DISEASES OF THE DIGESTIVE SYSTEM (AP)
Adams, F. M. **1899:** HOMŒOPATHIC PAMPHLET SERIES (P)
AFH **1925:** HOMŒOPATHY: A PAMPHLET FOR THE PEOPLE (P)
AFH **1946:** A QUALIFYING COURSE FOR LAYMEN (P)
Aggarwal, Devika **1990:** THE APPLIED REPERTORY (R)
Agrawal, M. L. **1985:** THE MATERIA MEDICA OF THE HUMAN MIND (MM)
Agrawal, V. R. **1980:** REPERTORY OF DESIRES AND AVERSIONS (R)
AIH **1846:** THE TRANSACTIONS OF THE AMERICAN INSTITUTE OF HOMŒOPATHY (MM)
AIH **1876:** TRANSACTIONS OF THE WORLD'S HOMŒOPATHIC CONVENTION UNDER THE AUSPICES OF THE AMERICAN INSTITUTE OF HOMŒOPATHY. VOL. 2. HISTORY OF HOMŒOPATHY (H)
AIH **1894:** SEMI CENTENNIAL SECTION ON MATERIA MEDICA AND THERAPEUTICS (PR)
AIH **1913:** EDUCATIONAL REPORT OF THE COUNCIL ON MEDICAL EDUCATION (H)
AIH **1916:** HOSPITALS AND SANITARIUMS OF THE HOMŒOPATHIC SCHOOL OF MEDICINE (H)
Allen, H. C. **1879:** THERAPEUTICS OF INTERMITTENT FEVER (T)
Allen, H. C. **1898:** KEYNOTES TO THE MATERIA MEDICA (MM)
Allen, H. C. **1902:** THERAPEUTICS OF FEVERS (T)
Allen, H. C. **1910:** THE MATERIA MEDICA OF THE NOSODES (MM)
Allen, J. H. **1902:** DISEASES AND THERAPEUTICS OF THE SKIN (T)
Allen, J. H. **1908:** THE CHRONIC MIASMS: PSORA AND PSEUDO PSORA (PR)
Allen, J. H. **1908:** THE CHRONIC MIASMS: SYCOSIS (PR)
Allen, J. V. **1887:** REPERTORY TO HAEMORRHAGES OF THE BOWELS (R)
Allen, J. V. **1889:** REPERTORY TO LABOR AND AFTER PAINS (R)
Allen, Karen B. **1994:** A TUTORIAL AND WORKBOOK FOR THE HOMEOPATHIC REPERTORY (O)
Allen, T. F. **1874:** THE ENCYCLOPEDIA OF PURE MATERIA MEDICA; A RECORD OF THE POSITIVE EFFECTS OF DRUGS UPON THE HEALTHY HUMAN ORGANISM (10 volumes) (MM)
Allen, T. F. **1876:** OPHTHALMIC THERAPEUTICS (T)
Allen, T. F. **1880:** THE SYMPTOM REGISTER (R)
Allen, T. F. **1889:** HANDBOOK OF MATERIA MEDICA AND HOMŒOPATHIC THERAPEUTICS (MM)
Allen, T. F. **1892:** A PRIMER OF MATERIA MEDICA (MM)
Allen, T. F. **1894:** POCKET CHARACTERISTICS (MM)
Allen, William A. **1883:** REPERTORY TO THE SYMPTOMS OF INTERMITTENT FEVER (R)
Altschul **1864:** REAL-LEXICON (PH)
Ameke, Wilhelm **1885:** HISTORY OF HOMŒOPATHY: ITS ORIGINS; ITS CONFLICTS (H)
Anderson, David, Chernin, Dennis, Buegel, Dale **1978:** HOMEOPATHIC REMEDIES FOR PHYSICIANS, LAYMEN, AND THERAPISTS (D)
Anonymous **1838:** PHARMACOPOEA UNIVERSALIS (PH)
Anonymous **1846:** A MANUAL OF HOMŒOPATHIC COOKERY (O)
Anonymous **1870:** BRITISH HOMŒOPATHIC PHARMACOPŒIA (PH)
Anonymous **1874:** A MANUAL OF HOMŒOPATHIC VETERINARY PRACTICE DESIGNED FOR HORSES, ALL KINDS OF DOMESTIC ANIMALS, AND FOWLS (V)
Anonymous **1876:** UNITED STATES HOMŒOPATHIC PHARMACOPOEIA (PH)
Anonymous **1882:** AMERICAN HOMŒOPATHIC PHARMACOPŒIA (PH)
Anonymous **1886:** SEXUAL ILLS AND DISEASES; A POPULAR MANUAL (D)
Anonymous **1901:** DEUTSCHES HOMÖOPATHISCHES ARZNEIBUCH (PH)
Anonymous **1965:** THE GIFT THAT GREW. THE HISTORY OF THE GENESEE HOSPITAL (H)
Anshutz, E. P. **1900:** NEW, OLD, AND FORGOTTEN REMEDIES (MM)

Anshutz, E. P. **1903:** DOGS. HOW TO CARE FOR THEM (V)
Arndt, Hugo R. **1885:** A SYSTEM OF MEDICINE BASED UPON THE LAW OF HOMŒOPATHY (AP)
Ashwell, Lawrence T. **c. 1880:** COMPANION TO BRITISH AND AMERICAN HOMŒOPATHIC PHARMACOPŒIAS, ARRANGED IN THE FORM OF A DICTIONARY (PH)
Assilem, Melissa **1994:** THE MAD HATTER'S TEA PARTY (MM)
Assorted authors **c. 1945:** WHY I BECAME A HOMŒOPATH (B)
Assorted authors **1998:** FUNDAMENTAL RESEARCH ON ULTRA HIGH DILUTIONS (O)
Baehr, Bernard **1869:** THE SCIENCE OF THERAPEUTICS ACCORDING TO THE PRINCIPLES OF HOMŒOPATHY (T)
Bailey, Philip **1995:** HOMEOPATHIC PSYCHOLOGY (MM)
Baker, Wyrth Post; Young, William W. ; Neiswander, Alan **1974:** INTRODUCTION TO HOMEOTHERAPEUTICS (MM)
Baker, Wyrth Post, editor **1974:** COMPENDIUM OF HOMEOTHERAPEUTICS (PH)
Bakshi, J. P. S. **1999:** THE PHOENIX REPERTORY (R)
Baldwin, C. A. **1925:** HAHNEMANN'S ORGANON OF THE ART OF HEALING RESTATED
Banerjea, S. K. **1983:** ESSENTIAL THEORY GUIDE TO MATERIA MEDICA (MM)
Banerjea, S. K. **1984:** SYNOPTIC MEMORIZER (MM)
Bannan, Robert **1994:** THE COLLECTED WRITINGS OF C. M. BOGER (O)
Barker, J. Ellis **1931:** MIRACLES OF HEALING AND HOW THEY ARE DONE (P)
Barker, J. Ellis **1934:** NEW LIVES FOR OLD: HOW TO CURE THE INCURABLE (P)
Barker, J. Ellis **1939:** MY TESTAMENT OF HEALING (P)
Barrett, Stephen and Herbert, Victor **1994:** THE VITAMIN PUSHERS (CR)
Barthel, Horst and Klunker, Will **1973:** THE SYNTHETIC REPERTORY (R)
Barthel, Horst **1986:** CHARACTERISTICS OF THE HOMEOPATHIC MATERIA MEDICA (MM)
Bartlett, Clarence **1923:** A TREATISE ON THE PRACTICE OF MEDICINE (AP)
Bastide, Madeleine **1997:** SIGNALS AND IMAGES (O)
Baur, J; Gypser, K-H; Keller, G.; Thomas, P. W. **1984:** BIBLIOTHECA HOMŒOPATHICA (O)
Bayes, William **1871:** APPLIED HOMŒOPATHY OR SPECIFIC RESTORATIVE MEDICINE (T)
Beach, James S. **1870:** VETERINARY HOMŒOPATHY (V)
Becker, Alexander C. **1847:** DISEASES OF THE EYE TREATED HOMŒOPATHICALLY (T)
Bedayn, Greg **1991:** LACHESIS; METAPHOR AS MEDICINE (MM)
Bedayn, Greg **1993:** METAPHORIC NATURALIS: (MM)
Bell, James B. **1869:** HOMŒOPATHIC THERAPEUTICS OF DIARRHEA (T)
Bellavite, Paolo and Signorini, Andrea **1995:** HOMEOPATHY: A FRONTIER IN MEDICAL SCIENCE (O)
Bennett, F. J. **1935:** SPEEDY DOG CURES (V)
Benson, Ruel **1908:** A NURSERY MANUAL (D)
Berjeau, J. Ph. **1869:** THE HOMŒOPATHIC TREATMENT OF SYPHILIS, GONORRHOEA, SPERMATORRHOEA AND URINARY DISEASES (T)
Berridge, Edward W. **1869:** A REPERTORY OF THE SYMPTOMS OF THE EYES AND HEAD (R)
Berridge, Edward W. **1873:** COMPLETE REPERTORY TO THE HOMŒOPATHIC MATERIA MEDICA/ DISEASES OF THE EYES (R)
Bhanja, K. C. **1947:** MASTER KEY TO HOMŒOPATHIC MATERIA MEDICA (MM)
Biddis, K. J. **1975:** HOMEOPATHY IN VETERINARY PRACTICE (V)
Bidwell, Glenn **1915:** HOW TO USE THE REPERTORY (O)
Biegler, Joseph A. **1885:** DOMESTIC GUIDE TO HOMOEOPATHIC TREATMENT, ALSO THE HYGENIC MEASURES REQUIRED IN THE MANAGEMENT OF EPIDEMIC CHOLERA (D)
Bier, August **1925:** WHAT SHALL BE OUR ATTITUDE TOWARD HOMŒOPATHY? (PR)
Bittinger, Rev. B. F. **1900:** AN HISTORIC SKETCH OF THE MONUMENT ERECTED IN WASHINGTON CITY (The History of the Hahnemann Monument) (H)
Blackie, Margery **1976:** THE PATIENT NOT THE CURE: THE CHALLENGE OF HOMŒOPATHY (P)
Blackie, Margery **1986:** CLASSICAL HOMEOPATHY (O)
Blackwood, A. L. **1902:** DISEASES OF THE LUNGS (AP)
Blackwood, A. L. **1906:** MANUAL OF MATERIA MEDICA, THERAPEUTICS, AND PHARMACOLOGY (MM)
Blatchford, Thomas W. **1842:** HOMŒOPATHY (CR)

Bodman, Frank **1990:** INSIGHTS INTO HOMEOPATHY (O)
Bœhm, Carl Ludwig **1857:** THE HOMOEOPATHIC CATTLE DOCTOR (V)
Bœhm, Carl Ludwig **1861:** REPERTORY OF THE VETERINARY HEALING ART ACCORDING TO PRINCIPLES (V)
Boehm, Carl Ludwig **1867:** DIE HOMÖOPATHISCHEN THIER ARZNEIMITTEL (V)
Boericke and Tafel **1880:** SAFETY IN CHOLERA TIMES (T)
Boericke and Tafel **1915:** CATALOGUE OF THE HOMŒOPATHIC BOOKS OF BOERICKE AND TAFEL (O)
Boericke, F. E. **1878:** THREE LECTURES ON HOMŒOPATHIC PHARMACEUTICS (PH)
Boericke, Felix A. and Anshutz, E. P. **1907:** THE ELEMENTS OF HOMŒOPATHIC THEORY, MATERIA MEDICA, PRACTICE, AND PHARMACY (O)
Boericke, Garth **1929:** A COMPEND OF THE PRINCIPLES OF HOMŒOPATHY FOR STUDENTS OF MEDICINE (PR)
Boericke, Garth **1939:** MATERIA MEDICA CARDS (MM)
Boericke, Garth **1950:** HOMEOPATHY (D)
Boericke, Oscar **1906:** HOMŒOPATHIC MATERIA MEDICA WITH REPERTORY (R)
Boericke, William and Dewey, Willis A. **1888:** THE TWELVE TISSUE REMEDIES (MM)
Boericke, William **1896:** A COMPEND OF THE PRINCIPLES OF HOMEOPATHY (PR)
Boericke, William **1901:** MATERIA MEDICA (MM)
Boger, Cyrus M. **1893:** REPERTORY OF SYMPTOMS OF THE OVARIES (R)
Boger, Cyrus M. **1898:** THE HOMŒOPATHIC THERAPEUTICS OF DIPHTHERIA (T)
Boger, Cyrus M. **1905:** CHARACTERISTIC AND REPERTORY OF BÖNNINGHAUSEN (R)
Boger, Cyrus M. **1910:** TIMES OF THE REMEDIES (R)
Boger, Cyrus M. **1915:** THE SYNOPTIC KEY (MM)
Boger, Cyrus M. **1926:** THE GENERAL ANALYSIS (R)
Boger, Cyrus M. **1932:** ADDITIONS TO KENT'S REPERTORY (R)
Bond, Annette **1997:** PROVING OF TUNGSTEN (MM)
Bönninghausen, C. von **1832:** REPERTORY OF ANTIPSORIC MEDICINES (R)
Bönninghausen, C. von **1834:** HOMŒOPATHY— A TEXT-BOOK FOR THE EDUCATED, NON-MEDICAL PUBLIC (P)
Bönninghausen, C. von **1836:** REPERTORY OF MEDICINES THAT ARE NOT ANTIPSORIC (R)
Bönninghausen, C. von **1846:** THE THERAPEUTIC POCKET BOOK (R)
Bönninghausen, C. von **1854:** THE SIDES OF THE BODY AND DRUG AFFINITIES (R)
Bönninghausen, C. von **1870:** HOMŒOPATHIC TREATMENT OF HOOPING COUGH (T)
Bönninghausen, C. von **1873:** THERAPEUTICS OF INTERMITTENT FEVERS (T)
Bönninghausen, C. von **1900:** A SYSTEMATIC, ALPHABETIC REPERTORY OF HOMŒOPATHIC REMEDIES (R)
Bönninghausen, C. von **1908:** BÖNNINGHAUSEN'S LESSER WRITINGS (PR)
Bopp, H. J. **1985:** HOMEOPATHY (CR)
Borland, Douglas **1939:** CHILDREN'S TYPES (T)
Borland, Douglas **1939:** INFULENZAS (T)
Borland, Douglas **1939:** PNEUMONIAS (T)
Borland, Douglas **c.1944:** DIGESTIVE DRUGS (MM)
Borland, Douglas **1950:** HOMEOPATHY FOR MOTHER AND INFANT (D)
Borland, Douglas **1950:** HOMŒOPATHY FOR MOTHER AND INFANT (T)
Borland, Douglas **c. 1950:** CHILDREN'S TYPE: (D)
Borland, Douglas and Priestman, Kathleen **1981:** HOMEOPATHY IN PRACTICE (T)
Bowditch, Henry I. **1887:** THE PAST, PRESENT, AND FUTURE TREATMENT OF HOMŒOPATHY, ECCLECTICISM, AND KINDRED DELUSIONS (CR)
Boyce, Captain William **1880:** ELECTRICITY: ITS NATURE AND FORMS, WITH A STUDY ON ELECTRO-THERAPEUTICS (O)
Boyd, Linn J. **1936:** A STUDY OF THE SIMILE IN MEDICINE (PR)
Boyle, C. C. **1897:** REPERTORY OF THERAPEUTICS OF THE EYE (R)
Bradford, T. L. **1892:** HOMŒOPATHIC BIBLIOGRAPHY (H)
Bradford, T. L. **1895:** THE LIFE AND LETTERS OF DR. SAMUEL HAHNEMANN (B)

Bradford, T. L. **1897**: THE PIONEERS OF HOMŒOPATHY (B)
Bradford, T. L. **1898**: HISTORY OF THE HOMŒOPATHIC MEDICAL COLLEGE OF PENNSYLVANIA (H)
Bradford, T. L. **1900**: THE LOGIC OF FIGURES OR COMPARATIVE RESULTS OF HOMŒOPATHIC AND OTHER TREATMENTS (H)
Bradford, T. L. **1901**: INDEX TO PROVINGS (O)
Breyfogle, William L. **1869**: EPITOME OF HOMEOPATHIC MEDICINES (MM)
Brigham, Gershom Nelson **1882**: PHTHISIS PULMONALIS; OR, TUBERCULAR CONSUMPTION (T)
Broackes, W. **1841**: DISEASES OF THE ALIMENTARY CANAL AND CONSTIPATION, TREATED HOMŒOPATHICALLY (T)
Broussalian, George **1969**: CARD REPERTORY (R)
Bryant, Joel **1851**: A POCKET MANUAL (D) (R)
Buchner, Joseph Benedict **1840**: HOMOOPATHISCHE ARZNEIBEREITUNGSLEHRE (PH)
Buffam, J. E. **1883**: DISEASES AND INJURIES OF THE EYE (AP)
Buffam, Joseph H. **1896**: MANUAL OF THE ESSENTIAL DISEASES OF THE EYE AND EAR (AP)
Burgher, J. C. **1888**: SEMI-CENTENNIAL CELEBRATION OF THE INTRODUCTION OF HOMŒOPATHY WEST OF THE ALLEGHENY MOUNTAINS (H)
Burnett, J. C. **1878**: NATRUM MUR AS A TEST OF THE DOCTRINE OF DRUG DYNAMIZATION (MM)
Burnett, J. C. **1879**: GOLD AS A REMEDY IN DISEASE (MM)
Burnett, J. C. **1880**: CURABILITY OF CATARACTS WITH MEDICINES (T)
Burnett, J. C. **1880**: ON THE PREVENTION OF HARE-LIP, CLEFT PALATE, AND OTHER CONGENITAL DEFECTS (T)
Burnett, J. C. **1881**: ECCE MEDICUS, OR HAHNEMANN AS A MAN AND AS A PHYSICIAN, AND THE LESSONS OF HIS LIFE (B)
Burnett, J. C. **1881**: THE MEDICINAL TREATMENT OF DISEASES OF THE VEINS (T)
Burnett, J. C. **1885**: VALVULAR DISEASE OF THE HEART FROM A NEW STANDPOINT (T)
Burnett, J. C. **1886**: DISEASES OF THE SKIN FROM THE ORGANISMIC STANDPOINT (T)
Burnett, J. C. **1887**: DISEASES OF THE SPLEEN (T)
Burnett, J. C. **1888**: FEVERS AND BLOOD POISONING, AND THEIR TREATMENT WITH SPECIAL REFERENCE TO THE USE OF PYROGENIUM (T)
Burnett, J. C. **1888**: FIFTY REASONS FOR BEING A HOMŒOPATH (PR)
Burnett, J. C. **1888**: TUMOURS OF THE BREAST AND THEIR CURE (T)
Burnett, J. C. **1889**: CATARACT ITS NATURE AND CURE (T)
Burnett, J. C. **1889**: ON FISTULA AND ITS RADICAL CURE BY MEDICINES (T)
Burnett, J. C. **1889**: ON NEURALGIA: ITS CAUSES AND REMEDIES (T)
Burnett, J. C. **1890**: CONSUMPTION AND ITS CURE BY ITS OWN VIRUS (T)
Burnett, J. C. **1891**: THE GREATER DISEASES OF THE LIVER (T)
Burnett, J. C. **1892**: RINGWORM: ITS CONSTITUTIONAL NATURE AND CURE (T)
Burnett, J. C. **1893**: CURABILITY OF TUMOURS (T)
Burnett, J. C. **1895**: DELICATE, BACKWARD, PUNY AND STUNTED CHILDREN (T)
Burnett, J. C. **1895**: GOUT AND ITS CURE (T)
Burnett, J. C. **1896**: ORGAN DISEASES OF WOMEN (T)
Burnett, J. C. **1897**: VACCINOSIS AND ITS CURE BY THUJA (T)
Burnett, J. C. **1898**: CHANGE OF LIFE IN WOMEN (T)
Burnett, J. C. **1901**: ENLARGED TONSILS CURED BY MEDICINE (T)
Burt, William **1869**: CHARACTERISTIC MATERIA MEDICA (MM)
Bush, Christian **1846**: THE HOMŒOPATHIC FARRIER (V)
Butler, John **1882**: ELECTRICITY IN SURGERY (O)
Butler, Kurt **1992**: A CONSUMER'S GUIDE TO ALTERNATIVE MEDICINE (CR)
Butler, William Morris **1911**: MENTAL DISEASES AND THEIR HOMŒOPATHIC TREATMENT (T)
Campbell, Anthony **1984**: THE TWO FACES OF HOMŒOPATHY (H)
Candegabe, Eugenio **1989**: COMPARATIVE MATERIA MEDICA (MM)
Carleton, Bukk **1895**: A MANUAL OF GENITO-URINARY AND VENEREAL DISEASES (AP)
Carleton, Bukk **1898**: A PRACTICAL TREATISE ON THE SEXUAL DISORDERS OF MEN (AP)
Carleton, Bukk **1898**: MEDICAL AND SURGICAL DISEASES OF THE KIDNEYS AND URETERS (AP)

Carleton, Bukk G. and Coles, Howard **1903**: A CLASSIFIED INDEX OF THE HOMŒOPATHIC MATERIA MEDICA FOR UROGENITAL DISEASES (T)
Carleton, Bukk G. **1905**: A TREATISE ON UROLOGICAL AND VENEREAL DISEASES (AP)
Carleton, Edmund **1913**: HOMŒOPATHY IN MEDICINE AND SURGERY (T)
Carter, Francois **1919**: THERAPEUTICS OF THE RESPIRATORY ORGANS (T)
Case, Erastus E. **1916**: SOME CLINICAL EXPERIENCES (T)
Caspari, Carl **1825**: HOMÖOPATHISCHES DISPENSATORIUM FÜR AERZTE UND APOTHEKER (PH)
Caspari, Carl **1826**: HOMÖOPATHISCHER HAUS-UND REISEARZT (Homœopathic Domestic and Traveling Physician)(D)
Caspari, Carl **1829**: DISPENSATORIUM HOMŒOPATHICUM (PH)
Caspari, Carl **1852**: HOMEOPATHIC DOMESTIC PHYSICIAN (D)
Castro, Miranda **1990**: THE COMPLETE HOMEOPATHY HANDBOOK (D)
Castro, Miranda **1993**: HOMEOPATHY FOR PREGNANCY, BIRTH, AND YOUR BABY'S FIRST YEAR (D)
Catellan, A. **1853**: NOUVELLE PHARMACOPÉE HOMŒOPATHIQUE (PH)
Chand, Diwan Harish and Schmidt, Pierre **1980**: THE FINAL GENERAL REPERTORY (R)
Chapman, Beryl **1976**: HOMEOPATHIC TREATMENT FOR BIRDS (V)
Chatroux, Sylvia Seroussi **1998**: MATERIA POETICA (MM)
Chavanon, Paul and Levannier, René **1977**: EMERGENCY HOMEOPATHY AND FIRST AID (T)
Chepmell, Edward D. **1868**: HINTS FOR THE PRACTICAL STUDY OF THE HOMŒOPATHIC METHOD, IN THE ABSENCE OF ORAL INSTRUCTION WITH CASES FOR CLINICAL COMMENT (O)
Chitkara, H. L. **1994**: COMPREHENSIVE HOMEOPATHIC MATERIA MEDICA OF THE MIND (MM)
Choudhuri, N. M. **1916**: A STUDY ON MATERIA MEDICA (MM)
Clark, George Henry **1884**: COUGH AND EXPECTORATION (R)
Clark, George Hardy **1901**: ABC MANUAL OF MATERIA MEDICA (MM)
Clarke, John Henry **1885**: THE PRESCRIBER; A DICTIONARY OF THE NEW THERAPEUTICS (T)
Clarke, John Henry **1888**: ODIUM MEDICUM AND HOMŒOPATHY: THE "TIMES" CORRESPONDENCE (H)
Clarke, John Henry **1890**: DICTIONARY OF DOMESTIC MEDICINE (D)
Clarke, John Henry **1896**: HEART REPERTORY (R)
Clarke, John Henry **1899**: CATARRH, COLDS, AND GRIPPE (T)
Clarke, John Henry **1900**: A DICTIONARY OF PRACTICAL MATERIA MEDICA in 3 Volumes (MM)
Clarke, John Henry **1904**: CLINICAL REPERTORY OF MATERIA MEDICA (R)
Clarke, John Henry **1904**: LIFE AND WORK OF JAMES COMPTON BURNETT (B)
Clarke, John Henry **1904**: THOMAS SKINNER (B)
Clarke, John Henry **1905**: HOMŒOPATHY EXPLAINED (P)
Clarke, John Henry **1908**: THE CURE OF TUMOURS BY MEDICINES (T)
Clarke, John Henry **1915**: GUNPOWDER AS A WAR REMEDY (MM)
Clarke, John Henry **1927**: CONSTITUTIONAL MEDICINE WITH ESPECIAL REFERENCE TO THE THREE CONSTITUTIONS OF VON GRAUVOGL (PR)
Clay, Joseph **1932**: DISEASES OF THE NOSE AND THROAT (AP)
Cleave, Egbert **1873**: CLEAVE'S BIOGRAPHICAL CYCLOPEDIA (B)
Cleveland, C. L. **1888**: SALIENT MATERIA MEDICA AND THERAPEUTICS (MM)
Close, Stuart N. **1924**: THE GENIUS OF HOMŒOPATHY (PR)
Cockburn, Samuel **1857**: MEDICAL REFORM: BEING AN EXAMINATION INTO THE PREVAILING SYSTEMS OF MEDICINE (PR)
Conger, A. B. **1867**: RINDPEST (V)
Cook, Trevor **1981**: SAMUEL HAHNEMANN THE FOUNDER OF HOMEOPATHIC MEDICINE (B)
Cooke, Nicholas Francis **1873**: INSTRUCTIONS FOR THE USE OF N. F. COOKE'S FAMILY MEDICINES (O)
Cooper, R. Le Hunte **1927**: THE CANCER PROBLEM SOME DEDUCTIONS BASED ON CLINICAL EXPERIENCE (T)
Copeland, Royal S. **1909**: THE SCIENTIFIC REASONABLENESS OF HOMŒOPATHY (PR)
Cordasco, Francisco **1991**: HOMŒOPATHY IN THE UNITED STATES A BIBLIOGRAPHY OF HOMŒOPATHIC MEDICAL IMPRINTS, 1825-1925 (O)

Coulter, Catherine R. **1986:** PORTRAITS OF HOMEOPATHIC MEDICINES VOL. I (MM)
Coulter, Catherine R. **1988:** PORTRAITS OF HOMEOPATHIC MEDICINES VOL. II (MM)
Coulter, Catherine R. **1989:** PORTRAITS OF INDIFFERENCE (MM)
Coulter, Catherine R. **1998:** PORTRAITS OF HOMEOPATHIC MEDICINES VOL. III (MM)
Coulter, Catherine R. **2000:** NATURE AND HUMAN PERSONALITY (MM)
Coulter, Harris L. **1972:** HOMŒOPATHIC MEDICINE (P)
Coulter, Harris L. **1973:** DIVIDED LEGACY: A HISTORY OF THE SCHISM IN MEDICAL THOUGHT. SCIENCE AND ETHICS IN AMERICAN MEDICINE, 1800-1914 (H)
Coulter, Harris L. **1973:** HOMŒOPATHIC INFLUENCES IN 19TH CENTURY ALLOPATHIC MEDICINE (H)
Coulter, Harris L. **1975:** DIVIDED LEGACY: A HISTORY OF THE SCHISM IN MEDICAL THOUGHT. THE PATTERNS EMERGE: HIPPOCRATES TO PARACELSUS (H)
Coulter, Harris L. **1977:** DIVIDED LEGACY: A HISTORY OF THE SCHISM IN MEDICAL THOUGHT. PROGRESS AND REGRESS: J. B. VAN HELMONT TO CLAUDE BERNARD (H)
Coulter, Harris L. **1992:** THE CONTROLLED CLINICAL TRIAL AN ANALYSIS (O)
Coulter, Harris L. **1994:** DIVIDED LEGACY TWENTIETH CENTURY MEDICINE THE BACTERIOLOGICAL ERA (H)
Cowperthwaite, Allen Corson **1878:** AN ELEMENTARY TEXTBOOK OF MATERIA MEDICA (MM)
Cox, Donovan and Hyne Jones, T. W. **1976:** BEFORE THE DOCTOR COMES (D)
Crockett, Peter **1995:** THE UNFOLDED ORGANON: A PRÉCIS OF HAHNEMANN'S SIXTH EDITION
Crook, Alan **1996:** A CHRISTIAN'S GUIDE TO HOMŒOPATHY (O)
Culp, Richard **1993:** CHRISTIAN COMMON SENSE AND MEDICAL CONTROVERSY (O)
Curie, Paul F. **1839:** DOMESTIC HOMŒOPATHY (D)
Curie, Paul F. **1847:** GENERAL REPERTORY (R)
Currim, Ahmed N. **1996:** GUIDE TO KENT'S REPERTORY (O)
Cushing, A. M. **1872:** LEUCORRHŒA, ITS CONCOMITANT SYMPTOMS AND ITS HOMŒOPATHIC TREATMENT (T)
Cushing, A. M. **1872:** REPERTORY OF LEUCORRHŒA (R)
Cushing, A. M. **1884:** REJECTED (H)
Custis, Marvin A. **1896:** THE PRACTICE OF MEDICINE; A CONDENSED MANUAL FOR THE BUSY PRACTITIONER (T)
D'Castro, J. Benedict **1989:** ENCYCLOPEDIA OF REPERTORIES (O)
Dake, Jabez **1859:** ACUTE DISEASES AND THEIR HOMEOPATHIC TREATMENT (D)
Dake, Jabez **1886:** THERAPEUTIC METHODS; AN OUTLINE OF PRINCIPLES OBSERVED IN THE ART OF HEALING (T)
Day, Christopher **1984:** HOMEOPATHIC TREATMENT OF SMALL ANIMALS (V)
Day, Christopher **1995:** HOMEOPATHIC TREATMENT OF BEEF AND DAIRY CATTLE (V)
De Charms, Rev. Richard **1850:** HAHNEMANN AND SWEDENBORG (O)
De Horatiis **1845:** HOMÖOPATHISCHE PHARMACOPOE (PH)
De Schepper, Luc **1999:** HAHNEMANN REVISITED A TEXTBOOK OF CLASSICAL HOMEOPATHY FOR THE PROFESSIONAL (PR)
Dearborn, Frederick M. **1923:** AMERICAN HOMŒOPATHY IN THE WORLD WAR (H)
Dearborn, Frederick M. **1937:** THE METROPOLITAN HOSPITAL (H)
Dearborn, Henry M. **1903:** DISEASES OF THE SKIN (AP)
Demarque, Denis, et. al. **1986:** HOMEOPATHIC PRACTICE IN CHILDHOOD DISORDERS (T)
Deventer, Ludwig **1860:** HOMÖOPATHISCHE PHARMACOPÖE (PH)
Dewey, Willis A. **1894:** ESSENTIALS OF MATERIA MEDICA (MM)
Dewey, Willis A. **1898:** ESSENTIALS OF HOMŒOPATHIC THERAPEUTICS (T)
Dewey, Willis A. **1901:** PRACTICAL HOMŒOTHERAPEUTICS (T)
Dhawale, M. L. **1967:** PRINCIPLES AND PRACTICE OF HOMŒOPATHY VOLUME 1 (PR)
Dickie, Perry **1903:** HAY FEVER ITS PREVENTION AND CURE (T)
Dienst, George E. **1906:** WHAT TO DO FOR THE HEAD (T)
Dienst, George E. **1907:** WHAT TO DO FOR THE STOMACH (T)
Diffenbach, William **1909:** HYDROTHERAPY (O)
Diffenbach, William **1928:** RADIUM (MM)

Dimitriadis, George **2000:** THE BÖNNINGHAUSEN REPERTORY; THERAPEUTIC POCKET BOOK METHOD (R)
Dinges, Martin **1996:** WELTGESCHICHTE DER HOMÖOPATHIE LÄNDER—SCHULEN—HEILKUNDIGE (H)
Dockx, Rene and Kokelenberg, Guy **1988:** KENT'S COMPARATIVE REPERTORY OF THE HOMŒOPATHIC MATERIA MEDICA (T)
Dodd, Gloria **1985:** ANIMAL EMERGENCY HANDBOOK (V)
Dooley, Timothy **1995:** HOMEOPATHY BEYOND FLAT EARTH MEDICINE (P)
Dorvault, F. **1859:** BEKNOPTE HANDLEIDING, VOOR DE HOMEOPATHISCHE PHARMACIE (PH)
Douglas, James S. **1853:** HOMŒOPATHIC TREATMENT OF INTERMITTENT FEVER (T)
Douglas, James S. **1860:** PRACTICAL HOMEOPATHY (D)
Douglas, M. E. **1896:** A REPERTORY OF TONGUE SYMPTOMS (R)
Douglas, M. E. **1901:** CHARACTERISTICS OF MATERIA MEDICA (MM)
Drake, Olin M. **1894:** REPERTORY OF FOOT SWEATS (R)
Drake, Olin M. **1897:** REPERTORY OF WARTS AND CONDYLOMATA (R)
Dudgeon, R. E. **1850:** PATHOGENIC CYCLOPEDIA (R)
Dudgeon, R. E. **1854:** LECTURES ON THE THEORY AND PRACTICE OF HOMŒOPATHY (H) (PR)
Dudgeon, R. E. **1859:** REPERTORY OF THE HOMŒOPATHIC MATERIA MEDICA (CYPHER REPERTORY) (R)
Duncan, T. C. **1878:** HOW TO BE PLUMP (O)
Duncan, T. C. **1898:** A HANDBOOK OF THE DISEASES OF THE HEART AND THEIR HOMŒOPATHIC TREATMENT (T)
Dunham, Carroll **1877:** THE SCIENCE OF THERAPEUTICS. (PR)
Dunham, Carroll **1878:** LECTURES ON MATERIA MEDICA (MM)
Dunsford, Harris **1838:** THE PATHOGENIC EFFECTS OF SOME OF THE PRINCIPAL HOMŒOPATHIC REMEDIES (MM)
Dunsford, Harris **1842:** PRACTICAL ADVANTAGES OF HOMŒOPATHY, ILLUSTRATED BY NUMEROUS CASES (P)
Eastman, Arthur M. **1917:** REMINICINCES OF CONSTANTINE HERING (B)
Eggert, William **1879:** UTERINE AND VAGINAL DISCHARGES (R)
Eising, Nuala **1997:** PROVING OF GRANITE, MARBLE, LIMESTONE (MM)
Eizayaga, Francisco **1991:** TREATISE ON HOMEOPATHIC MEDICINE (PR)
Elliott, Charles S. **1897:** LECTURES ON NERVOUS AND MENTAL DISEASES (AP)
Enz, Elizabeth **1911:** PATHOGENIC MATERIA MEDICA (MM)
Epps, John **1839:** DOMESTIC HOMEOPATHY (D)
Everest, Rev. Thomas R. **1835:** A POPULAR VIEW OF HOMŒOPATHY (P)
Faber, Herman **1915:** CONSTANTINE HERING A BIOGRAPHICAL SKETCH (B)
Fahnestock, J. C. **1901:** A MANUAL OF HOMŒOPATHIC MATERIA MEDICA (MM)
Farley, Robert H. **1950:** PUNCH CARD SPINDLE REPERTORY (R)
Farrington, Ernest A. **1874:** SUPPLEMENT TO GROSS' COMPARATIVE MATERIA MEDICA (MM)
Farrington, Ernest A. **1887:** A CLINICAL MATERIA MEDICA (MM)
Farrington, Harvey **1955:** HOMEOPATHY AND HOMEOPATHIC PRESCRIBING (O)
Field, Richard **1922:** SYMPTOM REGISTER (a card repertory) (R)
Fincke, Bernhardt **1865:** ON HIGH POTENCIES AND HOMŒOPATHICS (PR)
Fischer, Charles E. **1895:** A HANDBOOK ON THE DISEASES OF CHILDREN AND THEIR HOMŒOPATHIC TREATMENT (T)
Fischer, Charles E. and MacDonald, T. L. **1895:** A HOMŒOPATHIC TEXTBOOK OF SURGERY (AP)
Fishbein, Morris **1932:** FADS AND QUACKERY IN HEALING (CR)
Flexner, Abraham **1910:** MEDICAL EDUCATION IN THE UNITED STATES AND CANADA: A REPORT TO THE CARNEGIE FOUNDATION FOR THE ADVANCEMENT OF TEACHING (H)
Forbes, John **1846:** HOMŒOPATHY, ALLOPATHY, AND THE YOUNG PHYSIC (CR)
Foster, Steven and Duke, James A. **1990:** A FIELD GUIDE TO MEDICINAL PLANTS (PH)
Foubister, Donald **1958:** THE CARCINOSIN DRUG PICTURE (MM)
Foubister, Donald **1986:** TUTORIALS ON HOMŒOPATHY (O)
Franklin, Edward C. **1867:** THE SCIENCE AND ART OF SURGERY (AP)

Freligh, Martin **1853:** THE HOMŒOPATHIC PRACTICE OF MEDICINE (D)
Freligh, Martin **1856:** THE HOMOEOPATHIC POCKET COMPANION (D)
Freligh, Martin **1859:** HOMŒOPATHIC MATERIA MEDICA (MM)
Gaier, Harald **1991:** THORSONS' ENCYCLOPAEDIC DICTIONARY OF HOMEOPATHY (O)
Gallavardin, J. P. **c. 1890:** PSYCHISME ET HOMOEOPATHIE (R)
Gallivardin, J. P. **1890:** THE HOMŒOPATHIC TREATMENT OF ALCOHOLISM (T)
Garrett, Ray **1987:** CATCHING GOOD HEALTH WITH HOMEOPATHIC MEDICINE (P)
Gatchell, Charles **1883:** KEY NOTES OF MEDICAL PRACTICE (AP)
Gatchell, Charles **1891:** THE POCKET MEDICAL DICTIONARY (O)
Gatchell, Charles **1899:** POCKET BOOK OF MEDICAL PRACTICE (T)
Gemmell, David **1987:** EVERYDAY HOMOEOPATHY A SAFE GUIDE FOR SELF-TREATMENT (D)
Gentry, William **1890:** THE RUBRICAL AND REGIONAL TEXTBOOK OF THE HOMEOPATHIC MATERIA MEDICA, WITH SECTIONS ON URINE AND THE URINARY ORGANS (MM)
Gentry, William **1890:** GENTRY'S CONCORDANCE REPERTORY OF THE MATERIA MEDICA (R)
Genzke, Carl Ludwig **1837:** HOMOEOPATHIC MATERIA MEDICA FOR VETERINARIANS (V)
Gevitz, Norman **1988:** OTHER HEALERS: UNORTHODOX MEDICINE IN AMERICA (H)
Ghose, Sarat Chandra **1935:** LIFE OF MAHENDRA LAL SIRCAR (B)
Ghose, Sarat Chandra **1944:** DRUGS OF HINDOOSTAN (MM)
Gibson, Douglas **1987:** STUDIES OF HOMEOPATHIC REMEDIES (MM)
Gibson, Douglas **c. 1970:** FIRST AID HOMEOPATHY IN ACCIDENTS AND AILMENTS (D)
Gibson, Robin and Gibson, Shelia **1987:** HOMŒOPATHY FOR EVERYONE; WHAT IT IS, HOW IT DEVELOPED, HOW IT CAN HELP YOU, WHERE YOU CAN FIND TREATMENT (P)
Gilchrest, J. Grant **1873:** THE HOMEOPATHIC TREATMENT OF SURGICAL DISEASES (T)
Gladwin, Frederica E. **1974:** THE PEOPLE OF THE MATERIA MEDICA WORLD (MM)
Gollman, William **1855:** THE HOMŒOPATHIC GUIDE IN ALL DISEASES OF THE URINARY AND SEXUAL ORGANS, INCLUDING THE DERANGEMENTS CAUSED BY ONANISM AND SEXUAL EXCESSES (T)
Goodno, William C. **1894:** THE PRACTICE OF MEDICINE (AP)
Goullon, H. **1865:** HOMÖPATHISCHEN PHARMACOPOE AUFGENOMMENEN PFLANZEN (PH)
Gram, Hans Burch **1825:** THE CHARACTERISTICS OF HOMŒOPATHIA (P)
Gramm, Theodore J. **1888:** REPERTORY OF THE URINARY SYMPTOMS (R)
Grandgeorge, Didier **1998:** THE SPIRIT OF HOMEOPATHIC MEDICINES (MM)
Granier, Michel **1859:** CONFERENCES UPON HOMŒOPATHY (PR)
Grauvogl, Eduard von **1870:** TEXTBOOK OF HOMŒOPATHY (PR)
Gregg, Rollin R. **1879:** AN ILLUSTRATED REPERTORY OF PAINS IN CHEST, SIDES AND BACK (R)
Gregg, Rollin R. **1880:** DIPHTHERIA; ITS CAUSES, NATURE, AND TREATMENT (T)
Grimmer, Arthur H. **1996:** THE COLLECTED WORKS OF ARTHUR HILL GRIMMER (O)
Grossinger, Richard **1993:** HOMEOPATHY AN INTRODUCTION FOR SKEPTICS AND BEGINNERS (P)
Gruner, C. E. **1845:** HOMÖOPATHISCHE PHARMACOPOE (PH)
Gruner, C. E. **1850:** NEW HOMŒOPATHIC PHARMACOPOEIA AND POSOLOGY (PH)
Gruner, C. E. **1855:** HOMEOPATHIC PHARMACOPŒIA (PH)
Guernsey, Egbert **1853:** HOMEOPATHIC DOMESTIC PRACTICE (D)
Guernsey, Egbert **1855:** GENTLEMAN'S HANDBOOK OF HOMEOPATHY (D)
Guernsey, Henry N. **1867:** THE APPLICATION OF THE PRINCIPLES AND PRACTICE OF HOMŒOPATHY TO OBSTETRICS, AND DISORDERS PECULIAR TO WOMEN AND YOUNG CHILDREN (T)
Guernsey, Henry N. **1882:** PLAIN TALKS ON AVOIDED SUBJECTS (O)
Guernsey, Henry N. **1887:** KEYNOTES TO THE MATERIA MEDICA (MM)
Guernsey, J. C. **1889:** REPERTORY TO HERING'S CONDENSED MATERIA MEDICA (R)
Guernsey, William Jefferson **1879:** TRAVELLER'S MEDICAL REPERTORY AND FAMILY ADVISOR FOR HOMŒOPATHIC TREATMENT OF ACUTE DISEASES (D)
Guernsey, William Jefferson **1879:** A REPERTORY OF MENSTRUATION (R)
Guernsey, William Jefferson **1882:** A REPERTORY OF HAEMORRHOIDS (R)
Guernsey, William Jefferson **1883:** A REPERTORY OF DESIRES AND AVERSIONS (R)
Guernsey, William Jefferson **1885:** A CARD REPERTORY FOR DIPHTHERIA (R)

Guernsey, William Jefferson **1889**: REPERTORY TO MASTITIS (R)
Guernsey, William Jefferson **1889**: GUERNSEY'S BÖNNINGHAUSEN (R)
Guernsey, William Jefferson **1892**: A REPERTORY FOR DIPHTHERIA (R)
Guernsey, William Jefferson **1892**: THE HOMŒOPATHIC THERAPEUTICS OF HAEMORRHOIDS (T)
Gumpert, Martin **1945**: HAHNEMANN; THE ADVENTUROUS CAREER OF A MEDICAL REBEL (B)
Gunavante, S. W. **1982**: INTRODUCTION TO HOMŒOPATHIC PRESCRIBING (PR)
Günther, F. A. **1847**: NEW MANUAL OF HOMOEOPATHIC VETERINARY MEDICINE (V)
Gutman, William **1940**: THE LITTLE HOMEOPATHIC PHYSICIAN (D)
Gutmann, Salomo **1833**: DIE DYNAMIK DER ZAHNHEILKUNDE BEARBEITET NACH DEN GRUNDSÄTZEN DEN HOMÖOPATHIE (T)
Gypser, K-H. **1987**: KENT'S MINOR WRITINGS ON HOMŒOPATHY (PR)
Gypser, K-H. **1998**: HERINGS MEDIZINISCHE SCHRIFTEN (O)
Gypser, K-H. **2000**: BÖNNINGHAUSENS THERAPEUTISCHES TASCHENBUCH (R)
Haehl, Richard **1922**: SAMUEL HAHNEMANN, HIS LIFE AND WORK (B)
Hafner, Arthur W. **1993**: DIRECTORY OF DECEASED AMERICAN PHYSICIANS 1804-1929 (B)
Hagero, H. **1861**: MEDICAMENTA HOMOEOPATHICA ET ISOPATHICA OMNIA, AD ID TEMPUS A MEDICIS AUT EXAMINATA AUT USU RECEPTA (PH)
Hahnemann, Samuel **1810**: ORGANON DER RATIONELLEN HEILKUNDE (first edition)
Hahnemann, Samuel **1811-1821**: THE MATERIA MEDICA PURA (MM)
Hahnemann, Samuel **1817**: THE SYMPTOM DICTIONARY (handwritten) (R)
Hahnemann, Samuel **1819**: ORGANON DER HEILKUNST (second edition)
Hahnemann, Samuel **1824**: ORGANON DER HEILKUNST (third edition)
Hahnemann, Samuel **1828**: THE CHRONIC DISEASES; THEIR PECULIAR NATURE AND THEIR HOMŒOPATHIC CURE (MM)
Hahnemann, Samuel **1829**: ORGANON DER HEILKUNST (fourth edition)
Hahnemann, Samuel **1833**: ORGANON DER HEILKUNST (fifth edition)
Hahnemann, Samuel **1833**: THE HOMŒOPATHIC MEDICAL DOCTRINE OR THE ORGANON OF THE HEALING ART (first English)
Hahnemann, Samuel **1836**: THE ORGANON OF HOMŒOPATHIC MEDICINE (first American)
Hahnemann, Samuel **1843**: THE ORGANON OF HOMŒOPATHIC MEDICINE (second American)
Hahnemann, Samuel **1849**: ORGANON OF MEDICINE (Dudgeon translation)
Hahnemann, Samuel **1852**: THE LESSER WRITINGS OF SAMUEL HAHNEMANN (PR)
Hahnemann, Samuel **1865**: ORGANON DER HEILKUNST (Lutze edition)
Hahnemann, Samuel **1876**: ORGANON OF THE ART OF HEALING (Wesselhoeft Translation)
Hahnemann, Samuel **1889**: THE ORGANON (Fincke Translation)
Hahnemann, Samuel **1896**: DEFENSE OF THE ORGANON (PR)
Hahnemann, Samuel **1913**: THE ORGANON OF RATIONAL HEALING (Wheeler translation)
Hahnemann, Samuel **1921**: ORGANON DER HEILKUNST (sixth German)
Hahnemann, Samuel **1922**: THE ORGANON OF MEDICINE (sixth English/Boericke)
Hahnemann, Samuel **1970**: THE ORGANON OF MEDICINE (5th and 6th combined)
Hahnemann, Samuel **1979**: THE ORGANON OF MEDICINE (Kurt Hochstetter)
Hahnemann, Samuel **1982**: THE ORGANON OF MEDICINE (Naudé, Kunzli, Pendelton translation)
Hahnemann, Samuel **1991**: KRANKENJOURNAL (O)
Hahnemann, Samuel **1992**: ORGANON DER HEILKUNST (full 6th in German)
Hahnemann, Samuel **1994**: THE ORGANON OF MEDICINE with explanation by Joseph Reves
Hahnemann, Samuel **1996**: THE ORGANON OF THE MEDICAL ART (Decker/O'Reilly translation)
Hale, Edwin M. **1862**: A MONOGRAPH ON GELSEMIUM (MM)
Hale, Edwin M. **1864**: NEW REMEDIES (MM)
Hale, Edwin M. **1866**: A SYSTEMATIC TREATISE ON ABORTION (T)
Hale, Edwin M. **1878**: ON STERILITY (T)
Hale, Edwin M. **1884**: THE CAT AND ITS DISEASES (V)
Hale, Edwin M. **1898**: SAW PALMETTO (MM)
Hamilton, Donald **1999**: HOMEOPATHIC CARE FOR CATS AND DOGS A COMPREHENSIVE GUIDE (V)
Hamilton, Edward **1852**: FLORA HOMŒOPATHICA (MM) (PH)

Hamlyn, Edward **1979:** THE HEALING ART OF HOMOEOPATHY; THE ORGANON OF SAMUEL HAHNEMANN
Hammerton, George **1890:** THE HOMŒOPATHIC VETERINARY DOCTOR (V)
Hammond, Christopher **1991:** HOW TO USE HOMOEOPATHY (D)
Hanchett, Henry G. **1887:** THE ELEMENTS OF MODERN DOMESTIC MEDICINE (D)
Handley, Rima **1990:** A HOMEOPATHIC LOVE STORY (B)
Handley, Rima **1997:** IN SEARCH OF THE LATER HAHNEMANN (B)
Hart, Charles Porter **1876:** REPERTORY OF NEW REMEDIES (R)
Hartlaub, C. G. C. **1826:** SYSTEMATIC DESCRIPTION OF THE PURE EFFECTS OF REMEDIES (R)
Hartmann, Franz **1829:** HOMÖOPATHISCHE PHARMAKOPÖE FÜR AERZTE UND APOTHEKER (PH)
Hartmann, Franz **1831:** SPECIAL THERAPY OF ACUTE AND CHRONIC DISEASES (T)
Hartmann, Franz **1841:** PRACTICAL OBSERVATIONS ON SOME OF THE CHIEF HOMEOPATHIC REMEDIES (MM)
Hartmann, Franz **1853:** DISEASES OF CHILDREN AND THEIR HOMŒOPATHIC TREATMENT (T)
Hartmann, Franz **1857:** SPECIAL THERAPEUTICS ACCORDING TO HOMŒOPATHIC PRINCIPLES, VOLUME 3: MENTAL DISEASES (T)
Hayfield, Robin **1993:** HOMEOPATHY FOR COMMON AILMENTS (D)
Helmuth, William Tod **1855:** SURGERY, AND ITS ADAPTATION TO HOMŒOPATHIC PRACTICE (AP)
Helmuth, William Tod **1879:** A SYSTEM OF SURGERY (AP)
Helmuth, William Tod **1879:** SCRATCHES OF A SURGEON (O)
Helmuth, William Tod **1882:** SUPRAPUBIC LITHOTOMY (AP)
Helmuth, William Tod **1892:** WITH THE "POUSSE CAFÉ;" BEING A COLLECTION OF POST-PRANDIAL VERSES (O)
Hempel, C. J. **1846:** THE HOMEOPATHIC DOMESTIC PHYSICIAN (D)
Hempel, C. J. **1853:** THE COMPLETE REPERTORY (R)
Hempel, C. J. **1854:** ORGANON OF SPECIFIC HOMEOPATHY (O)
Hempel, C. J. **1859:** A NEW AND COMPREHENSIVE SYSTEM OF MATERIA MEDICA AND THERAPEUTICS (MM)
Hempel, C. J. **1874:** THE SCIENCE OF HOMŒOPATHY (PR)
Henderson, William **1854:** HOMEOPATHY FAIRLY REPRESENTED (O)
Henriques, Nicola **1998:** CROSSROADS TO CURE THE HOMEOPATH'S GUIDE TO THE SECOND PRESCRIPTION (PR)
Henshaw, George Russell **1980:** A SCIENTIFIC APPROACH TO HOMEOPATHY (O)
Hering, Carl **1918:** CHRONOLOGY OF EVENTS IN THE LIFE OF CONSTANTINE HERING, MD (B)
Hering, Constantine **1835:** THE HOMŒOPATHIST OR DOMESTIC PHYSICIAN (D)
Hering, Constantine **1838:** REPERTORY TO THE MANUAL (R)
Hering, Constantine **1867:** DR. H GROSS' COMPARATIVE MATERIA MEDICA (MM)
Hering, Constantine **1873:** MATERIA MEDICA VOL. 1 (MM)
Hering, Constantine **1873:** THE TREATMENT OF TYPHOID FEVERS, WITH A FEW ADDITIONS (T)
Hering, Constantine **1875:** ANALYTICAL THERAPEUTICS (R)
Hering, Constantine **1877:** CONDENSED MATERIA MEDICA (MM)
Hering, Constantine **1879:** THE GUIDING SYMPTOMS OF THE MATERIA MEDICA (MM)
Hering, Rudolph **1919:** CONSTANTINE HERING— AN APPRECIATION (B)
Herrick, Nancy **1998:** ANIMAL MINDS, HUMAN VOICES (MM)
Herscu, Paul **1991:** THE HOMEOPATHIC TREATMENT OF CHILDREN (MM)
Herscu, Paul **1996:** STRAMONIUM (MM)
Herscu, Paul **1999:** THE HERSCU LETTER (PR)
Heysinger, Isaac W. **1897:** THE SCIENTIFIC BASIS OF MEDICINE (PR)
Higgins, S. B. **1873:** OPHIDIANS; ZOOLOGICAL ARRANGEMENT OF THE DIFFERENT GENERA (O)
Hill, B. L. **1855:** THE HOMŒOPATHIC PRACTICE OF SURGERY AND OPERATIVE SURGERY (AP)
Hiusmans, Bart **1996:** QUICK REMEDY INDEX TO THE HOMEOPATHIC MATERIA MEDICA (O)
Hobhouse, Rosa Waugh **1933:** LIFE OF CHRISTIAN SAMUEL HAHNEMANN (B)
Holcomb, A. W. **1894:** SENSATIONS AS IF (R)
Holcomb, A. W. **1895:** REPERTORY OF SPASMS AND CONVULSIONS (R)
Holcombe, William H. **1879:** ON THE TREATMENT, DIET, AND NURSING OF YELLOW FEVER (T)

Holcombe, William H. **1894:** THE TRUTH ABOUT HOMŒOPATHY (PR)
Holden, George Parker **1897:** A PRACTICAL WORKING HANDBOOK IN THE DIAGNOSIS AND TREATMENT OF THE DISEASES OF THE GENITO-URINARY SYSTEM AND SYPHILIS (AP)
Holmes, Oliver Wendell **1842:** HOMŒOPATHY AND ITS KINDRED DELUSIONS (CR)
Holmes, Oliver Wendell **1861:** CURRENTS AND COUNTERCURRENTS IN MEDICAL SCIENCE (CR)
Holt, Daniel **1845:** VIEWS ON HOMŒOPATHY (P)
Hooker, Worthington **1850:** LESSONS FROM THE HISTORY OF MEDICAL DELUSIONS (CR)
Hooker, Worthington **1851:** HOMŒOPATHY; AN EXAMINATION OF ITS DOCTRINES AND EVIDENCES (CR)
Hooker, Worthington **1852:** THE TREATMENT DUE FROM THE MEDICAL PROFESSION TO PHYSICIANS WHO BECOME HOMŒOPATHIC PRACTITIONERS (CR)
Hopkins, Branson **1995:** HOMŒOPATHY SOME THINGS ARE NOT WHAT THEY THEY SEEM (CR)
Horvilleur, Alain **1986:** THE FAMILY GUIDE TO HOMEOPATHY (D)
Houghton, Henry M. **1885:** LECTURES ON CLINICAL OTOLOGY (T)
Houghton, Jacquelyn and Halahan, Elisabeth **1994:** THE PROVING OF LAC HUMANUM (MM)
Hoyne, Temple **1868:** REPERTORY OF THE NEW REMEDIES (R)
Hoyne, Temple **1878:** CLINICAL THERAPEUTICS (MM)
Hoyne, Temple **1883:** VENEREAL AND URINARY DISEASES (AP)
HPCUS **1982:** HPUS SUPPLEMENT A (PH)
HPCUS **1991:** THE HOMŒOPATHIC PHARMACOPŒIA OF THE UNITED STATES, REVISION SERVICE (PH)
HPCUS **1994:** HPUS ABSTRACTS 1994 (PH)
Hubbard, Elizabeth Wright **1977:** A BRIEF STUDY COURSE IN HOMEOPATHY (PR)
Hughes, Richard **1867:** A MANUAL OF PHARMACODYNAMICS (MM)
Hughes, Richard **1869:** A MANUAL OF THERAPEUTICS (T)
Hughes, Richard **1900:** REPERTORY OF THE CYCLOPEDIA OF DRUG PATHOGENESY (R)
Hughes, Richard and Dake, Jabez P. editors **1885:** A CYCLOPEDIA OF DRUG PATHOGENESY (MM)
Hull, A. Gerald **1841:** HULL'S JAHR; A NEW MANUAL OF HOMŒOPATHIC PRACTICE (R)
Humphreys, Frederick **1856:** HUMPHREYS' MANUAL OF SPECIFIC HOMEOPATHY (D)
Humphreys, Frederick **1860:** MANUAL OF VETERINARY SPECIFIC HOMŒOPATHY (V)
Humphreys, Frederick **1872:** HUMPHREYS' HOMEOPATHIC MENTOR (D)
Humphreys, Frederick **1885:** HUMPHREYS' VETERINARY GUIDE (V)
Hunt, DeForest **1880:** THE HOMŒOPATHIC TREATMENT OF DIPHTHERIA (T)
Hunter, Francis **1984:** HOMEOPATHIC FIRST AID TREATMENT FOR PETS (V)
Hurndall, John Sutcliffe **1886:** DOGS IN HEALTH AND DISEASE (V)
Hurndall, J. S. **1895:** HOMŒOPATHY IN VETERINARY PRACTICE (V)
Hurndall, J. S. **1896:** VETERINARY HOMŒOPATHY IN ITS APPLICATION TO THE HORSE (V)
Hutchinson, J. W. **1924:** 700 RED-LINE SYMPTOMS (MM)
Idarius, Betty **1996:** HOMEOPATHY CHILDBIRTH MANUAL (D)
Ikenze, Ifeoma **1998:** MENOPAUSE AND HOMEOPATHY A GUIDE FOR WOMEN IN MID-LIFE (D)
Imhäuser, Hedwig **1988:** HOMEOPATHY IN PEDIATRIC PRACTICE (T)
Ivins, Horace F. **1893:** DISEASES OF THE NOSE AND THROAT (AP)
Jacobs, P. H. **1891:** THE POULTRY DOCTOR (V)
Jahr, G. H. G. **1834:** JAHR'S MANUAL (R)
Jahr, G. H. G. **1834:** MANUAL OF HOMEOPATHIC MEDICINE (MM)
Jahr, G. H. G. **1836:** JAHR'S MANUAL OF HOMEOPATHIC MEDICINE (MM)
Jahr, G. H. G. **1840:** NOUVELLE PHARMACOPÉE ET POSOLOGIE HOMOEOPATHIQUE (PH)
Jahr, G. H. G. **1842:** NEW HOMŒOPATHIC PHARMACOPOEIA AND POSOLOGY (PH)
Jahr, G. H. G. **1847:** NEUVA FARMACOPEA Y POSOLOGIA HOMEOPATICA, O MODO DE PREPARAR LOS MEDICAMENTOS HOMEOPATICOS Y DE ADMINISTRAR LAS DOSIS. (PH)
Jahr, G. H. G. **1850:** JAHR'S CLINICAL GUIDE OR POCKET REPERTORY (T)
Jahr, G. H. G. **1850:** ALPHABETICAL REPERTORY OF THE SKIN SYMPTOMS (R)
Jahr, G. H. G. **1850:** NEW HOMŒOPATHIC PHARMACOPOEIA AND POSOLOGY (PH)
Jahr, G. H. G. **1853:** JAHR AND POSSART'S NEW MANUAL OF HOMŒOPATHIC MATERIA MEDICA, ACCOMPANIED BY AN ALPHABETIC REPERTORY (R)

Jahr, G. H. G. **1853:** NOUVELLE PHARMACOPÉE HOMŒOPATHIQUE (PH)
Jahr, G. H. G. **1856:** DISEASES OF FEMALES, AND INFANTS AT THE BREAST (T)
Jahr, G. H. G. **1869** THERAPEUTIC GUIDE (T)
Jeanes, Jacob **1838:** HOMŒOPATHIC PRACTICE OF MEDICINE (T)
Jervis, Horace B. **1929:** TREATMENT OF CANINE DISTEMPER WITH THE POTENTIZED VIRUS (V)
Jimenez, Marcos **1948:** PRACTICAL HOMEOPATHIC REPERTORY IN COLORED AND PERFORATED CARDS (R)
Jiminez-Nuñez, Enrique **1920:** CARD REPERTORY (R)
Johnson, Isaac D. **1871:** THERAPEUTIC KEY; OR PRACTICAL GUIDE FOR THE TREATMENT OF ACUTE DISEASES (T)
Johnson, Isaac D. **1879:** A GUIDE TO HOMEOPATHIC PRACTICE (D)
Johnson, J. W. **1879:** HOMŒOPATHIC VETERINARY HANDBOOK (V)
Johnston, Linda **1991:** EVERYDAY MIRACLES HOMEOPATHY IN ACTION (P)
Jonas, Wayne and Jacobs, Jennifer **1996:** HEALING WITH HOMEOPATHY THE NATURAL WAY TO PROMOTE RECOVERY AND RESTORE HEALTH (D)
Jones, Samuel A. **1880:** THE GROUNDS OF A HOMŒOPATH'S FAITH (PR)
Jones, Samuel A. **1898:** THE PORCELAIN PAINTER'S SON A FANTASY (B)
Jones, Stacy **1887:** THE MEDICAL GENIUS A GUIDE TO THE CURE (T)
Jones, Stacy **1894:** BEE-LINE REPERTORY (R)
Jones, Stacy **1895:** PRESCRIPTION CARD (O)
Jones, Stacy **1904:** THE MNEMONIC SIMILIAD (MM)
Joslin, Benjamin Franklin **1849:** THE HOMŒOPATHIC TREATMENT OF CHOLERA (T)
Joslin, Benjamin Franklin **1850:** THE PRINCIPLES OF HOMŒOPATHY IN FIVE LECTURES (PR)
Jouanny, Jacques **1980:** ESSENTIALS OF HOMEOPATHIC MATERIA MEDICA (MM)
Jouanny, Jacques **1980:** THE ESSENTIALS OF THERAPEUTICS (T)
Jouanny, Jacques **1997:** PHARMACOLOGY AND HOMEOPATHIC MATERIA MEDICA (MM)
Jousset, Pierre **1901:** PRACTICE OF MEDICINE CONTAINING THE HOMŒOPATHIC TREATMENT OF DISEASES (AP)
Jousset, Marc and Leon-Simon, Vincent **1898:** PHARMACOPÉE HOMŒOPATHIQUE FRANÇAISE (PH)
Julian, O. A. **1971:** MATERIA MEDICA OF NEW REMEDIES (MM)
Julian, O. A. **1977:** TREATISE ON DYNAMIZED IMMUNOLOGY (T)
Julian, O. A. **1981:** DICTIONARY OF MATERIA MEDICA (MM)
Jütte, Robert **1998:** CULTURE, KNOWLEDGE, AND HEALING HISTORICAL PERSPECTIVES OF HOMEOPATHIC MEDICINE IN EUROPE AND NORTH AMERICA (H)
Kamthan, P. S. **1955:** MARASMUS AND RICKETS (T)
Kaufman, Martin **1971:** HOMEOPATHY IN AMERICA: THE RISE AND FALL OF A MEDICAL HERESY (H)
Kayne, Stephen **1997:** HOMEOPATHIC PHARMACY AN INTRODUCTION AND HANDBOOK (PH)
Kent, James Tyler **1879:** SEXUAL NEUROSES (O)
Kent, James Tyler **1897:** A REPERTORY OF HOMŒOPATHIC MATERIA MEDICA (R)
Kent, James Tyler **1900:** LECTURES ON HOMŒOPATHIC PHILOSOPHY (PR)
Kent, James Tyler **1905:** LECTURES ON MATERIA MEDICA (MM)
Kent, James Tyler **1926:** NEW REMEDIES; CLINICAL CASES, LESSER WRITINGS, APHORISMS, AND PRECEPTS (PR)
Kent, James Tyler **1987:** KENT'S MINOR WRITINGS ON HOMŒOPATHY ; K-H Gypser, editor (PR)
Kimball, Samuel A. **1888:** A REPERTORY OF GONORRHEA (R)
King, John C. **1879:** A REPERTORY OF HEADACHES (R)
King, John C. **1879:** HEADACHES AND THEIR CONCOMITANT SYMPTOMS (T)
King, William Harvey **1904:** MEDICAL UNION NUMBER SIX (O)
King, William Harvey **1905:** HISTORY OF HOMŒOPATHY AND ITS INSTITUTIONS IN AMERICA (B) (H)
Kirschmann, Anne **1999:** A VITAL FORCE; WOMEN PHYSICIANS AND PATIENTS IN AMERICAN HOMEOPATHY 1850-1930 (H)
Kishore, Jugal **1959:** CARD REPERTORY (R)
Knerr, Calvin **1896:** A REPERTORY OF THE GUIDING SYMPTOMS (R)

Knerr, Calvin **1940:** LIFE OF HERING (B)
Koehler, Gerhard **1986:** THE HANDBOOK OF HOMEOPATHY; ITS PRINCIPLES AND PRACTICE (PR)
Köhler, Hermann A. **1883:** MEDIZINAL PFLANZEN (PH)
Kreisberg, Joel **1997:** HOMEOPATHIC HANDBOOK FOR POISON IVY AND POISON OAK (T)
Kruzel,Thomas **1992:** HOMEOPATHIC EMERGENCY GUIDE (T)
Kulkarni, V. M. **1930:** MATERIA MEDICA IN VERSE (MM)
Künzli, Jost **1987:** REPERTORIUM GENERALE (R)
Lafitte, P. J. **1842:** PURE SYMPTOMATOLOGY OR SYNOPTIC PATTERN OF ALL THE MATERIA MEDICA PURA (R)
Laurie, Joseph **1841:** HOMOEOPATHIC DOMESTIC MEDICINE (D)
Laurie, Joseph **1852:** ELEMENTS OF HOMŒOPATHIC PRACTICE OF PHYSIC (T)
Lawrence, Frederic Mortimer **1901:** PRACTICAL MEDICINE (AP)
Leckridge, Bob **1997:** HOMEOPATHY IN PRIMARY CARE (T)
Lederman, Jeff **1997:** CRIES OF THE WILD; A WILDLIFE REHABILITATOR'S JOURNAL (V)
Lee, Edmund Jennings **1884:** COUGH AND EXPECTORATION (R)
Lee, Edmund Jennings **1889:** REPERTORY OF THE CHARACTERISTIC SYMPTOMS OF THE HOMŒOPATHIC MATERIA MEDICA (R)
Lees, Hans **1975:** CARD REPERTORY (R)
Leeser, Otto **1935:** TEXTBOOK OF MATERIA MEDICA (MM)
Leo-Wolf, William **1835:** REMARKS ON THE ABRACADABRA OF THE NINETEENTH CENTURY (CR)
Lessell, Colin **1983:** THE DENTAL PRESCRIBER (T)
Lessell, Colin **1995:** A TEXTBOOK OF DENTAL HOMOEOPATHY (T)
Lilienthal, Samuel **1878:** HOMŒOPATHIC THERAPEUTICS (T)
Lippe, Adolph **1854:** KEY TO THE MATERIA MEDICA OR COMPARATIVE PHARMACODYNAMICS (MM)
Lippe, Adolph **1866:** TEXTBOOK OF MATERIA MEDICA (MM)
Lippe, Constantine **1879:** REPERTORY TO THE MORE CHARACTERISTIC SYMPTOMS OF THE MATERIA MEDICA (R)
Lockie, Andrew **1989:** THE FAMILY GUIDE TO HOMEOPATHY THE SAFE FORM OF MEDICINE FOR THE FUTURE (D)
Lockie, Andrew and Geddes, Nicola **1995:** THE COMPLETE GUIDE TO HOMEOPATHY (P)
Logan, Robin **1998:** THE HOMEOPATHIC TREATMENT OF ECZEMA (T)
Lord, I. S. P. **1871:** ON INTERMITTENT FEVER AND OTHER MALARIOUS DISEASES (T)
Lutze, Arthur **1862:** MANUAL OF HOMEOPATHIC THEORY AND PRACTICE DESIGNED FOR THE USE OF PHYSICIANS AND FAMILIES (D)
Lutze, F. H. **1898:** REPERTORY FACIAL AND SCIATIC NEURALGIAS (R)
Lutze, F. H. **1898:** THERAPEUTICS OF FACIAL AND SCIATIC NEURALGIA WITH CLINICAL CASES AND REPERTORIES (T)
Lutze, F. H. **1916:** DISEASES OF THE RESPIRATORY ORGANS (R)
Lux, Wilhelm **1837:** ZOOIASIS, OR HOMŒOPATHY IN ITS APPLICATION TO THE DISEASES OF ANIMALS (V)
MacAdam, E. Wallace **1938:** CARROLL DUNHAM HIS LIFE AND WORKS (B)
MacFarlan, Donald **1936:** CONCISE PICTURES OF DRUGS PERSONALLY PROVEN (MM)
Macfarlan, Malcolm **1894:** PROVINGS AND CLINICAL OBSERVATIONS WITH HIGH POTENCIES (MM)
Mack, Charles S. **1888:** SIMILIA SIMILIBUS CURANTUR? ADDRESSED TO THE MEDICAL PROFESSION (PR)
Mack, Charles S. **1904:** ARE WE TO HAVE A UNITED MEDICAL PROFESSION (H)
MacLeod, George **1977:** TREATMENT OF HORSES BY HOMEOPATHY (V)
MacLeod, George **1981:** HOMEOPATHY FOR PETS (V)
MacLeod, George **1981:** TREATMENT OF CATTLE BY HOMEOPATHY (V)
MacLeod, George **1983:** VETERINARY MATERIA MEDICA WITH REPERTORY (V)
MacLeod, George **1983:** HOMEOPATHIC TREATMENT OF DOGS (V)
MacLeod, George **1990:** CATS HOMEOPATHIC REMEDIES (V)
MacLeod, George **1991:** TREATMENT OF GOATS BY HOMEOPATHY (V)

MacLeod, George **1994:** PIGS A HOMEOPATHIC APPROACH TO THE TREATMENT AND PREVENTION OF DISEASES (V)
Majumdar, P. C. **1883:** THERAPEUTICS OF CHOLERA (T)
Malan, H. V. **1852:** FAMILY GUIDE TO THE ADMINISTRATION OF HOMOEOPATHIC REMEDIES (D)
Malcom, John and Moss, Oscar **1895:** COMPARATIVE MATERIA MEDICA (MM)
Male, Ronald **1985:** THE BIBLE AND HOMEOPATHY A DEFENCE OF PURIST HOMEOPATHIC MEDICINE (O)
Mathur, Kailash Narain **1972:** SYSTEMATIC MATERIA MEDICA (MM)
Maury, E. A. **1965:** DRAINAGE IN HOMŒOPATHY (DETOXIFICATION) (T)
Maury, E. A. **1974:** WINE IS THE BEST MEDICINE (O)
McCabe, Vinton **1997:** LET LIKE CURE LIKE (P)
McCabe, Vinton **2000:** PRACTICAL HOMEOPATHY (D)
McGavack, Thomas Hodge **1932:** THE HOMEOPATHIC PRINCIPLE IN THERAPEUTICS (PR)
McIntyer, E. R. **1903:** STEPPING STONES TO NEUROLOGY A MANUAL FOR THE STUDENT AND GENERAL PRACTITIONER (AP)
McKenzie, C. Frazer **c. 1945** THE MIRACLE OF HOMŒOPATHY (P)
McMichael, Arkell **1892:** COMPENDIUM OF MATERIA MEDICA, THERAPEUTICS, AND REPERTORY OF THE DIGESTIVE SYSTEM (MM)
McNeil, A. **1881:** A TREATISE ON DIPHTHERIA (T)
Medical Investigation Club of Baltimore **1895:** PATHOGENIC MATERIA MEDICA (MM)
Metcalf, James W. **1853:** HOMEOPATHIC PROVINGS (MM)
Millard, Henry B. **1863:** A GUIDE FOR EMERGENCIES (D)
Mills, Walter Sands **1915:** PRACTICE OF MEDICINE (AP)
Millspaugh, Charles F. **1884:** AMERICAN MEDICINAL PLANTS (PH)
Millspaugh, Charles F. **1885:** REPERTORY OF ECZEMA (R)
Minton, Henry **1883:** UTERINE THERAPEUTICS (T)
Mirilli, José Antonio **1998:** THEMATIC REPERTORY AND MATERIA MEDICA OF THE MIND SYMPTOMS (T)
Mirman, Jacob **1994:** WHAT THE HELL IS HOMEOPATHY? (P)
Mitchel, G. Ruthven **1975:** HOMŒOPATHY; THE FIRST AUTHORITATIVE STUDY OF ITS PLACE IN MEDICINE TODAY (H)
Mitchel, Kristen M. **1989:** HER PREFERENCE WAS TO HEAL WOMEN'S CHOICE OF HOMEOPATHIC MEDICINE IN THE NINETEENTH CENTURY UNITED STATES (H)
Mitchell, Clifford **1898:** RENAL THERAPEUTICS (AP)
Mohr, Charles **1879:** THE INCOMPATIBLE REMEDIES (MM)
Monroe, Andrew Leight **1882:** MATERIA MEDICA MEMORIZER (MM)
Moore, James **1857:** OUTLINES IN VETERINARY HOMŒOPATHY (V)
Moore, James **1863:** THE DISEASES OF DOGS AND THEIR HOMŒOPATHIC TREATMENT (V)
Moore, James **1892:** "INCURABLE" DISEASES OF BEAST AND FOWL (V)
Morgan, Alonzo Richard **1899:** REPERTORY OF THE URINARY ORGANS (R)
Morgan, Samuel **1891:** THE TEXT BOOK FOR DOMESTIC PRACTICE (D)
Morrison, Roger **1993:** THE DESKTOP GUIDE (MM)
Morrison, Roger **1998:** THE DESKTOP COMPANION TO PHYSICAL PATHOLOGY (T)
Morrow, H. C. **1897:** THE BED FEELS HARD (R)
Moskowitz, Richard **1980:** HOMŒOPATHIC REASONING: (P)
Moskowitz, Richard **1992:** HOMEOPATHIC MEDICINES FOR PREGNANCY AND CHILDBIRTH (T)
Mouzin, Ph. **1835:** PHARMACOPÉE HOMŒOPATHIQUE (PH)
Mure, Benoit **1853:** PROVINGS OF THE PRINCIPAL ANIMAL AND VEGETABLE POISONS OF THE BRAZILIAN EMPIRE (MM)
Murphy, Robin **1993:** THE HOMEOPATHIC MEDICAL REPERTORY (R)
Murphy, Robin **1995:** LOTUS MATERIA MEDICA (MM)
Nash, E. B. **1899:** LEADERS IN THERAPEUTICS (MM)
Nash, E. B. **1900:** LEADERS IN TYPHOID (T)
Nash, E. B. **1901:** REGIONAL LEADERS (MM)
Nash, E. B. **1907:** SULPHUR AND COMPARISONS (MM)

Nash, E. B. **1907:** HOW TO TAKE THE CASE AND FIND THE SIMILLIMUM (O)
Nash, E. B. **1909:** LEADERS IN RESPIRATORY ORGANS (T)
Nash, E. B. **1911:** THE TESTIMONY OF THE CLINIC (T)
Nauman, Eileen **1998:** HELP! AND HOMEOPATHY WHAT TO DO IN AN EMERGENCY BEFORE 911 ARRIVES (D)
Neatby, Edwin A. and Stonham, Thomas George **1927:** MANUAL OF HOMŒOTHERAPEUTICS (MM)
Neel, Edith K. **1902:** CATS. HOW TO CARE FOR THEM (V)
Neidhard, Charles **1860:** ON THE EFFICACY OF CROTALUS HORRIDUS IN YELLOW FEVER, ALSO IN MALIGNANT, BILIOUS, AND REMITTENT FEVERS (T)
Neidhard, Charles **1874:** ON THE UNIVERSALITY OF THE HOMŒOPATHIC LAW OF CURE (PR)
Neidhard, Charles **1888:** PATHOGENIC AND CLINICAL REPERTORY OF THE MOST PROMINENT SYMPTOMS OF THE HEAD, WITH THEIR CONCOMITANTS AND CONDITIONS (R)
Neiswander, Allan **1986:** HOMEOPATHIC GUIDE FOR THE FAMILY (D)
Neustaedter, Randall **1986:** MANAGEMENT OF OTITS MEDIA WITH EFFUSION IN HOMEOPATHIC PRACTICE (T)
Neustaedter, Randall **1991:** HOMEOPATHIC PEDIATRICS ASSESSMENT AND CASE MANAGEMENT (AP)
Neustaedter, Randall **1996:** THE VACCINE GUIDE MAKING AN INFORMED CHOICE (O)
Nicholls, Philip A. **1988:** HOMŒOPATHY AND THE MEDICAL PROFESSION (H)
Noack, Alphons **1843:** MANUAL OF HOMŒOPATHIC MATERIA MEDICA (MM)
Noirot, L. **1835:** PHARMACOPÉE HOMŒOPATHIQUE (PH)
Norton, Arthur B. **1892:** OPHTHALMIC DISEASES AND THERAPEUTICS (T)
Norton, George S. **1876:** OPHTHALMIC THERAPEUTICS (T)
O'Connor, Joseph **1898:** NERVOUS DISEASES WITH HOMŒOPATHIC TREATMENT (T)
Oliver, Ian **1999:** HOMŒOPATHY BEFORE HAHNEMANN THE FORGOTTEN MEN (H)
Ortega, Proceso Sanchez **1980:** NOTES ON THE MIASMS OR HAHNEMANN'S CHRONIC DISEASES (PR)
Palen, Gilbert and Clay, Joseph **1929:** THE PRACTITIONER OTOLOGY (AP)
Palmer, A. B. **1880:** HOMŒOPATHY WHAT IS IT? (CR)
Pancoast, Seth **1877:** THE KABBALA; OR THE TRUE SCIENCE OF LIGHT (O)
Panelli, Cav. Francesco **1878:** A TREATISE ON TYPHOID FEVER (T)
Panos, Maesimund B. and Heimlich, Jane **1980:** HOMEOPATHIC MEDICINE AT HOME (D)
Panos, Maesimund B. and Desrosiers, Della P. **1989:** THE HOMEOPATHIC RECORDER AND PROCEEDINGS OF THE INTERNATIONAL HAHNEMANNIAN ASSOCIATION, CUMULATIVE INDICES 1881-1958 (O)
Patel, Ramanlal **1978:** AUTOVISUAL REPERTORY (R)
Patersimilias **1949:** SONG OF SYMPTOMS (MM)
Peebles, Elinore **1952:** THE PLACE OF HOMŒOPATHY IN MODERN MEDICINE (P)
Perkins, Daniel C. **1888:** THE HOMŒOPATHIC TREATMENT OF RHEUMATISM (T)
Perko, Sandra **1997:** HOMEOPATHY FOR THE MODERN PREGNANT WOMAN AND HER INFANT (T)
Perko, Sandra **1999:** THE HOMEOPATHIC TREATMENT OF INFLUENZA (T)
Phatak, S. R. **1963:** THE CONCISE REPERTORY (R)
Phatak, S. R. **1977:** MATERIA MEDICA OF HOMEOPATHIC REMEDIES (MM)
Pierce, Willard Ide **1895:** COUGH BY LYING (R)
Pierce, Willard Ide **1907:** COUGH BETTER AND WORSE (R)
Pierce, Willard Ide **1911:** PLAIN TALKS ON MATERIA MEDICA (MM)
Pinchuck, Tony and Clark, Richard **1984:** MEDICINE FOR BEGINNERS (O)
Pitcairn, Richard H. and Pitcairn, Susan Hubble **1982:** DR. PITCAIRN'S COMPLETE GUIDE TO NATURAL HEALTH FOR DOGS AND CATS (V)
Pratt, Noel **1980:** HOMEOPATHIC PRESCRIBING (T)
Price, Eldridge C. **1904:** A PHILOSOPHY OF THERAPEUTICS (PR)
Puddephatt, Noel **1944:** THE HOMEOPATHIC MATERIA MEDICA AND HOW IT SHOULD BE STUDIED (MM)
Puddephatt, Noel and Smith, Marjorie Kincaid **1976:** SIGNPOSTS TO THE REMEDIES (MM)

Pugh, J. S. **1929:** CORRECTIONS TO KENT'S REPERTORY(R)
Pulford, Alfred **1898:** REPERTORY OF RHEUMATISM, SCIATICA, AND ETC. (R)
Pulford, Alfred **1926:** FORTY-ONE YEARS OF HOMEOPATHY (B)
Pulford, Alfred **1939:** A REPERTORY OF LEUCORRHOEA (R)
Pulford, Alfred and Pulford, Dayton **1928:** LEADERS IN PNEUMONIA (T)
Pulford, Alfred and Pulford, Dayton **1936:** KEYS TO HOMEOPATHIC MATERIA MEDICA (MM)
Pulford, Alfred and Pulford, Dayton **1944:** MATERIA MEDICA OF GRAPHIC DRUG PICTURES (MM)
Pulte, Joseph Hypolyte **1850:** THE HOMOEOPATHIC DOMESTIC PHYSICIAN (D)
Pulte, Joseph Hypolyte **1853:** WOMAN'S MEDICAL GUIDE (D)
Pursell, James P. **1911:** POULTRY SENSE A TREATISE ON THE MANAGEMENT AND CARE OF CHICKENS (V)
Quin, Frederick Foster Hervey **1834:** PHARMACOPŒIA HOMŒOPATHICA (PH)
Rae, Julius H. **1877:** ON THE APPLICATION OF ELECTRICITY AS A THERAPEUTIC AGENT (O)
Raja, Vincenzo la **1829:** ELEMENTI DI FARMACOIPEA OMIOPATICA ESTRATTI DALLA MATERIA MEDICA DI S. HAHNEMANN (PH)
Ransom, Steven **1999:** HOMOEOPATHY WHAT ARE WE SWALLOWING? (CR)
Rau, Gottlieb Ludwig **1837:** ORGANON DER SPECIFISCHEN HEILKUNST (O)
Raue, Charles G. **1868:** SPECIAL PATHOLOGY AND DIAGNOSTICS, WITH THERAPEUTIC HINTS (T)
Raue, Charles G. **1870:** ANNUAL RECORD OF HOMŒOPATHIC LITERATURE (H)
Raue, Charles G. **1884:** A MEMORIAL TO CONSTANTINE HERING (B)
Reese, David Meredith **1838:** HUMBUGS OF NEW YORK (CR)
Rehman, Abdur **1997:** REMEDY RELATIONSHIPS (O)
Reichenbach, Ludwig **1856:** HOMÖOPATHISCHEN HAUS UND SCHIFFSARZT (D)
Remsen, J. B. F. **1857:** PROFESSOR REMSEN'S HOMŒOPATHIC FAMILY GUIDE FOR TRAVELLERS, ETC. (D)
Retzek, Heli O. **1995:** THE COMPLETE MATERIA MEDICA OF THE MIND (MM)
Reves, Joseph **1993:** 24 CHAPTERS ON HOMEOPATHY (PR)
Ribot, Th. **1909:** DISEASES OF THE PERSONALITY (AP)
Roberts, Herbert A. **1936:** THE PRINCIPLES AND ART OF CURE BY HOMŒOPATHY (PR)
Roberts, Herbert A. **1937:** SENSATIONS AS IF (R)
Roberts, Herbert A. **1939:** THE RHEUMATIC REMEDIES (T)
Roberts, Herbert A. **1941:** THE STUDY OF REMEDIES BY COMPARISON (MM)
Roberts, H. A. and Wilson, Annie C. **1935:** THE PRINCIPLES AND PRACTICALITY OF BÖNNINGHAUSEN'S THERAPEUTIC POCKET BOOK (R)
Robinson, Karl **1980:** HOMŒOPATHY QUESTIONS AND ANSWERS (P)
Rogers, Naomi **1998:** AN ALTERNATIVE PATH THE MAKING AND RE-MAKING OF HAHNEMANN MEDICAL COLLEGE AND HOSPITAL OF PHILADELPHIA (H)
Rollink, A. von **1836:** HOMÖOPATHISCHE PHARMACOPÖE (PH)
Rosenberg, A. Von **1909:** POCKET BOOK OF VETERINARY MEDICAL PRACTICE (V)
Rosenstein, I. G. **1840:** THEORY AND PRACTICE OF HOMŒOPATHY (PR)
Ross, A. C. Gordon **1977:** THE AMAZING HEALER ARNICA, AND A DOZEN OTHER HOMŒOPATHIC REMEDIES (D)
Royal London Homœpathic Hospital **1949:** ROYAL LONDON HOMŒOPATHIC HOSPITAL CENTENARY (H)
Royal, George **1920:** TEXTBOOK OF HOMEOPATHIC MATERIA MEDICA (MM)
Royal, George **1928:** HOMŒOPATHIC THERAPY OF THE DISEASES OF THE BRAIN AND NERVES (T)
Royal, George **1930:** A HANDY BOOK OF REFERENCE (T)
Rückert, Ernst Ferdinand **1831:** SYSTEMATIC PRESENTATION OF ALL HOMŒOPATHIC MEDICINES (R)
Rückert, Ernst Ferdinand **1839:** PERCEPTION AND CURE OF THE MOST IMPORTANT DISEASES OF THE HORSE (V)
Ruddock, E. Harris **c. 1864:** STEPPING STONES TO HOMEOPATHY AND HEALTH (D)
Ruddock, E. Harris **1878:** POCKET MANUAL OF HOMŒOPATHIC VETERINARY MEDICINE (V)
Ruoff, A. Joseph Fredericus **1838:** REPERTORIUM FÜR DIE HOMÖOPATHISCHE PRAXIS (R)
Rush, John **1854:** THE HANDBOOK OF VETERINARY HOMŒOPATHY (V)

Rushmore, Edward **1895:** REPERTORY OF SCARLET FEVER (R)
Russell, Rutherford **1865:** CLINICAL LECTURES ON THE TREATMENT OF RHEUMATISM, EPILEPSY, ASTHMA, FEVER (T)
Sankaran, P. **1965:** CARD REPERTORY (R)
Sankaran, P. **1996:** THE ELEMENTS OF HOMEOPATHY (MM) (O)
Sankaran, Rajan **1991:** THE SPIRIT OF HOMEOPATHY (PR)
Sankaran, Rajan **1994:** THE SUBSTANCE OF HOMEOPATHY (PR)
Sankaran, Rajan **1997:** THE SOUL OF REMEDIES (MM)
Sankaran, Rajan **1998:** PROVINGS (MM)
Sankaran, Rajan **2000:** THE SYSTEM OF HOMEOPATHY (PR)
Santee, Ellis M. **1890:** REPERTORY OF CONVULSIONS (R)
Sarkar, B. K. **1968:** ESSAYS ON HOMEOPATHY (O)
Sastry, G. S. R. **1981:** SEQUELAE (R)
Sault, David **1990:** A MODERN GUIDE AND INDEX TO THE MENTAL RUBRICS IN KENT'S REPERTORY (O)
Schadde, Anne **1997:** PROVING OF OZONE (MM)
Schaeffer, J. C. **1856:** NEW MANUAL OF HOMŒOPATHIC VETERINARY MEDICINE (V)
Schmid, Georg **1846:** HOMOOPATHISCHE ARZNEILBEREITUNG UND GABENGRÖSSE (PH)
Schoen, Allen M. and Wynn, Susan G. **1998:** COMPLEMENTARY AND ALTERNATIVE VETERINARY MEDICINE PRINCIPLES AND PRACTICE (V)
Scholten, Jan **1993:** HOMEOPATHY AND MINERALS (MM)
Scholten, Jan **1996:** HOMEOPATHY AND THE ELEMENTS (MM)
Schröter, Fr. **1878:** POULTRY PHYSICIAN (V)
Schroyens, Frederik **1993:** THE SYNTHESIS REPERTORY (R)
Schroyens, Frederik **1995:** 1001 SMALL REMEDIES (MM)
Schuster, Bernd **1997:** PROVING OF BAMBOO (MM)
Schuster, Bernd **1999:** PROVING OF COLA NITIDA (MM)
Schwabe, Willmar **1872:** PHARMACOPOEA HOMÖOPATHICA POLYGLOTTA (PH)
Schweitzer, Wolfgang **1991:** IKONOGRAPHIE SAMMLUNG, DOKUMENTATION, HISTORIE, UND LEGENDEN DER BILDER DES HOFRATES, DR. MED. HABIL. C. F. S. HAHNEMANN (B)
Shadman, Alonzo **1958:** WHO IS YOUR DOCTOR AND WHY? (P)
Shannon, S. F. **1893:** COMPLETE REPERTORY TO THE TISSUE REMEDIES OF SCHÜSSLER (R)
Sharp, William **1852:** SHARP'S TRACTS ON HOMŒOPATHY (P)
Shedd, P. W. **1907:** THE LIBRARY OF HOMŒOPATHIC CLASSICS, Volume I (MM)
Shedd, P. W. **1908:** CLINICAL REPERTORY (R)
Shepherd, Dorothy **1945:** HOMEOPATHY FOR THE FIRST AIDER (D)
Shepherd, Dorothy **1946:** MAGIC OF THE MINIMUM DOSE (P)
Shepherd, Dorothy **1951:** A PHYSICIAN'S POSY (MM)
Shepherd, Dorothy **1967:** HOMŒOPATHY IN EPIDEMIC DISEASES (T)
Sheppard, K. **1960:** TREATMENT OF CATS BY HOMEOPATHY (V)
Sheppard, K. **1963:** TREATMENT OF DOGS BY HOMEOPATHY (V)
Sherr, Jeremy **1986:** SCORPION (MM)
Sherr, Jeremy **1992:** PROVING OF HYDROGEN (MM)
Sherr, Jeremy **1993:** THE PROVING OF CHOCOLATE (MM)
Sherr, Jeremy **1994:** THE DYNAMICS AND METHODOLOGY OF HOMOEOPATHIC PROVINGS (O)
Sherr, Jeremy **1997:** DYNAMIC PROVINGS (MM)
Shiloh, Jana **1987:** CURING COLIC AND LACTOSE INTOLERANCE (D)
Shinghal, J. N. **1970:** QUICK BEDSIDE PRESCRIBER (T)
Simmons, B. **1892:** NOTES ON SCIATICA (R)
Simpson, James Y. **1854:** HOMŒOPATHY; ITS TENETS AND TENDENCIES, THEORETICAL, THEOLOGICAL, and THERAPEUTICAL (CR)
Singh, Hari **1990:** SYNTHETIC MATERIA MEDICA OF THE MIND (MM)
Skinner, Thomas **1876:** HOMŒOPATHY IN ITS RELATION TO THE DISEASES OF WOMEN (T)
Small, Alvan Edward **1854:** MANUAL OF HOMEOPATHIC PRACTICE (D)
Smith, A. Dwight **1955:** HOMŒOPATHY A RATIONAL AND SCIENTIFIC METHOD (P)

Smith, A. Dwight **1960:** THE HOME PRESCRIBER (D)
Smith, Constance Babington **1986:** CHAMPION OF HOMŒOPATHY; THE LIFE OF MARGERY BLACKIE (B)
Smith, Dean T. **1906:** BEFORE AND AFTER SURGICAL OPERATIONS (T)
Smith, Henry M. **1879:** LIST OF MEDICINES MENTIONED IN HOMŒOPATHIC LITERATURE (PH)
Smith, Trevor **1982:** HOMOEOPATHIC MEDICINE A DOCTORS GUIDE TO REMEDIES FOR COMMON AILMENTS (D)
Smith, Trevor **1983:** THE ENCYCLOPEDIA OF HOMŒOPATHY (O)
Smith, Trevor **1984:** A WOMAN'S GUIDE TO HOMOEOPATHIC MEDICINE (D)
Smith, Trevor **1984:** THE HOMOEOPATHIC TREATMENT OF EMOTIONAL ILLNESS (D)
Snader, Edwin **1888:** REPERTORY OF HEART SYMPTOMS (R)
Snelling, Frederick **1861:** HULL'S JAHR (R)
Soler-Medina, Alberto **1989:** REPERTORY OF PREGNANCY, PARTURITION, AND PUERPERIUM (R)
Speight, Phyllis **1983:** HOMEOPATHIC REMEDIES FOR CHILDREN (D)
Speight, Phyllis **1985:** HOMEOPATHY FOR WOMEN'S AILMENTS (D)
Stapf, Ernst **1846:** ADDITIONS TO THE MATERIA MEDICA PURA (MM)
Stearns, Guy Beckley **1931:** PHYSICS OF HIGH DILUTIONS (PR)
Stearns, Guy Beckley and Evia, Edgar D. **1942:** A NEW SYNTHESIS (PR)
Stens, Wilhelm **1863:** DIE THERAPIE UNSERER ZEIT (P)
Stephens, Philetus J. **1875:** A RECORD OF THE SURGICAL CLINICS OF WILLIAM TOD HELMUTH, MD, HELD AT THE NEW YORK HOMŒOPATHIC MEDICAL COLLEGE DURING THE SESSION OF 1874-75 (AP)
Stephenson, James **1963:** HAHNEMANNIAN PROVINGS (MM)
Stephenson, James **1976:** A DOCTORS' GUIDE TO HELPING YOURSELF WITH HOMEOPATHIC REMEDIES (D)
Subotnick, Stephen **1991:** SPORTS AND EXERCISE INJURIES (D)
Suits, Adelaide **1985:** BRASS TACKS THE ORAL BIOGRAPHY OF A 20TH CENTURY PHYSICIAN (B)
Swan, Samuel **1888:** CATALOGUE OF MORBIFIC PRODUCTS, NOSODES, AND OTHER REMEDIES, IN HIGH POTENCIES: (O)
Swan, Samuel **1888:** A MATERIA MEDICA CONTAINING PROVINGS AND CLINICAL VERIFICATIONS OF NOSODES AND MORBIFIC PRODUCTS (MM)
Swayne, Jeremy **2000:** INTERNATIONAL HOMEOPATHIC DICTIONARY (O)
Tagen, C. H. Von **1881:** BILIARY CALCULI (AP)
Talcott, Selden H. **1901:** MENTAL DISEASES AND THEIR MODERN TREATMENT (T)
Tarbell, John A. **1849:** THE POCKET HOMEOPATHIST AND FAMILY GUIDE (D)
Tarbell, John A. **1856:** HOMŒOPATHY SIMPLIFIED (D)
Temple, John Taylor **1853:** DR. J. T. TEMPLE'S REPLY TO PROF. PALLEN'S ATTACK ON HOMŒOPATHY IN HIS VALEDICTORY ADDRESS BEFORE THE ST. LOUIS UNIVERSITY (O)
Teste, Alphonse **1853:** THE HOMEOPATHIC MATERIA MEDICA, ARRANGED SYSTEMATICALLY AND PRACTICALLY (MM)
The Committee on Pharmacopœia of the American Institute of Homœopathy **1897:** THE PHARMACOPŒIA OF THE AMERICAN INSTITUTE OF HOMEOPATHY (PH)
The Committee on Pharmacopœia of the American Institute of Homœopathy **1914 :** THE HOMŒOPATHIC PHARMACOPŒIA OF THE UNITED STATES (PH)
The Committee on Pharmacopœia of the American Institute of Homœopathy **1964:** THE HOMŒOPATHIC PHARMACOPŒIA OF THE UNITED STATES (PH)
The Committee on Pharmacopœia of the American Institute of Homœopathy **1979:** THE HOMŒOPATHIC PHARMACOPŒIA OF THE UNITED STATES (PH)
The O. O. & L. Society **1906:** TEST DRUG PROVING (MM)
Thompson, Michael **1996:** AMBRA GRISEA ROAD TO HOMEOPATHIC PRACTICE, VOL. I (MM)
Tischner, R. **1939:** GESCHICHTE DER HOMÖOPATHIE (H) (B)
Treuherz, Francis **1995:** HOMŒOPATHY IN THE IRISH POTATO FAMINE (H)
Trinks, Carl Friedrich Gottfried **1843:** MANUAL OF HOMŒOPATHIC MATERIA MEDICA (MM)
Tyler, Margaret **1912:** A CARD REPERTORY (R)
Tyler, Margaret **c. 1939:** POINTERS TO THE COMMON REMEDIES (T)

Tyler, Margaret **1942:** HOMEOPATHIC DRUG PICTURES (MM)
Ullman, Dana **1988:** HOMEOPATHY MEDICINE FOR THE 21ST CENTURY (P)
Ullman, Dana **1992:** HOMEOPATHIC MEDICINE FOR CHILDREN AND INFANTS (D)
Ullman, Dana **1995:** CONSUMER'S GUIDE TO HOMEOPATHY (D)
Ullman, Dana and Cummings, Stephen **1984:** EVERYBODY'S GUIDE TO HOMEOPATHIC MEDICINES (D)
Ullman, Robert and Reichenberg-Ullman, Judyth **1995:** PATIENTS GUIDE TO HOMEOPATHIC MEDICINE (P)
Ullman, Robert and Reichenberg-Ullman, Judyth **1996:** RITALIN FREE KIDS: (P)
Ullman, Robert and Reichenberg-Ullman, Judyth **1997:** HOMEOPATHIC SELF CARE THE QUICK AND EASY GUIDE FOR THE WHOLE FAMILY (D)
Ullman, Robert and Reichenberg-Ullman, Judyth **1999:** PROZAC FREE: (P)
VanDenburg, M. W. **1916:** THERAPEUTICS OF THE RESPIRATORY SYSTEM (T)
Vandenburgh, Federal **1857:** THE UNCERTAINTY OF HUMAN TESTIMONY. CONCLUSIONS NOT JUDGMENT. A LETTER TO THE HONORABLE WILLIAM KENT (O)
Vandenburgh, Federal **1865:** THE GEOMETRY OF VITAL FORCES (O)
Vannier, Leon **1992:** TYPOLOGY IN HOMŒOPATHY (PR)
Vannier, Leon **c. 1955** HOMŒOPATHY HUMAN MEDICINE (PR)
Vargo, Kay **1975:** WHAT IS HOMŒOPATHY? (P)
Verdi, Tullio S. **1870:** MATERNITY A POPULAR TREATISE FOR YOUNG WIVES AND MOTHERS (D)
Verdi, Tullio S. **1893:** SPECIAL DIAGNOSIS AND HOMŒOPATHIC TRATMENT OF DISEASE FOR POPULAR USE (D)
Verkade, Tineke **1997:** HOMŒOPATHIC HANDBOOK FOR DAIRY FARMING (V)
Vermeulen, Frans **1992:** THE SYNOPTIC MATERIA MEDICA (MM)
Vermeulen, Frans **1994:** CONCORDANT MATERIA MEDICA (MM)
Vermeulen, Frans **1996:** THE SYNOPTIC MATERIA MEDICA, VOL. II (MM)
Verna, P. N. **1995:** ENCYCLOPEDIA OF HOMEOPATHIC PHARMACOPOEIA (PH)
Verspoor, Rudolph and Smith, Patricia **1995:** HOMEOPATHY RENEWED (PR)
Verspoor, Rudolph and Decker, Stephen **1999:** HOMEOPATHY RE-EXAMINED BEYOND THE CLASSICAL PARADIGM (PR)
Villers, A. von and Thümen, F. von **1893:** DIE PFLANZEN DES HOMÖOPATHICHEN ARZNEISCHATZES (PH)
Vithoulkas, George **1971:** HOMEOPATHY MEDICINE OF THE NEW MAN (P)
Vithoulkas, George **1974:** ADDITIONS TO KENT'S REPERTORY (R)
Vithoulkas, George **1978:** THE SCIENCE OF HOMŒOPATHY (PR)
Vithoulkas, George **1988:** ESSENCES OF MATERIA MEDICA (MM)
Vithoulkas, George **1991:** A NEW MODEL OF HEALTH AND DISEASE (PR)
Vithoulkas, George **1992:** MATERIA MEDICA VIVA VOLUME 1 (MM)
Voegeli, Adolph **1979:** HOMOEOPATHIC PRESCRIBING; REMEDIES FOR THE HOME AND SURGERY (D)
Walker, Kaetheryn **1996:** HOMEOPATHIC FIRST AID FOR ANIMALS (V)
Walker, Mahlon **1878:** TERATOLOGY, OR THE SCIENCE OF MONSTERS (O)
Ward, James William **1910:** THE AGNOSTIC IN MEDICINE (PR)
Ward, James William **1925:** THE PRINCIPLES AND SCOPE OF HOMŒOPATHY (PR)
Ward, James William **1939:** THE UNABRIDGED DICTIONARY OF SENSATIONS AS IF (R)
Watson, Ian **1991:** A GUIDE TO THE METHODOLOGIES OF HOMEOPATHY (PR)
Watt, Frank **1949:** A PHILOSOPHY OF HEALING AND A PRACTICAL PRESENTATION OF HOMŒOPATHIC PRINCIPLES (P)
Weber, Georg Adolph **1830:** SYSTEMATIC DESCRIPTION OF ANTIPSORIC REMEDIES (R)
Weber, George P. F. **1854:** CODEX DES MEDICAMENTS HOMŒOPATHIQUES OU PHARMACOPÉE (PH)
Weiner, Michael and Goss, Kathleen **1982:** THE COMPLETE BOOK OF HOMEOPATHY (P)
Weir, John **1923:** THE TREND OF MODERN MEDICINE (PR)
Weir, John **1927:** THE PRESENT-DAY ATTITUDE OF THE MEDICAL PROFESSION TOWARDS HOMŒOPATHY (H)

Wershub, Leonard Paul **1967:** ONE HUNDRED YEARS OF MEDICAL PROGRESS A HISTORY OF NY MEDICAL COLLEGE AND FLOWER HOSPITAL (H)
Westcott, Giri **1994:** HOMEOPATHY UNVEILED AN EXPLANATION OF HOW IT REALLY WORKS (P)
Wheeler, Charles E. **1914:** THE CASE FOR HOMŒOPATHY (PR)
Wheeler, Charles E. **1919:** AN INTRODUCTION TO THE PRINCIPLES AND PRACTICE OF HOMŒOPATHY (MM)
Whitmont, Edward **1980:** PSYCHE AND SUBSTANCE (PR)
Whitmont, Edward **1993:** THE ALCHEMY OF HEALING (PR)
Wichmann, Jorg and Bolte, Anglica **1997:** NATURAL RELATIONSHIP OF REMEDIES (O)
Widenmann, G. **1830:** MEDICAMENTORUM HOMŒOPATHICIS (PH)
Williams, Theo D. **1884:** AMERICAN HOMŒOPATHIC DISPENSATORY (PH)
Wilsey, E. H. **1897-1899:** REPERTORY OF THE BACK (R)
Wilson, John Eastman **1916:** DISEASES OF THE NERVOUS SYSTEM (AP)
Wilson, Thomas P. **1871:** THE REJECTED ADDRESS. MAN'S TRUE RELATION TO NATURE; HIS ORIGIN, CHARACTER AND DESTINY (O)
Winans, J. E. **1887:** A COUGH TIME TABLE (R)
Winans, W. W. **1897:** NOTES ON MATERIA MEDICA LECTURES (MM)
Winkler, Eduard **1836:** ABBILDUNGEN DER ARZNEIGEWÄCHSE WELCHE HOMÖOPATISCH GEPRÜFT WORDEN SIND UND ANGEWENDET WERDEN (PH)
Winkler, Eduard **1836:** AUSFÜHRLICHE BESCHREIBUNG SÄMMTLICHER ARZNEIGEWÄCHSE, WELCHE HOMÖOPATHISCH GEPRÜFT WORDEN SIND UND ANGEWENDET WERDEN. FUR HOMÖOPATHIKER ZUR BENUTZUNG BEIM EINSAMMELN DER ARZNEIKÖRPER AUS DEM PFLANZENREICHE (PH)
Winston, Julian **1983:** SOME NOTES AND OBSERVATIONS (H)
Winston, Julian **1999:** THE FACES OF HOMŒOPATHY AN ILLUSTRATED HISTORY OF THE FIRST 200 YEARS (B) (H)
Winterburn, George W. **1886:** REPERTORY OF THE MOST CHARACTERISTIC SYMPTOMS (R)
Wolff, Hans Gunther **1991:** YOUR HEALTHY CAT HOMEOPATHIC MEDICINES FOR COMMON FELINE AILMENTS (V)
Wolff, M. A. A. **1890:** THE HOMŒOPATHC CURE OF DOMESTIC ANIMALS (V)
Wood, James C. **1894:** A TEXTBOOK OF GYNECOLOGY (AP)
Wood, James C. **1917:** CLINICAL GYNECOLOGY (AP)
Wood, James C. **1924:** THE VALUE AND LIMITATIONS OF HOMŒOPATHY (PR)
Wood, James C. **1942:** AN OLD DOCTOR OF THE NEW SCHOOL (B)
Wood, Matthew **1990:** THE MAGICAL STAFF; THE VITALIST TRADITION IN WESTERN MEDICINE (H)
Woodbury, Benjamin **1917:** MATERIA MEDICA FOR NURSES (T)
Woodhouse, Charles **1868:** HOMOEOPATHIC HOME AND SELF TREATMENT OF DISEASE. FOR THE USE OF FAMILY AND TRAVELLERS (D)
Woods, H. Fergie **1950:** ESSENTIALS OF HOMEOPATHIC TREATMENT (D)
Woods, H. Fergie **c. 1960:** HOMEOPATHIC TREATMENT IN THE NURSERY (D)
Worcester, Samuel **1880:** REPERTORY TO THE MODALITIES (R)
Worthington, A. **1887:** PRACTICAL GUIDE TO HOMEOPATHY (D)
Wright, Elizabeth **1928:** TEN REMEDIES INDICATED IN THE TREATMENT OF SCARLET FEVER (T)
Yamini, Sally **1999:** RHYMING REMEDIES (MM)
Yasgur, Jay **1990:** A DICTIONARY OF HOMEOPATHIC MEDICAL TERMINOLOGY (O)
Yasgur, Jay **1996:** CUMULATIVE INDEX TO THE HOMŒOPATHIC PHYSICIAN (O)
Yeldham, Stephen **1864:** HOMŒOPATHY IN VENEREAL DISEASES (T)
Yingling, William A. **1895:** ACCOUCHEUR'S EMERGENCY MANUAL (T)
Yingling, William A. **1895:** REPERTORY OF APPENDICITIS (R)
Zandvoort, Roger van **1992:** THE COMPLETE REPERTORY (R)
Zandvoort, Roger van **1995:** THE COMPLETE REPERTORY (R)
Zaren, Ananda **1994:** CORE ELEMENTS OF THE MATERIA MEDICA OF THE MIND (MM)

Glossary

There are several words used within these pages that I thought might be in need of an expanded definition...

AIH: The American Instuitute of Homœopathy, the first USA medical organization founded in 1844.

Aphorisms: Generally, this refers to the specific numbered paragraphs in the body of Hahnemann's *Organon*.

Fascicles: The individual sections of a book, made up of one or more *signatures* (see below). For example, the pages containing only the first chapter are the "fascicles" for that chapter. Derived from the Latin for "bundle"— the same derivation as "Fascist" (after the bundle of sticks wrapped around an axe that were the symbol of authority of Roman magistrates).

IHA: The International Hahnemannian Association, founded in 1880.

Interleaved: A book where there is a blank page inserted between each page, giving room for additions or comments to be hand-written. Some books were available from the publishers in this fashion. More often, the owner had the book taken apart, new leaves added, and then the book re-bound and new boards (covers) put in place.

Octavo, Quarto, Folio, etc.: These are measurements of the size of the book. The words denote how many times the paper is folded to produce the finished page size. A tabloid newspaper is, generally, printed on a sheet that, when folded once, produces a "folio" sized signature consisting of two sheets or four large pages.
If that size is then folded again, it has four leaves that produce a signature of eight pages. This is a "Quarto" sized book— often abbreviated as "4to." One more fold produces eight leaves and a signature of 16 pages. This is an Octavo sized book— "8vo."
The chart below summarizes the sizes and nomenclature relating to book sizes.

Signature: The grouping of printed pages, folded. The signatures are stitched together to form the book. The book is then trimmed to size and cased, i.e., the spine and boards (covers) are added.

Slipcase: A box, made from thin wood or cardboard, and coved in leather or fabric. The box is open on the tall side to allow a book to slip in.

NOMENCLATURE FOR BOOK SIZES

old name	size (inches)	new name	abbr.
folio	12 x 19	folio	fo
quarto	9.5 x 12	quarto	4to
octavo	6 x 9	octavo	8vo
imperial octavo	8.25 x 11.5		
super octavo	6.5 x 10		
medium octavo	6.125 x 9.25		
crownoctavo	5.375 x 8		
duodecimo	5 x 7.375 (4.5 x 7)	twelve mo	12vo
sextodecimo	4 x 6.75	sixteen mo	16mo
octodecimo	4 x 6.5		18mo
trigesimo secundo	3.5 x 5.5	thirty-two mo	32mo
quartragesimo octavo	2.25 x 4	forty-eight mo	48mo
sexigesimo quarto	2 x 3 or less	sixty-four mo	64mo

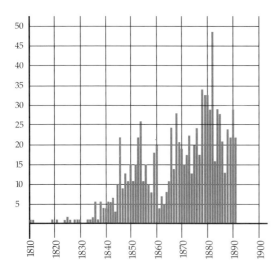

958 titles from Bradford
(books published until 1891)

When I began graphing the books I realized that it needed to be put into perspective. Between the years of 1810 and 1891 I have charted (in this work) about 340 books. The actual number of books published between those times was almost three times that amount. Bradford, whose *Bibliography* covered that exact time frame, listed over 3,000 published works. I went through Bradford's *Bibliography* and charted just those works that were books— eliminating all the journal reprints, addresses, etc. I found 958 books listed.

Since there is no accurate record of books through the 1930s I will assume that as we approach the 1920s, my graphing begins to reflect more closely the actual number of books published although it would be higher at the earlier end (toward 1892) and closer to the graph presented below toward 1920.

Between 1930 and 1960, the graph is fairly accurate. There were very few books published during that time and most have been included.

Between 1970 and 2000 the graph is probably a bit shallow, but only by a few percent since a large number of the books published during that time have been included. It might have no more than 20% added to it.

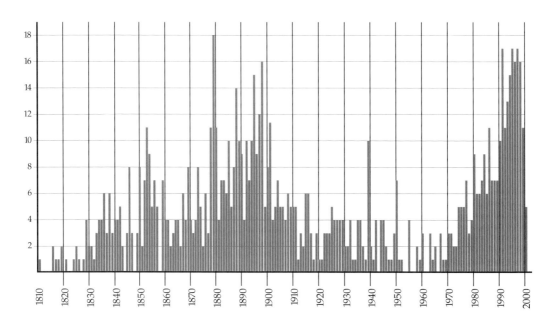

Number of books by year
(only those books in this work)

Some final thoughts about the literature

When we survey the literature of homœopathy, it is amazing to realize that many of these books are over 100 years old. As each book was written, more information was added to the body of knowledge. The statement made by Jahr in 1868 concerning the amount of information the beginner needs to learn homœopathy is even more pertinent today than when it was written. The amount of information we have available is overwhelming.

Through the graces of several publishers in India, many of these older books, which otherwise would have been lost, have been republished. Although the physical quality of these Indian editions often leaves much to be desired, the content of the books has been preserved.

It is interesting that some of the reprints are of old material that is of marginal usefulness, e.g., Bryant's *Pocket Guide* that was first printed in 1851 and certainly has been exceeded in scope by many other domestic guides.

When looking at the graphing of the books included in this volume, I was struck by some interesting details:

First, how close the Bradford graph is to my book graph. The curve is similar, although the vertical scale changes.

Second, how few books were actually published on the subject each year, compared to how many we know about and use. Of the 64 books I have listed that were published between 1870 and 1879, almost half (31) are still in print.

Third, how some of the high spots on the graph are the result of a few authors. Burnett contributed two or three titles a year to our library. The high point in 1939, amid a general drop in titles, can be attributed to three titles by Douglas Borland, one by Tyler, one by Roberts, and one by Ward. And all of them are still in print.

Fourth, the amazing resurgence of publication in the last ten years. I do not believe that this rise in the graph is simply because it is at this time I have chosen to graph the material. There *has* been a resurgence of all the literature: the major new repertories, the many books on new provings, more domestic manuals, more philosophy texts. More of these have been added to the literature in the last 20 years than in the 80 years prior.

It is of interest to note how few of the history books (Bradford's *Pioneers of Homeopathy*, Bradford's *Logic of Figures*, Ameke's *History*) have been reprinted. It seems as if the interest is in the practice of the system. But without knowing the history or having any access to material which discusses it, we have no living record of where we are now and how we got here.

I see many practitioners who are learning to use the books, but are not always taking the time to become deeply familiar with them. How many practitioners have read *Chronic Diseases*? How many, for that matter, have read and pondered the *Organon*? How many have read the introduction in any of the books? There is important information tucked in the books which is being bypassed. There appears to be a desire to master the technique without the understanding of the content and context. It is a problem common to many disciplines— to look for the final product without involving oneself in the process; to want to use the equipment without reading the instruction manual.

This brings us back to the question of experience. Although information is contained in the books, believing what they say without experiencing the system (again, content and context) can lead to poor practice. This problem was of concern to Hering when he wrote, in 1867, "Experience shows how ready such [homœopathic practitioners] are to take for granted what another has made up for sale. The same confidence they place in Jahr, the conscientious, over careful, anxious, rather pedantic, and very industrious man, they place in Noack and Trinks who are arbitrary, full of errors, ruled by prejudice and malignity more than the love of truth."

Another problem with the literature, often overlooked, concerns the question of language. One basic concern is that of translation. Has the language of the original been adequately translated? If not, there is one level of meaning lost. Another concern is that while the symptoms are given in the words of the patient, the labeling of diseased states (something difficult to avoid) is in the language of the last two centuries. We live in different times than Hering and Kent. Society has changed. For example, with the advent of the working woman, the entire picture of *Sepia* has changed in subtle ways. When Tyler says, "You can see this type everywhere— just look out the window," she was talking about her window in England in the l930s not about a window in California in the new century. Work is needed to bring the literature of homœopathy into the new millennium. Yet it must be done with care. The tendency of our modern language to speak in broad generalities ("you know… like… I feel so out of it") does not help us in our work. Homœopathy requires precision and specifics.

When I surveyed the literature I was amazed at the amount of work that was generated by these authors, and the kinships that were developed. It was a small fraternity, and they all knew each other. They were all searching for the same answers. When one got close, the others were informed. The intensity must have been mind-boggling! And they were doing it without the benefit of faxes, telephones, e-mail or the web–based internet.

We now find ourselves having more and more information available plus access to world-wide communication that is unlike anything before. Where it used to take months for someone's work on the east coast of the USA to come to the attention of the community on the west coast, not to mention the UK and the Continent, now the information can be around the world literally in seconds.

This ability to access new information so quickly is both a blessing and a curse. A blessing because it *can* be done, and a curse because, as in the classic game of "telephone," the information passed on is often mis–heard or incomplete, or both. The new frontiers are now easier to explore but with it comes the responsibility of comprehending and sticking to the basic principles.

It is easy to look back at the literature from the turn of the 19th century and draw forth from it the "classics." It is not so easy to look at the literature of the last 15 years and say, with certainty, "This book will still be useful at the turn of the century" or to pick which ones will come up a cropper. Only time will sort the wheat from the chaff. The good books always remain those which help cure patients based upon "easily comprehensible principles." All we have to do is to remember to "hew to the line and let the chips fall where they may."

For those who would like to explore some of the literature that is not readily available in reprinted books, several internet sites have posted journal articles, books, and other writing quoted here.

http://homeoint.org
http:/www.homeopathy.ca/journal.htm
http://www.wholehealthnow.com
http:/www.minutus.com
http:/www.similibus.com
http:/www.simillimum.com
http:/www.homeopathic.co.nz/archives.htm

About the Author

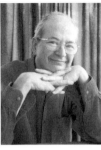

Julian Winston was introduced to homœopathy by Raymond Seidel, MD, HMD, shortly after moving to Philadelphia PA to assume a position as an Associate Professor of Design at The University of the Arts in 1969.

Julian attended the National Center for Homeopathy summer school at Millersville in 1980, became registrar of the program in 1981, and dean of the program in 1988. He was elected to the board of directors of the NCH in 1982, and became the editor of the NCH's newsletter, *Homeopathy Today*, in 1984.

In 1992, on a visit to New Zealand he met Gwyneth Evans, the principal of the Wellington College of Homœopathy. They married in 1994, and he moved to New Zealand in 1995.

They live in Tawa, just outside of Wellington, with his over 2,000 homœopathic books, 4,000 remedies, and a large amount of homœopathic ephemera.

He became board member emeritus of the National Center for Homeopathy in 1997. He continues to edit *Homeopathy Today* and edits *Homœopathy NewZ*, a small newsletter devoted to things homœopathic in New Zealand.

In 1999, he wrote and published *The Faces of Homœopathy: An Illustrated History of the First 200 Years*.

He can be reached at:
PO Box 51-156
Tawa, Wellington, NZ
e-mail: <jwinston@actrix.gen.nz>